VITAMINS AND HORMONES

VOLUME 38

VITAMINS AND HORMONES

ADVANCES IN RESEARCH AND APPLICATIONS

Edited by

PAUL L. MUNSON
University of North Carolina
Chapel Hill, North Carolina

EGON DICZFALUSY
Karolinska Sjukhuset
Stockholm, Sweden

JOHN GLOVER
University of Liverpool
Liverpool, England

ROBERT E. OLSON
St. Louis University
St. Louis, Missouri

Consulting Editors

ROBERT S. HARRIS
32 Dwhinda Road
Newton, Massachusetts

KENNETH V. THIMANN
University of California, Santa Cruz
Santa Cruz, California

JOHN A. LORAINE
University of Edinburgh
Edinburgh, Scotland

IRA G. WOOL
University of Chicago
Chicago, Illinois

Volume 38
1980

ACADEMIC PRESS   A Subsidiary of Harcourt Brace Jovanovich, Publishers

New York   London   Toronto   Sydney   San Francisco

ACADEMIC PRESS, INC.
111 Fifth Avenue, New York, New York 10003

United Kingdom Edition published by
ACADEMIC PRESS, INC. (LONDON) LTD.
24/28 Oval Road, London NW1 7DX

LIBRARY OF CONGRESS CATALOG CARD NUMBER: 43–10535

ISBN 0–12–709838–0

PRINTED IN THE UNITED STATES OF AMERICA

80 81 82 83   9 8 7 6 5 4 3 2 1

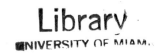

Contents

Systemic Mode of Action of Vitamin A

J. GANGULY, M. R. S. RAO, S. K. MURTHY, AND K. SARADA

Aldosterone Action in Target Epithelia

DIANA MARVER

Thyroid-Stimulating Autoantibodies

D. D. ADAMS

Role of Cyclic Nucleotides in Secretory Mechanisms and Actions of Parathyroid Hormone and Calcitonin

E. M. BROWN AND G. D. AURBACH

Recent Approaches to Fertility Control Based on Derivatives of LH-RH

ANDREW V. SCHALLY, AKIRA ARIMURA, AND DAVID H. COY

Sexual Differentiation of the Brain

GÜNTER DÖRNER

Contributors to Volume 38

Numbers in parentheses indicate the pages on which the authors' contributions begin.

D. D. ADAMS, *Autoimmunity Research Unit, Medical Research Council of New Zealand, University of Otago Medical School, Dunedin, New Zealand* (119)

AKIRA ARIMURA, *The Veterans Administration Medical Center, Department of Medicine, School of Medicine, Tulane University, New Orleans, Louisiana 70146* (257)

G. D. AURBACH, *Metabolic Diseases Branch, National Institute of Arthritis, Metabolism, and Digestive Diseases, National Institutes of Health, Bethesda, Maryland 20205* (205)

E. M. BROWN, *Division of Endocrinology, Peter Bent Brigham Hospital, Boston, Massachusetts 02115* (205)

DAVID H. COY, *The Veterans Administration Medical Center, Department of Medicine, School of Medicine, Tulane University, New Orleans, Louisiana 70146* (257)

GÜNTER DÖRNER, *Institute of Experimental Endocrinology, Humboldt University, 1040 Berlin, German Democratic Republic* (325)

J. GANGULY, *Department of Biochemistry, Indian Institute of Science, Bangalore 560 012, India* (1)

DIANA MARVER, *Departments of Internal Medicine and Biochemistry, University of Texas Health Science Center, Dallas, Texas 75235* (55)

S. K. MURTHY, *Department of Biochemistry, Indian Institute of Science, Bangalore 560 012, India* (1)

M. R. S. RAO, *Department of Biochemistry, Indian Institute of Science, Bangalore 560 012, India* (1)

K. SARADA,* *Department of Biochemistry, Indian Institute of Science, Bangalore 560 012, India* (1)

ANDREW V. SCHALLY, *The Veterans Administration Medical Center, Department of Medicine, School of Medicine, Tulane University, New Orleans, Louisiana 70146* (257)

*Present address: Department of Pharmacology, University of Texas Medical School, Texas Medical Center, Houston, Texas 77030.

Preface

Vitamins and Hormones, Volume 38, begins with a review on the systemic mode of action of vitamin A by J. Ganguly and colleagues. The systemic mode of action of vitamin A, in contrast to its visual action, is still unknown and a subject of continuing research and much controversy. Dr. Ganguly and his co-authors carefully review the development of research related to the somatic function of vitamin A in analogy with developments in understanding the mode of action of steroid hormones. Since the fat-soluble vitamins resemble the steroid hormones in many of their biological properties, this approach is revealing.

The rest of the volume is made up of five reviews of topics in endocrinology. The preponderance of reviews on hormones in this serial publication over reviews on vitamins in recent years reflects the current balance of scientific concentration between these two subjects.

The review of aldosterone actions in target epithelia, especially on Na^+ transport, by Diana Marver includes the nature and role of the cytoplasmic receptor; increases in RNA, total protein, and specific proteins; enhancement of end organ responses to antidiuretic hormone; relation to secretion of H^+ and K^+; the permease and ATP hypotheses; target cells in kidney and toad bladder; and antagonists.

D. D. Adams recounts some of the intellectual adventures involved in the acquisition of our present understanding of the nature of the thyroid-stimulating autoantibodies, the bases for their occurrence, and their mechanisms of action. The historical approach is utilized, clinical implications are highlighted, and there are extrapolations to autoimmune diseases in general.

E. M. Brown and G. D. Aurbach review the role of cyclic nucleotides, principally cyclic AMP, in the mechanisms of secretion and in the actions of parathyroid hormone and calcitonin. There is much evidence to link cyclic AMP to these two hormones, but how their striking effects on bone and kidney are related to cyclic nucleotides remains to be elucidated.

Nobel Laureate Andrew V. Schally, Akira Arimura, and David H. Coy review and evaluate recent approaches to fertility control based on derivatives of LH-RH, which include antibodies and analogs, some superactive and others antagonistic to LH-RH. Depending on the dose level and schedule, the superactive analogs may either enhance or, paradoxically, suppress fertility. The studies reviewed provide basic information on reproductive physiology and on the pharmacology of LH-RH and its many synthetic analogs and supply leads toward further advances in the direction of more effective population control measures.

In the final chapter of the volume, Günter Dörner reviews the provocative, still developing subject of the sexual differentiation of the brain. After a detailed presentation of much animal experimentation and some clinical studies, the author advances the controversial hypothesis that "sexual deviations in the human may be based, at least in part, on discrepancies between the genetic sex and a sex-specific androgen level during brain differentiation."

The international character of *Vitamins and Hormones* is again exemplified in Volume 38. If both authors and editors are considered, four continents and six countries are represented. May this tradition continue!

The Editors join in thanking the authors of the reviews in this volume for their outstanding contributions.

PAUL L. MUNSON
EGON DICZFALUSY
JOHN GLOVER
ROBERT E. OLSON

VITAMINS AND HORMONES

VOLUME 38

Systemic Mode of Action of Vitamin A

J. GANGULY, M. R. S. RAO, S. K. MURTHY, AND K. SARADA*

Department of Biochemistry, Indian Institute of Science, Bangalore, India

I. INTRODUCTION

By the late 1950s the major pathways of metabolism in animal tissues were worked out. Many of them contained enzymes that were shown to require cofactors derived from the water-soluble vitamins. These findings led to attempts during the 1960s to identify similar enzyme systems requiring the fat-soluble vitamins. In particular, vitamin A was implicated in the action of a number of enzymes whose activities appeared to be depressed in vitamin A deficiency. Workers in

*Present address: Department of Pharmacology, University of Texas Medical School, Texas Medical Center, Houston, Texas 77030.

1

several laboratories reported that a variety of enzyme activities including ATP-sulfurylase, sulfotransferase, 3β-hydroxy-Δ^5-steroid dehydrogenase, L-gulonolactone oxidase, codeine demethylase, and p-hydroxyphenylpyruvate oxidase were affected in the tissues of animals deprived of vitamin A. It was also shown in a few laboratories that addition of vitamin A, *in vitro,* to the reaction mixture could restore the lost activity in some of these enzyme systems, particularly ATP-sulfurylase and sulfotransferase. At the same time, other laboratories failed to notice any effects of vitamin A deficiency in enzyme systems like ATP-sulfurylase, gulonolactone oxidase, and the steroid dehydrogenase. These contradictory claims were reviewed at a meeting held at the Massachusetts Institute of Technology (Cambridge, Massachusetts) in 1968, when it was generally agreed that such divergence of claims must be due to the wide disparity in the methods employed in different laboratories for obtaining the vitamin A-deficient animals (Spencer, 1969; Pitt, 1971). At the same time the general opinion was expressed that there was no evidence that vitamin A participates directly as a coenzyme in various enzyme systems. The question of involvement of vitamin A in membrane functions and in electron transport systems has been summarized by Pitt (1971).

It has been recognized from many studies that vitamin A is essential for several physiological functions in animals, namely, (a) vision, (b) growth, (c) reproduction, and (d) proper maintenance of the integrity of epithelial cells. It is rather difficult to imagine the role of a particular compound, required in small amounts, in such diverse areas of physiology of the animal. In such cases, it would be logical to assume that the compound might function at a fundamental point common to all the affected physiological functions. Indeed, if the manifestations of vitamin A deficiency in an animal are critically analyzed from this viewpoint, a focal point for the participation of vitamin A emerges.

II. EFFECTS OF VITAMIN A DEFICIENCY

A. VISION

Probably the only physiological function of vitamin A that is understood with a certain amount of clarity is its participation in the visual processes where cis-trans isomers of retinal function in Wald's visual cycle. This particular process is well documented and therefore will not be discussed here. In terms of understanding the function of vitamin

A, the amount of the vitamin involved in the visual cycle is only a very small fraction of the total amount of the vitamin in the rest of the animal body. It is possible that the involvement of retinal in the opsin–rhodopsin system represents a special adaptation of the major physiological function of vitamin A and is a variant of photosensitive systems that are extensively found in lower organisms.

In vitamin A deficiency the outer segments of the rods lose their opsin, leading to their eventual degeneration. The initial changes in this process consist of swelling and fragmentation of the disk membranes of the rods into distended vesicles and tubules. With the progress of the deficiency the entire structure becomes filled with tubules and vesicles, while the outer segment loses its normal shape and becomes spherical. Eventually the outer segment disappears completely and the lysosome-like structures present in the surrounding pigment epithelial cells seem to be involved in this process. It is possible to regenerate the rods even at this stage by supplementation with vitamin A. But, if the deficiency is allowed to continue further, leading to disintegration of the cones, recovery is virtually impossible and the end result is total blindness. Electron microscopic examination has revealed that vitamin A deficiency also causes extensive changes in the ultrastructure of the visual cells, ultimately leading to their total degeneration (Brammer and White, 1969). It is thus clear that vitamin A plays a vital role not only in dark adaptation, but also in the maintenance of the integrity of the visual cells as well as in their normal regeneration.

B. GROWTH

Growth results from the increase in cell number and/or cell mass, and may be associated with the appearance of differentiated functions. The process of growth begins with the fusion of the sperm with the egg giving rise to the zygote. Development of the fetus or the embryo is a typical example of extremely rapid growth, and it involves proliferation as well as differentiation of numerous types of cells. The process of growth continues in an animal postnatally until adulthood is attained, although the rate of growth progressively decreases with age. Even in an adult animal cell division actually never ceases, although the rates vary significantly from tissue to tissue. Thus, while the liver cells of an adult animal regenerate extremely slowly, the epithelial cells undergo constant *in situ* division and differentiation at a rather rapid rate.

One of the most pronounced effects of deprivation of vitamin A is retardation and ultimate cessation of growth. When weanling rats are put on a vitamin A-free diet they continue to grow until their initial reserves of vitamin A are exhausted, whereupon they cease to grow and attain the weight-plateau stage of the deficiency. After this stage they rapidly lose weight and ultimately die. At the terminal stages of the deficiency most of the epithelial cells, particularly those of the intestine and of the respiratory systems, become susceptible to infection. These points were clearly brought out by the interesting work of Bieri (1969) with germ-free rats. In these experiments, as compared to those with rats raised on a vitamin A-deficient diet under conventional conditions, rats maintained under germfree conditions took a much longer time to reach the weight-plateau stage, and once they reached such a stage they continued to live for a considerable length of time without gaining or losing significant amounts of weight. On the other hand, when given some supplements of vitamin A, these rats promptly resumed growth, reached a fresh weight plateau, and thereafter again maintained their weight for a long time. These experiments thus clearly showed that the growth of the rat is directly dependent upon the supply of vitamin A and that rats actually do not die of vitamin A deficiency but die owing to secondary effects of the deficiency, such as widespread infection. It was interesting, however, that extensive keratinization of the epithelial cells was noticed in these rats.

The effect of vitamin A deprivation on the growth of the chick embryo could be cited as another equally interesting example. It has been reported that, when fertilized eggs obtained from hens raised on a vitamin A-deficient diet and supplemented with retinoic acid were incubated, the embryo grew only up to 48 hours, after which it died. But, when methyl retinoate or retinol was injected into such eggs a good proportion of the embryos survived and hatched to baby chicks (Thompson, 1969). Other aspects of the effects of retinoic acid supplementation are discussed later.

C. Reproduction

1. *Males*

The pronounced effect of deprivation of vitamin A on the reproductive processes of both males and females of various species of animals is well established. Under normal circumstances the original stem cells of the seminiferous tubules undergo several mitotic divisions giving rise to spermatogonia, which in turn divide and differentiate, eventually yielding primary spermatocytes. These undergo meiosis producing spermatids, which contain haploid DNA and no longer divide, but differentiate into mature spermatozoa. Earlier work of Mason (1935) had shown that the testes of vitamin A-deficient rats are reduced to half the usual size with pronounced atrophy, while the germinal epithelium undergoes degenerative changes and the sperm do not develop beyond the spermatid stage. Subsequent histological examination of the testes of the vitamin A-deprived rats has revealed that even at the very mild state of the deficiency the germinal epithelium contains mostly spermatogonia with a few spermatocytes, and no spermatids are seen. It is important to point out here that at the acute stage of the deficiency the animal becomes very sick and susceptible to infection, so that the effects seen at such stages of the deficiency may not indicate the true effects of vitamin A deprivation. But, since such marked effects on spermatogenesis are noticed even at the very early stages of vitamin A depletion, when no other effects have set in, it is obvious that such effects are indeed due to an insufficient supply of vitamin A. This point has been further established by the use of retinoic acid. Thus, it has been repeatedly demonstrated that rats raised on a vitamin A-deficient diet supplemented with retinoic acid show normal growth and outwardly appear normal. Their testes, however, appear more like those of the vitamin A-deficient rats (Juneja *et al.*, 1964; Thompson *et al.*, 1964) in that the testes of the retinoate-supplemented rats also show poor development with marked atrophy and the germinal epithelium undergoes similar degenerative changes. Similarly, mostly spermatogonia, with a few spermatocytes but no spermatids, are found in the seminiferous tubules of the testes of these rats. It would therefore appear that even the initial steps of mitosis leading to the formation of spermatocytes from the spermatogonia are arrested in these rats.

2. *Females*

The effect of deprivation of vitamin A is less perceptible in rat ovaries, although the ovaries of vitamin A-deficient rats have been reported to be distinctly smaller (Moore, 1957). On the other hand, although the acutely deficient female rats fail to conceive when allowed to mate with normal males, mildly deficient ones become pregnant, but either resorb their fetuses or give birth to malformed offspring (Moore, 1957).

Nevertheless, the well known effect of vitamin A deprivation on the cycling patterns of the vaginal epithelial cells is probably one of the most pronounced effects in the females. Under normal circumstances the vaginal epithelial cells of the rat undergo cyclic changes over a period of 4 to 5 days under the influence of estrogens. With the onset of the deficiency these cells become cornified and remain in this state so that the animal appears to be in constant estrus (Mason and Ellison,

1935a,b). In fact, reversal of cornification of the vaginal cells has been widely accepted as a reliable bioassay procedure for the determination of vitamin A activity.

The retinoate-supplemented female rats also appear normal and conceive when allowed to mate with males of proved fertility, but the pregnancy is terminated by gestation resorption around day 14 of pregnancy (Juneja *et al.*, 1964; Thompson *et al.*, 1964). Takahashi *et al.* (1975) reported that the rate of cell division in both the placenta and fetus of retinoate-fed pregnant rats is markedly reduced around day 14 of their pregnancies.

The effect of retinoate supplementation is very pronounced in rat testes, and therefore it has been possible to demonstrate such effects rather readily by the usual histological techniques. It has not been easy, however, to demonstrate such effects in rat ovaries; nevertheless biological differences can be seen under stress conditions like pregnancy and unilateral ovariectomy. Thus Juneja *et al.* (1969) have shown that when rats are subjected to unilateral ovariectomy the consequent compensatory hypertrophy of the remaining ovary is markedly less in the retinoate-treated animals compared to the corresponding normal controls. These workers have further shown that the activity of the enzyme, 3β-hydroxy-Δ^5-steroid dehydrogenase (a key enzyme in the steroidogenic pathway that converts pregnenelone to progesterone) is also perceptibly lower in the hypertrophied ovaries (after unilateral ovariectomy) in the retinoate-fed rats. At the same time it was further shown that the ovaries of the retinoate-fed rats are less responsive to gonadotropin stimulus.

Soon after this work, an examination of the steroid contents of the ovaries and of the ovarian venous blood revealed that both synthesis and secretion of pregnenelone, progesterone, and 20α-hydroxyprogesterone are markedly less in the retinoate-supplemented pregnant rats (Ganguly *et al.*, 1971a,b; and Jayaram *et al.*, 1973) demonstrated that the activity of the cholesterol side-chain cleavage enzyme, which is a rate-limiting enzyme in the biosynthesis of steroids, is markedly affected in the testes and ovaries of the retinoate-fed rats. Further convincing evidence regarding the effect of retinoate-supplementation on steroid biogenesis in both male and female rats has recently been produced by Sarada *et al.* (1977). Thus it used to be widely accepted that retinoate-supplemented female rats maintain a normal estrous cycle and ovulate regularly. In fact, such a belief arose out of the consistent observation that the retinoate-supplemented female rats become pregnant when allowed to mate with normal males. The cycling pattern in types of vaginal epithelial cells from leukocytes at diestrus through small epithelial cells to the larger cornified or keratinized cells at estrus is determined by the concentrations of steroids in the circulating blood, which in turn reflect the activities of the ovaries. Since it has been demonstrated that the ovaries of the retinoate-supplemented rats function suboptimally (which leads to reduced synthesis of steroids), Sarada *et al.* (1977) investigated the blood progesterone levels, mating behavior, and vaginal cell cycles of such rats. Indeed, as expected, the blood progesterone levels of these rats were strikingly low and were almost comparable to those of vitamin A-deficient female rats. At the same time such effects were fully reflected in their mating behavior and vaginal cell cycles, in that they mated very irregularly and their vaginal cells were continuously cornified instead of showing the normal cycling pattern. Thus the evidence is rather striking that vitamin A deprivation or even retinoate supplementation exerts pronounced effects on the functioning of the ovaries. It may also be pointed out in this context that during the estrous cycle the thecal and granulosa cells of the ovaries undergo very active mitosis; therefore, this is yet another example of pronounced effects of vitamin A deprivation on a system undergoing active mitosis.

D. Epithelial Cells

The lesions caused by vitamin A deficiency in an animal are rather extensive and the earliest effects are noticed in the epithelial cells of the animal. A relationship exists between vitamin A and normal division and differentiation of epithelial cells. Some of the well known examples are discussed below.

Leaving aside the direct participation of vitamin A in the process of visual excitation, it is also essential for the maintenance of the various types of cells connected with the visual system. Deficiency of vitamin A leads not only to loss of scotopic vision, but also to xerophthalmia followed by keratomalacia. According to Wolbach and Howe (1925) the first histological change in xerophthalmia in rats is keratinization of the cornea and conjunctival epithelium, after which the mucus-secreting cells of the conjunctiva become overlaid with keratinized cells leading to a glossy appearance of the eyes. Some information is also available regarding the changes in the visual cells.

Observations made by several groups of workers have consistently indicated that vitamin A deficiency leads to keratinization of normally nonkeratinizing epithelia, as in paraocular and salivary glands, larynx, trachea, bronchi, and urogenital tracts in rats (Mori, 1922;

Wolbach and Howe, 1925; Parnel and Sherman, 1962). Out of a variety of such tissues, the pathological changes that are noticed in the tracheal epithelium of vitamin A-deficient rats and hamsters have been studied in some detail. Thus the epithelium of the trachea of normal rats consists of a pseudostratified heterogeneous population of basal cells, brush-border cells, ciliated cells, and goblet cells. Earlier work of Wolbach and Howe (1925) had indicated that during vitamin A deprivation the columnar epithelium of rat trachea undergoes progressive degenerative changes and is eventually replaced by keratinizing cells leading to extensive squamous metaplasia. More recently Wong and Buck (1971) provided electron microscope evidence for an actual decrease in the population of the ciliated and goblet cells of the tracheal epithelium of vitamin A-deficient rats, and Boren *et al.* (1974) reported that in hamster trachea vitamin A deficiency causes a marked increase in the number of basal cells with a simultaneous decrease in the population of ciliated cells. Yet another target of vitamin A function is the intestinal epithelium, which undergoes constant *in situ* replacement every 24–36 hours in rats. These epithelial cells are the first to be affected even at the mild stages of vitamin A deficiency, and at the acute stages of the deficiency, the epithelial lining of the intestine of rats is sloughed off. But, according to De Luca *et al.* (1969), the number of goblet cells (periodic acid–Schiff-staining cells) in the intestinal epithelium of such rats is significantly less, although the existing cells appear normal.

Studies with *in vitro* systems also have shown that vitamin A prevents keratinization of the epithelial cells. Thus Kahn (1954), who studied the influence of vitamin A on explants of normal and estrogen-treated rat vagina grown *in vitro,* noticed that keratinization was inhibited by vitamin A in the normal vagina, and its onset was delayed by the vitamin only in the cultures grown in the presence of estrone. Similar effects of addition of vitamin A to mouse vagina grown in chemically defined media were reported by Lasnitzki (1961), who also noticed that in such systems the addition of vitamin A stimulates proliferation of the new epithelium.

On the other hand, it has been reported that excess vitamin A causes conversion of some normally keratinizing epithelia to the columnar secretory type. Thus, when the skin of a 6- to 7-day-old chick embryo was cultured *in vitro* in the presence of excess vitamin A, the epithelium formed a mucin-secreting, often ciliated, membrane instead of the squamous, keratinizing epidermis that developed in similar explants grown in normal medium (Fell and Mellanby, 1953; Weiss and James, 1955).

Yet another point that deserves special mention in this context is that the keratinizing hyperplasia and hyperkeratosis of the epithelia usually found in experimental vitamin A deficiency may reflect its effect on the epithelial mitotic activity and the rates of replacement of the cells in these tissues. However, reports on the effects of hyper- and hypovitaminosis A on mitosis, both *in vivo* and *in vitro,* have not been very consistent. Thus, although Wolbach and Howe (1933) had found an increase in mitotic activity in the cornea of vitamin A-deficient rats, Friedenwald *et al.* (1945) had failed to notice any significant effect of the deficiency on the mitosis of the basal cells of the corneal epithelium of rats. On the other hand, Sherman (1961) and Parnell and Sherman (1962), who made a careful study of this particular aspect in rats, convincingly demonstrated that the mitotic activities of the corneal epithelium, tracheal epithelium, and epidermis progressively decrease with the progress of the deficiency and further showed that the decrease in the mitotic activities can be directly correlated with the decline in the serum vitamin A levels. It was, however, most significant that topical application of vitamin A on the skin or cornea effected an increase in the mitotic activity in the deficient tissue, while there was no such effect on the normal tissue. The observations reported in the literature regarding the effects of vitamin A deprivation on the various epithelial cells of an animal are summarized in Table I.

This extensive information leads to the general conclusion that vitamin A deprivation not only affects the mitotic activities of the epithelial cells, but probably affects also the normal course of differentiation of such cells. It has already been discussed that lesions caused by vitamin A deficiency in an animal are very extensive involving a wide variety of tissues and systems. Ganguly (1974) suggested that vitamin A might be required for normal proliferation and differentiation of epithelial and perhaps other cells. Indeed the available information lends strong support to this generalized concept about the role of vitamin A in regenerating tissue (Ganguly *et al.,* 1978a,b).

III. REQUIREMENT OF VITAMIN A IN SPECIFIC BIOLOGICAL EVENTS

A. REGENERATION OF RAT LIVER AFTER PARTIAL HEPATECTOMY

Regeneration of the liver cells in an adult rat is usually very slow, but rapid division of the cells can be induced in the tissue by partial hepatectomy involving removal of major portions of it. Such a system

TABLE I

SUMMARY OF THE OBSERVATIONS REPORTED ON THE EFFECTS OF VITAMIN A-NUTRITIONAL STATUS ON VARIOUS EPITHELIAL CELLS

Epithelium	Vitamin A deprivation	Vitamin A excess	Reference
Trachea of rats	Squamous metaplasia[a]	—	Wolbach and Howe (1925)
	Slight decrease in goblet and ciliated cells[b]	—	Wong and Buck (1971)
	Decrease in mitotic activity[a]	—	Sherman (1961)
Trachea of hamsters	Decrease in ciliated cells and increase in basal cells[a]	Increase in ciliated cells and slight decrease in mucous cells[a]	Boren et al. (1974)
Intestinal epithelium of rats	Decrease in goblet cells[a,b]	—	De Luca et al. (1969)
	Duration of cell cycle lengthened[c]	—	Zile et al. (1977)
Germinal epithelium			
Rat testes	Seminiferous epithelium sloughed off[a]	—	Mason (1935)
Rat vagina	Vaginal epithelium cornified[a]	—	Mason and Ellison (1935a,b)

Tissue/system	Effect		Reference
Mouse vagina in culture	—	Increased proliferation of epithelium[a]	Lasnitzki (1961)
Explants of chick embryo skin	—	Mucin-secreting membrane instead of squamous epithelium[a]	Fell and Mellanby (1953)
Corneal epithelium	Decrease in mitotic activity[a]	—	Parnell and Sherman (1962)
Estrogen-primed chick oviduct	Decrease in tubular gland cells[a]	—	Ganguly et al. (1978a)
	Poor growth	—	Joshi et al. (1976)
	Decrease in tubular gland cells, increase in goblet cells, and disorganization of rough endoplasmic reticulum[b]	—	Das et al. (1979)

[a] Histopathological observations.
[b] Electron microscopic observations.
[c] Biochemical observations.

has been widely recognized as a highly reproducible one for studies of rapid growth and cell proliferation. When a major portion of the liver is removed by surgery, the remaining mass of the liver undergoes compensatory hypertrophy and hyperplasia as a consequence of which the original liver mass and function are almost fully restored in course of time.

Extensive cytological and biochemical information is available regarding the changes that take place after partial removal of the liver. Immediately after surgery the hepatocytes dedifferentiate, and they return to the embryonic stage before the process of regeneration begins. Such a process becomes obvious from the appearance of the endoplasmic reticulum, which changes from the organized flat cisternae of the rough endoplasmic reticulum (RER) to the smooth structure. Synthesis of DNA, which is negligible in the normal liver, shows a striking increase at 12-18 hours after surgery, reaching a peak at 20-24 hours, which is followed by mitosis 6-8 hours later. In sharp contrast to such relatively slow changes in DNA synthesis, marked changes in RNA metabolism are perceptible at much earlier times. Thus, increased incorporation of labeled precursors into RNA starts even at 3-6 hours after the operation, maximum incorporation taking place at 12-30 hours after hepatectomy. Such changes in RNA synthesis correlate well with the changes in the template activity of the liver chromatin, which doubles at 4-6 hours, and parallel changes in the machinery for protein synthesis in the cells are also noticed. Such striking increase in the template activity of the liver chromatin would obviously suggest activation of transcription of specific sites of the DNA, which is necessary for the triggering of the process of cell proliferation.

Using regenerating rat liver as a typical system for artificially induced rapid cell proliferation, Jayaram et al. (1975) studied the effects of depletion of vitamin A on the rate of regeneration of the liver after partial hepatectomy. It was consistently observed by them that the extent of regeneration in terms of increase in net weight, and also in DNA, RNA, and protein contents, was markedly less in the deficient liver, when compared with the corresponding pair-fed controls (Table II). Supplementation of the deficient rats with retinyl acetate immediately after the surgery was fully effective in restoring the slower rate of regeneration to near normal patterns in terms of net weight and DNA content, while the RNA values showed a rather marked increase immediately after the supplementation. These observations were fully substantiated by temporal studies on the incorporation of [^{3}H]thymidine, [^{32}P]orthophosphate, and [^{14}C]amino acids into the DNA, total RNA, and total proteins, respectively, when it was found

TABLE II

EFFECT OF VITAMIN A-NUTRITIONAL STATUS ON THE REGENERATION OF RAT LIVER AFTER PARTIAL HEPATECTOMY[a,b]

Time of regeneration (hours)	Liver (gm)		DNA(mg)		RNA (mg)		Protein (mg)	
	Normal	Deficient	Normal	Deficient	Normal	Deficient	Normal	Deficient
0	2.5 ± 0.4	2.4 ± 0.3	4.4 ± 0.4	4.3 ± 0.3	24 ± 4	22 ± 2	450 ± 4	375 ± 25
24	3.9 ± 0.3	2.9 ± 0.5	5.4 ± 0.5	4.5 ± 0.4	30 ± 3	24 ± 2	550 ± 45	420 ± 30
48	4.2 ± 0.4	3.0 ± 0.6	6.8 ± 0.6	4.8 ± 0.5	37 ± 4	27 ± 2	800 ± 60	500 ± 50
72	5.0 ± 0.5	3.4 ± 0.4	7.8 ± 0.3	5.2 ± 0.5	44 ± 3	31 ± 3	920 ± 40	580 ± 50

[a]Adapted from Jayaram et al. (1975).

[b]Both retinyl acetate-supplemented and vitamin A-deficient rats were subjected to partial hepatectomy. The rats were sacrificed at the given intervals of time, and the liver weights, DNA, RNA, and protein contents were determined. Values are from at least five animals in each group. Results are expressed per liver per 100 gm body weight and ± SD.

that the incorporation of these precursors was consistently lower in the depleted liver undergoing regeneration (Jayaram, unpublished observations).

At the same time histological examination revealed that in the control livers the endoplasmic reticulum (ER) appeared "coarse," and the mitotic index was nearly zero before the hepatectomy. At 24 hours after hepatectomy, the mitotic index increased to 1–4%, and the ER appeared uniformly "fine," thereby indicating that the hepatocytes had returned to the embryonic type. At 48 hours of regeneration, however, the ER returned to the rough structure, and the mitotic index was reduced to 0–2%. On the other hand, in the deficient liver before hepatectomy the ER appeared to be mostly of the "fine" structure and the mitotic index was near zero, but here, at 24 hours after the operation the ER revealed "fine" structure and the mitotic index was lower—at 1–2% in some animals, while in some others there was virtually no mitotic activity. At 48 hours also, the ER continued to maintain the "fine" structure with virtually no improvement in the mitotic activity. Administration of retinyl acetate immediately after the operation restored these parameters to near normal patterns (Jayaram, unpublished observations). These experiments with the regenerating rat liver therefore clearly showed that rapid cell proliferation is markedly affected in the absence of vitamin A.

B. ESTROGEN-INDUCED DEVELOPMENT OF CHICK OVIDUCT

The mucosa of the magnum portion of the oviduct of immature chicks consists of a thin layer of pseudostratified columnar epithelial cells which rest upon a compact stroma of polygonal cells intermingled with collagen. In response to estrogen stimulation the columnar epithelial cells divide and differentiate into three distinct cell types: tubular gland cells, goblet cells, and ciliated cells; the stromal cells form the muscles that make up the oviduct wall.

The histological and ultrastructural changes that take place during the hormone-induced cytodifferentiation of the chick oviduct magnum have been studied in considerable detail by Kohler et al. (1969), by Palmiter and Wrenn (1971), and by Oka and Schimke (1969a,b). Some of the salient features of their findings are summarized as follows.

1. *Ultrastructure of the Surface Epithelium*

a. Protodifferentiated Cells and Tubular Gland Cells. The pseudostratified epithelial cells of the magnum of immature chicks contain sparse RER, large numbers of ribosomes, and no apparent secretory granules. Upon administration of estrogen the surface epithelium becomes uneven with budlike invagination of the lumen into the original epithelial layer and subepithelial stroma; at the same time the epithelial progenitor cells undergo initial mitosis, after which they differentiate into protodifferentiated cells containing pronounced RER, large numbers of polysomes, and small secretory granules at the apex. Some of these cells migrate downward into the stroma underlying the epithelium and differentiate into mature tubular gland cells. Essentially these protodifferentiated cells are intermediate between the progenitor cells and mature tubular gland cells and have the intrinsic capacity to differentiate in several directions.

b. Goblet Cells and Ciliated Cells. After the period of proliferation of the tubular gland cells, glandular development ceases to be an important event of the surface epithelial layer, and this happens at about day 7–9 of estrogen administration. At this stage the small cells located basally and containing electron-opaque cytoplasm as well as small crenated nuclei develop into intercalated cells called goblet cells. These cells contain large flocculent bodies with or without dense patches and synthesize avidin, when specifically stimulated by progesterone. They also synthesize mucin.

At the same time some of the larger cells located superficially at the surface epithelium develop into ciliated cells around day 7–9 of estrogen administration.

2. *The Subepithelial Region*

During the process of growth of the oviduct the protodifferentiated cells move down into the stromal space, replacing the stromal cells. The stromal cells in turn migrate to the oviduct perimeter and condense to form bundles of smooth muscles. The marked stromal edema seen during the early phases of estrogen treatment is eventually replaced by the tubular gland cells.

3. *Specialization of the Tubular Gland Cells*

The proliferation of the tubular gland cells is accelerated by intraglandular mitosis. These cells actively synthesize characteristic proteins including ovalbumin, conalbumin, ovomucoid, and lysozyme and contain well organized elongated profiles of RER, where synthesis of these secretory proteins apparently takes place. The vesiculated secretory proteins move into the Golgi zone and coalesce in the condensing vacuoles to form the mature secretory granules.

The chick oviduct system offers a special advantage with respect to the study of any role of vitamin A in the process of division and differentiation of cells in particular and growth in general. First, as discussed above, a great deal of background information is already available regarding the sequence of events leading to the appearance of different types of cells in the magnum of the chick oviduct after estrogen stimulation. Indeed, after estrogen treatment the oviduct of an immature chick undergoes very rapid growth; for example, within a span of 10 days of continuous estrogen treatment the gross weight of the oviduct magnum can increase from about 5–10 mg to about 1.5 gm, and during this process of very rapid growth the three distinct types of cells are formed from the previously indistinguishable primitive epithelial cells. These cells synthesize considerable amounts of the characteristic proteins, most of which are glycoproteins. Second, Joshi *et al.* (1973) have demonstrated that a freshly laid fertilized egg contains about 250 nmol of retinol, out of which about 135 nmol of the vitamin could be recovered from the residual yolk and liver of the bird at the time of hatch. Their results have further shown that the embryo uses up 68 nmol of the vitamin for its growth until the hatch, whereas the newly hatched bird uses about 108 nmol of the vitamin for its growth during the first 7 days, leaving only 27 nmol of the vitamin in its vitelline sac and liver. These results therefore have shown that vitamin A is used during the growth and development of the embryo and young bird. Therefore it follows that it should be fairly easy to make day-old birds deficient of vitamin A by placing them on a vitamin A-free diet. In fact, when day-old female chickens are put on a vitamin A-free diet, such birds become deficient in vitamin A in about 20 days. By treating such deficient birds with estrogen it should be possible to study any role of vitamin A in the development of the oviduct. Third, since it is well established that estrogens act at the level of chromatin and since vitamin A appears to be involved in division and differentiation of cells, it should be possible to use the oviduct system to study interactions, if any, between an estrogen and vitamin A in such processes.

4. *Effect of Vitamin A Deficiency on Estrogen-Induced Growth of the Oviduct Magnum of Immature Chicks*

When 2 mg of estradiol-17β benzoate (dissolved in 0.1 ml of peanut oil) were injected subcutaneously for 6 consecutive days into each of the vitamin A-deprived, retinoate-supplemented, or normal female chicks, the growth of the oviduct in terms of length, weight, total DNA, RNA, and proteins was markedly less in the depleted birds, compared to that for birds given supplements of retinyl acetate (Table III); retinoate supplementation was, however, only partially effective in reversing the effects of the deficiency. It was most interesting that, when

TABLE III

EFFECT OF VITAMIN A-NUTRITIONAL STATUS ON THE GROWTH AND DEVELOPMENT OF THE OVIDUCT MAGNUM OF YOUNG CHICKS AFTER STIMULATION WITH ESTROGEN[a,b]

Treatment	Oviduct		Magnum			
	Weight (gm)	Length (cm)	Weight (gm)	Protein (mg/mg DNA)	RNA (mg/mg DNA)	DNA (mg/gm tissue)
Vitamin A deprived	0.75 ± 0.034	8.9 ± 0.13	0.36 ± 0.023	85.38 ± 6.72	10.47 ± 0.52	0.88 ± 0.047
Retinoic acid after depletion	1.12 ± 0.042	11.0 ± 0.14	0.60 ± 0.014	90.29 ± 5.57	10.63 ± 0.33	0.92 ± 0.032
Retinyl acetate after depletion	1.35 ± 0.031	12.5 ± 0.18	0.72 ± 0.02	91.80 ± 2.85	10.66 ± 0.26	0.94 ± 0.019
Retinyl acetate from day 1 (normal)	1.49 ± 0.053	12.6 ± 0.32	0.81 ± 0.03	105.19 ± 4.26	11.34 ± 0.53	0.92 ± 0.036

[a] Adapted from Joshi et al. (1976).

[b] White Leghorn female chicks (1 day old) were kept on a vitamin A-deficient diet until they ceased to grow. At this stage the birds were distributed into several groups as follows: One of the groups continued to receive the deficient diet only, whereas two other groups received, in addition to the deficient diet, supplements of 40 μg of retinyl acetate per bird per day, or of 10 μg of retinoic acid per gram of the diet. At the same time the normal birds received the deficient diet together with 40 μg of retinyl acetate daily from day 1. At 2 days after the supplementation with vitamin A was started, all birds began to receive by intraperitoneal injection 2 mg of estradiol-17β benzoate (dissolved in 0.1 ml of peanut oil) per bird per day for 6 consecutive days, after which the birds were sacrificed and the oviduct magnum was analyzed.

expressed per gram of tissue, the DNA and RNA values did not reveal any significant differences within the groups. It is thus obvious that the increase in length and weight of the tissues actually reflected increase in cell population, which would certainly mean that cell proliferation was greatly affected in the deficient birds (Joshi *et al.*, 1976).

a. *Histological Studies.* Histological examination of the oviduct magnum of these birds revealed several striking effects of vitamin A deprivation, the most pronounced effect being on the formation of the tubular gland cells, both qualitatively and quantitatively. Thus, after 6 days of estrogen administration the epithelial lining of the control birds measured about 19.1 μm in height and invariably contained protodifferentiated cells at the subepithelial region; at the same time development of the tubular gland cells from the protodifferentiated cells was also distinctly noticeable in many areas. The lobules in these samples were large and well developed, and they contained about 39.2 acini per unit area (10.8 $\times$ 10^4 μm^2); the tubular gland cells in these acini were well formed and revealed the presence of condensed chromatin (Fig. 1). In sharp contrast, the epithelial lining was thicker (about 27.1 μm) in the corresponding vitamin A-deprived birds and contained

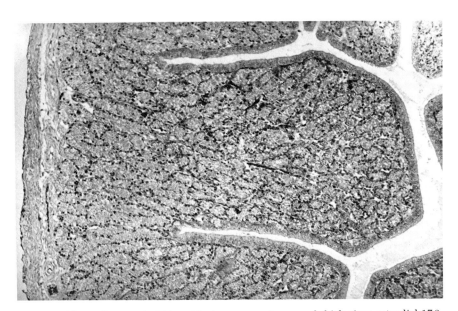

FIG. 1. Photomicrograph of the oviduct magnum of a normal chick given estradiol-17β benzoate for 6 consecutive days. Note that the lobe is packed with acini and that there is very little space in the lumen of the oviduct owing to healthy growth of the lobes from all sides. ×72.

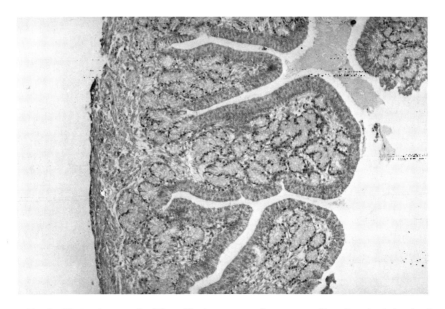

FIG. 2. Photomicrograph of the oviduct magnum of a corresponding vitamin A-deprived chick. Note that the lobes are distinctly smaller in size and that the acini are fewer, swollen, and elongated. Also note that, as compared to Fig. 1, the lining of the epithelium is much thicker. ×72.

several layers of protodifferentiated cells in the subepithelial region (Fig. 2). Even though tubular gland formation could be noticed in these samples, there were only 15.6 acini per unit area, and consequently marked stromal edema was quite conspicuous. Furthermore, the tubular gland cells appeared swollen and elongated (see also Fig. 8).

Examination of the mitotic activities revealed that, although the cells of the epithelium and of the glandular acini undergo active mitotic division in the control birds, no mitosis could be seen in the epithelial or acinar cells in the corresponding vitamin A-deprived birds.

It has already been discussed that after estrogen treatment the progenitor epithelial cells of the normal oviduct magnum differentiate into protodifferentiated cells; these, in turn, after luminal invagination move downward into the subepithelial region, giving rise to the tubular gland cells, the nuclei of which appear dense owing to condensed chromatin. On the other hand, even though tubular gland formation was clearly evident in the vitamin A-deprived birds, clumps of protodifferentiated cells were seen in many areas, and it appeared as though these protodifferentiated cells were trying to move into the subepithelial region without differentiating into tubular gland cells,

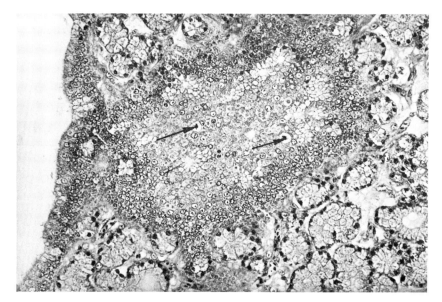

FIG. 3. Photomicrograph of the magnum of a retinoic acid-supplemented bird showing a cluster of protodifferentiated cells. Note the formation of acinar structures from these protodifferentiated cells, but without condensation of the nuclear chromatin. Mitosis of the protodifferentiated cells is also seen (light arrow). ×180.

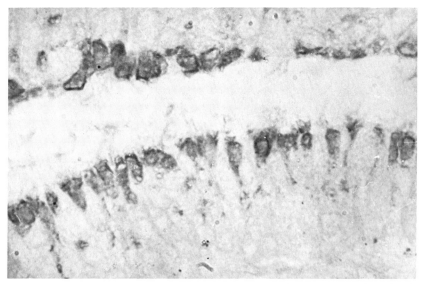

FIG. 4. Photomicrograph of the epithelium of the oviduct magnum of a vitamin A-deficient chick stained with alcian blue. Note thick staining along the epithelium facing the lumen. This was virtually absent in the normal tissue. ×720.

and at the same time their nuclear chromatin was not condensed. Such events were more striking in the retinoic acid-supplemented birds (Fig. 3). Thus, rather large clusters of such protodifferentiated cells were noticed in the subepithelial region of the oviduct magnum of these birds, and some of these cells formed acinar structures and occasionally showed mitosis. Owing to the apparent defect in the condensation of the nuclear chromatin, these cells failed to differentiate into normal tubular gland cells and consequently appeared as though they were disintegrating.

In contrast to such pronounced effects on the tubular gland cells there were distinctly more and prominent goblet cells in the epithelial region of the vitamin A-deprived birds, as compared to the normals. Thus, when sections of the magnum stained with alcian blue were examined under light and phase contrast microscopes, large numbers of intensely alcian blue-positive cells were seen facing the luminal side of the epithelium of the deficient birds (Fig. 4; see also Figs. 6 and 9); in sharp contrast such cells were rare in the normal controls, and at the same time showed only faint staining with alcian blue. Usually alcian blue specifically stains mucin-like materials, and therefore such heavy staining with this dye would obviously suggest the presence of large amounts of such materials in the deficient tissue. It has already been mentioned that the goblet cells synthesize and secrete mucins.

A summary of these histomorphological observations with respect to the effect of vitamin A deprivation on the estrogen-induced development of the chick oviduct is given in Table IV.

b. Electron Microscopic Observations. Electron microscopic examination of the oviduct magnum of the vitamin A-deprived and normal birds treated with estrogen revealed several remarkable differences. Thus, while there were very few protodifferentiated cells in the epithelium of the normal magnum on day 6 of estrogen administration (Fig. 5), large numbers of these cells were seen in the magnum of the deficient birds (Fig. 6). Furthermore, while there were very few small electron-opaque secretory granules in the protodifferentiated cells of the normal birds, in the deficient birds these granules were fairly large and were reminiscent of the mature secretory granules usually seen in the tubular gland cells. It will also be seen from Fig. 6 that, in addition to the secretory granules, flocculent bodies, which are characteristic of the goblet cells, were also prominent in the depleted birds (Das *et al.*, 1979).

Similar electron microscopic examination of the subepithelial region of the magnum fully substantiated our observations with light microscope. Thus, although the subepithelial region of the control birds was

TABLE IV

Effect of Vitamin A-Nutritional Status on the Histomorphological Patterns of the Magnum Portion of Estrogen-Primed Chick Oviduct[a]

| | Lobules | | Acini | | | | |
Treatment	Height of epithelium (μm)	Shape	Number per $10.8 \times 10^4 \ \mu m^2$	Mitosis	Chromatin	Protodiffer-entiated cells	Goblet cells
Vitamin A deficient	27.1	Swollen and elongated	15.6	Rare	Poor conden-sation	Abundant at epi-thelium	Abundant at epi-thelium
Retinyl acetate from day 1 (normal)	19.1	Well developed	39.2	Active	Thick	Few	Few

[a] Unpublished observations of J. Ganguly, P. S. Joshi, S. K. Murthy, E. Unni, and G. F. X. David.

packed with tubular gland cells (Fig. 7), in the corresponding vitamin A-depleted birds they were fewer with consequent marked stromal edema. Moreover, here also, as compared to the control birds, the acini in the magnum of the depleted birds were elongated (Fig. 8).

The RER has been recognized to be the seat of synthesis of secretory proteins. The RER in the tubular gland cells was well developed and was organized into flat cisternae in the normal birds, but in the depleted birds the RER was mostly vesicular (Das *et al.*, 1979). It will be discussed later that it has been consistently observed in several laboratories that vitamin A deprivation exerts a pronounced effect on the nature and synthesis of RNA in those cells of the animal that regenerate rapidly, and it has already been mentioned that Jayaram (unpublished observations) has noted a marked effect of vitamin A depletion on the appearance of the RER in regenerating rat liver after partial hepatectomy. It would thus appear that vitamin A depletion not only affects the formation of the tubular gland cells from the progenitor epithelial cells, but also affects the development of the RER.

As well as the decrease in the number of the tubular gland cells, the ciliated cells were fewer in the magnum of the depleted birds. This is in agreement with the earlier findings of Boren *et al.* (1974), who had reported that vitamin A deprivation leads to significant decrease in the number of ciliated cells in the tracheal epithelium of hamsters.

In striking contrast to the reduction in the population of the tubular gland cells and ciliated cells, there was a distinct increase in the number of goblet cells in the deficient magnum (Fig. 9). Such pronounced increase in the population of goblet cells in the chick oviduct is at variance with the earlier observations of De Luca *et al.* (1969), who had reported an actual decrease in the number of goblet cells in the small intestine of vitamin A-deficient rats, and of Boren *et al.* (1974), who could find no significant change in the population of goblet cells in the trachea of vitamin A-deficient hamsters. It should, however, be pointed out here that the system used by us was different from those used by the other two groups of workers in that, whereas De Luca *et al.* (1969) studied the changes in the cell population in the intestine of rats made deficient of vitamin A and Boren *et al.* (1974) in the trachea of vitamin A-deficient hamsters, in our work the effect of deprivation of vitamin A was studied in an avian species where very rapid division and differentiation of the cells of the oviduct magnum were induced by estrogen administration.

A summary of these electron microscopic observations regarding the effect of vitamin A deprivation on the estrogen-induced development of the chick oviduct is given in Table V.

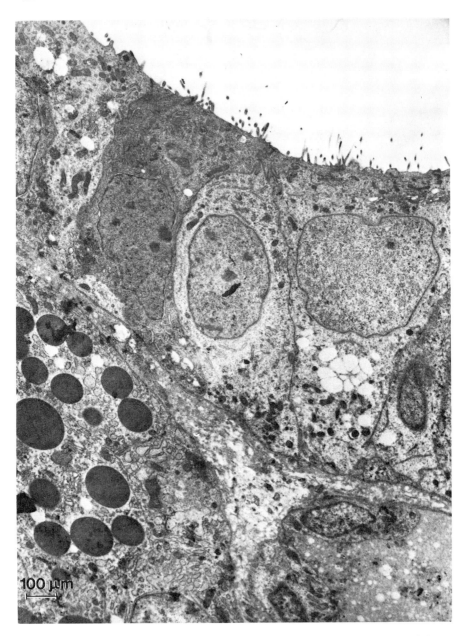

FIGS. 5 and 6. Electron micrographs of the epithelium of the magnum of normal (Fig. 5, left) and vitamin A-deficient (Fig. 6, right) chicks given estradiol-17β benzoate for 6 consecutive days. Note the presence of protodifferentiated cells containing secretory gran-

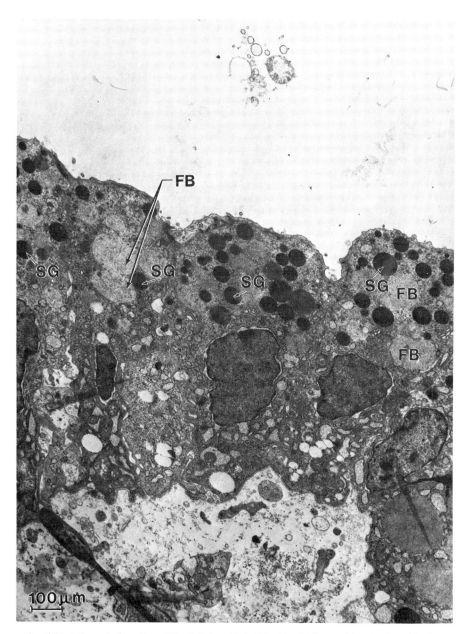

100 μm

ules (SG) at the apical portion of the deficient birds (Fig. 6), which are virtually absent in the normal birds (Fig. 5). Also note the presence of several flocculent bodies (FB) in such cells of the deficient tissue (Fig. 6), which are rarely seen in the normal tissue (Fig. 5). ×6930.

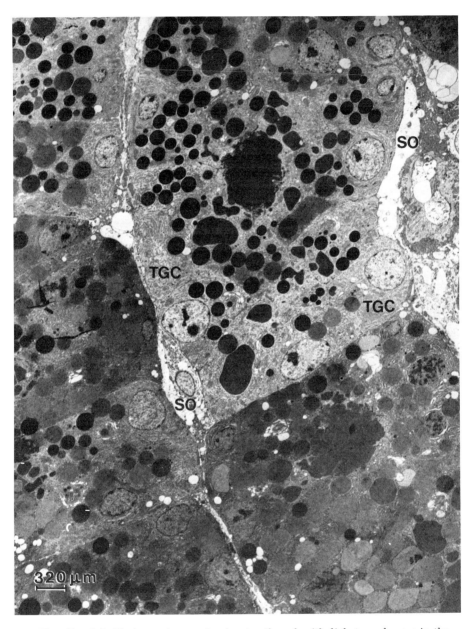

FIGS. 7 and 8. Electron micrographs showing the subepithelial stromal space in the normal (Fig. 7, left) and vitamin A-deprived (Fig. 8, right) chicks. Note that the stromal space is packed with the gland cells in the normal birds (Fig. 7) whereas stromal edema is

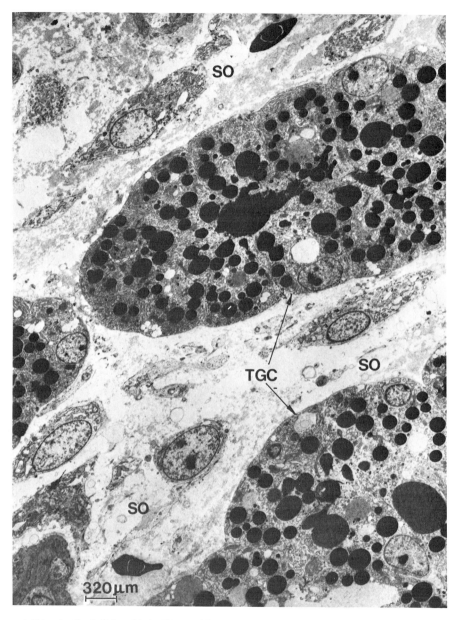

striking in the deficient birds (Fig. 8). Also note that, the acini are compact in the normal birds, but they are elongated in the deficient ones. TGC, tubular gland cells; SO, stromal edema. ×2240.

J. GANGULY ET AL.

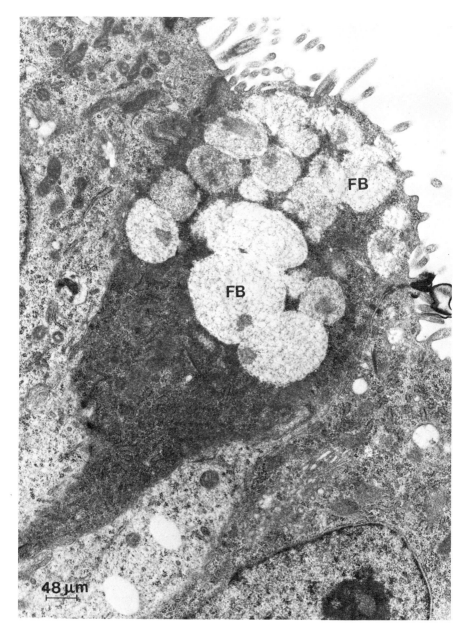

Fig. 9. Electron micrograph showing a typical goblet cell in the epithelial lining facing the lumen of the oviduct magnum of a vitamin A-deficient bird. Note that the flocculent bodies (FB) are prominent with or without electron-dense patches. ×14,840.

TABLE V

ULTRASTRUCTURAL OBSERVATIONS ON THE EFFECT OF VITAMIN A-DEPRIVATION ON THE ESTROGEN-INDUCED GROWTH OF THE MAGNUM OF CHICK OVIDUCT[a,b]

Sample	Retinyl acetate from day 1	Vitamin A depleted
Surface epithelium		
Protodifferentiated cells	Few	Significant numbers with abundant secretory granules
Goblet cells (clusters of inter-calated cells with flocculent, electron-opaque materials within)	Seen occasionally	Very prominent throughout the surface epithelium
Subepithelial region		
Stromal edema	Very little	Very prominent
Tubular glands		
Population	Abundant	Sparse
Size	Large	Small
Shape	Circular	Ellipsoidal
RER	Well developed	Vesicular
Stromal cells	Migrated to form smooth muscles	Abundant in subepithelial stromal space

[a]Adapted from Das et al. (1979).
[b]The pictures from retinoate-fed chicks were almost similar to those from deficient chicks.

It was mentioned previously that the temporal sequence of events during the normal process of development of the oviduct magnum is that the formation of the tubular gland cells is the major program of differentiation during the first 6 days of estrogen administration; only after this do the goblet cells start to appear in significant numbers, and they become prominent by day 9. But in the vitamin A-deprived birds clusters of goblet cells were very prominent and frequent throughout the surface epithelium even on day 6 of estrogen treatment (Fig. 4), and similar cells were rarely seen in the corresponding control birds. It was even more interesting that, whereas few secretory granules were seen in the protodifferentiated cells of the normal magnum (Fig. 5), in the depleted birds such cells not only contained large numbers of mature granules but also contained flocculent bodies, which are characteristic of the goblet cells (Fig. 6). It would be pertinent to mention in this context that during their work on the effect of progesterone administration together with estradiol, Palmiter and Wrenn (1971) also had noted the presence of such flocculent bodies in the protodifferentiated cells of the oviduct magnum, which had led them to conclude that in the presence of both the hormones the progenitor epithelial cells simul-

taneously differentiate in several directions owing to conflicting sig-
nals. It would thus appear that a similar situation arises in the absence
of an adequate supply of vitamin A in that, in the absence of retinol,
the programmed sequence of events that take place during the normal
process of estrogen-induced development of the magnum is disturbed,
thereby leading to simultaneous differentiation of some of the progenitor cells in different directions.

Therefore, it is clear that vitamin A deficiency affects both division
and differentiation of cells. Thus, whereas earlier work had shown
that, as compared to normal rats, the mitotic indices are significantly
lower in the cornea, trachea, and epidermis of the vitamin A-deficient
rats, more recent work with regenerating rat liver has demonstrated
that the regeneration is markedly less in the vitamin A-deprived rats.
Similarly earlier work had shown, consistently and conclusively,
marked effects of vitamin A deprivation on the differentiation of many
epithelial systems, the classic examples being spermatogenesis in the
males and vaginal cell cycles in the females, whereas our most recent
work with the chick oviduct has demonstrated similar striking effects
of vitamin A deprivation on the division and differentiation of the
various types of cells of the oviduct magnum.

IV. Effect of Vitamin A Deprivation on Biosynthesis of RNA and Proteins and on Glycosylation of Proteins

A. RNA and Protein Synthesis

Previous work with vitamin A-deficient rats did not lead to any
general agreement regarding a coenzymic role for the vitamin. Work in
a few other laboratories on the effect of vitamin A deficiency on RNA
metabolism and protein synthesis seems to have yielded more suggestive results. Thus, Yonemoto and Johnson (1967) had reported
that codeine demethylase activity in the microsomal fraction of the
liver of vitamin A-deficient rats is very low. The decrease in the
activity of the enzyme could be restored to normal levels by supplementation of the deficient animals with vitamin A. The restoration with vitamin A was sensitive to actinomycin D. Further support
for such an idea of participation of vitamin A in RNA metabolism came
from the work of Zachman (1967), who claimed that administration of
vitamin A stimulates RNA synthesis in the colon and intestinal mucosa of vitamin A-deficient rats, but not in the liver and kidneys of the
same animals. Similarly, according to Johnson *et al.* (1969) an injec-

tion of potassium retinoate into vitamin A-deficient rats induces marked increase in the synthesis of nuclear as well as total RNA in the liver and mucosa of such rats.

The effect of vitamin A deprivation on the different species of RNA in animal tissues has also been investigated. Thus, Johnson *et al.* (1969) claimed that the messenger-like RNA is the target of vitamin A function, whereas according to Kaufman *et al.* (1972) a high molecular weight RNA of the tracheal epithelium of hamsters is sensitive to vitamin A deprivation. At about the same time De Luca *et al.* (1971) reported that vitamin A deprivation affects the synthesis of rRNA and tRNA in the intestinal mucosa of rats. By using the system of rapid cell proliferation, that is, regeneration of rat liver following partial hepatectomy, Jayaram *et al.* (1975) found that the net increase in the RNA and DNA contents of the regenerating liver of the vitamin A-deprived rats was markedly lower than in the corresponding controls. Soon after this preliminary work, Jayaram (unpublished observations) observed that, after an intraperitoneal injection of [^{32}P]orthophosphate, incorporation of the radioactivity into the total RNA of the regenerating liver was significantly lower in the deficient rats, and later work of Jayaram and Ganguly (1977) on the analysis of different species of RNA in rat tissues revealed an increase in the oligonucleotide fraction at the expense of the rRNA and tRNA in the intestinal mucosa and testes, but not in the liver of deficient animals. In addition to such effects on the contents of the rRNA and tRNA, the deficiency also caused a reduction in the percentage of poly(A) in the RNA of the intestinal mucosa and testes, but not in the liver RNA, and incorporation of [^{32}P]orthophosphate was depressed in the testicular RNA of the deficient animals. Equally significant was the observation of Jayaram that the increase in the RNA polymerase activity of the nuclei isolated from the liver undergoing regeneration was lower in the vitamin A-deprived rats; this observation is in general agreement with the later findings of Tsai and Chytil (1978a,b), who reported that RNA synthesis is lower in the liver nuclei of vitamin A-deficient rats.

Thus all these observations made on the basis of different approaches, including analysis of the contents and rates of synthesis of total as well as different species of RNA, have consistently indicated a marked effect of vitamin A deprivation on the nature and synthesis of different types of RNA in those cells that undergo rapid regeneration. It remains, however, to be seen whether these effects of vitamin A deprivation on RNA synthesis reflect primary function of vitamin A or whether they reflect indirectly the primary events of vitamin A function at another level.

In addition to these studies on the effect of vitamin A deprivation on the synthesis of nucleic acids in animal tissues there have been some attempts to study the effect of the deficiency on protein synthesis. Thus De Luca *et al.* (1969) and De Luca and Wolf (1969) claimed that deficiency of vitamin A causes a decrease in the incorporation of [^{14}C]leucine into the proteins synthesized by the RER of the intestinal mucosa of rats, and De Luca and Wolf (1969) were able to trace such defects in protein synthesis to the "pH 5 fraction," which contains the aminoacyl-tRNA synthetases and tRNAs. But subsequent work of De Luca *et al.* (1971) indicated that, while vitamin A deficiency does not affect the aminoacyl-tRNA synthetases, it leads to an actual decrease in the tRNA contents of the intestinal mucosa of rats. Further information on the effects of vitamin A deprivation on tRNA of the intestinal mucosa of rats was subsequently made available by Jayaram and Ganguly (1977), who not only reported lower contents of tRNA in the deficient mucosa, but also observed that its charging capacity was also reduced. By using the aminoacyl-tRNA synthetases isolated from homologous tissues of normal animals, which eliminated any possible changes in the enzyme activity caused by the deficiency, these workers found that the amino acid acceptor activity of the tRNA of the testes and intestinal mucosa of the deficient rats was lower than in the corresponding control samples. It would be pertinent to point out in this context that, according to Krause *et al.* (1975), vitamin A deficiency markedly affects the tRNA methylase activities of rat testes.

B. Glycosylation of Proteins

Polyisoprenoid alcohols, called polyprenols, are widely distributed in both plant and animal systems. They vary in chain length depending upon the number of isoprene units they contain. Solanesol, an all-*trans*-nonaprenol was the first polyprenol to be isolated from tobacco leaves (Rowland *et al.*, 1956), the isolation of castaprenol from horse chestnut leaves by Wellburn *et al.* (1967) followed. Eventually a whole family of isoprenyl alcohols called dolichols was identified in yeast (Dunphy *et al.*, 1966) and in animal systems including pig liver (Dunphy *et al.*, 1967) and rat liver (Gough and Hemming, 1970).

Soon after the polyprenols were recognized, they were shown to act as lipid intermediates in the biosynthesis of the bacterial cell-wall polysaccharides. The essential features of the reactions involving polyprenols are that the phosphomonoester derivatives of the prenols accept a sugar moiety from an appropriate sugar nucleotide, which is followed by transfer of the sugar to an endogenous acceptor.

Such sugar-transfer reactions involving various polyprenols have been shown in yeast and in the plant systems also. At the same time it was also observed that membrane preparations obtained from a variety of animal tissues can catalyze the transfer of mannose from GDP-mannose to an endogenous lipid acceptor (Cacaam *et al.*, 1969), and in this particular case the lipid moiety was eventually identified as dolichol (Behrens *et al.*, 1971, 1973). The point that is most relevant to the present discussion is that, according to Waechter and Lennarz (1976), such biosynthesis of mannolipids can be effected by monophosphate derivatives of several polyprenols including betulaprenol, solanesol, and ficaprenol, with dolichol being most effective in this respect.

Retinol is a tetraprenol, and therefore by analogy it would certainly appear that this particular prenol also might be able to take part in similar sugar-transfer reactions. Indeed, such considerations have led to rather extensive work demonstrating participation of retinol in similar sugar-transfer reactions. Thus it has been claimed that deprivation of vitamin A affects the synthesis of certain glycopeptides and glycolipids in the intestinal mucosa (De Luca *et al.*, 1970b; 1973; Rossa *et al.*, 1971; Kleinman and Wolf, 1974) and corneal epithelium (Kim and Wolf, 1975) of rats and in the tracheal epithelium (Bonanni *et al.*, 1973) and liver (De Luca *et al.*, 1975) of hamsters.

During their attempts to demonstrate transfer of activated sugar to retinol, De Luca *et al.* (1970a) had found that a mannolipid is formed when GDP-mannose and retinol are incubated with a preparation containing membrane-bound polysomes isolated from the liver of mildly vitamin A-deficient rats. The lipid moiety of this complex was more polar than retinol, but was distinct from retinol or retinoic acid, and was called "polar metabolite of retinol." Later, by using GDP-mannose and ATP labeled with ^{32}P at different positions, De Luca *et al.* (1973) showed that in such reactions retinol is linked to the sugar moiety through a monophosphate diester bond; this indicated that the formation of retinyl phosphate is the primary step in the participation of retinol in glycosylation reactions. On the other hand, by incubating retinyl phosphate and [^{14}C]galactose with crude membrane fractions of mouse mastocytoma, Helting and Peterson (1972) claimed transfer of the labeled galactose from retinyl phosphate-[^{14}C]galactose into trichloroacetic acid-precipitable materials, and very recently Hassel *et al.* (1978) reported that administration of excess retinol to rats stimulates incorporation of [^{14}C]mannose into the liver mannosyl retinyl phosphate and dolichol mannosyl phosphate as also into liver glycoproteins by over 200% during a 20-minute labeling period. Finally, De

Luca (1977) claimed on the basis of his experiments that (a) retinyl phosphate occurs in the membranes of animal cells, (b) it can be formed biosynthetically, (c) mannosyl retinyl phosphate and galactosyl retinyl phosphate are formed biosynthetically from retinyl phosphate and the respective sugar, and (d) these compounds serve as natural intermediates in glycosylation reactions.

Chick oviduct is probably one of the most active tissues involved in the synthesis of several characteristic glycoproteins, including ovalbumin. Therefore in our laboratory extensive analysis was carried out of the different glycoproteins as well as of the protein-bound hexoses and hexosamines in the oviduct of normal and vitamin A-depleted chicks given daily injections of estradiol-17β benzoate for six consecutive days. Our results have shown significant increase in the levels of free hexoses and hexosamines in the oviduct of the depleted birds with a corresponding decrease in the protein-bound sugars. On the other hand, the ovalbumin contents per oviduct and [^{3}H]mannose incorporation into the total cytosol proteins as well as into the ovalbumin were lower in the depleted oviduct, while there was no significant difference in the carbohydrate contents per mg ovalbumin in the two groups of birds. These results therefore did not provide any definite indications regarding any role of retinol in the glycosylation of ovalbumin (Ganguly et al., 1978a,b). In addition to these observations of ours, there are several other points which have made it rather difficult for us to accept the idea that retinol plays any special role in sugar-transfer reactions and our views can be summarized as follows.

According to Waechter and Lennarz (1976), the role played by polyprenols in sugar-transfer reactions is rather nonspecific. In fact, De Luca et al. (1973) had reported that, even under those conditions where retinol participates in such reactions dolichol also does so with equal efficiency. This point assumes great significance, because the amounts of dolichol found in animal liver are usually vastly in excess of the amounts of retinol present in the same tissue. On the other hand, De Luca (1977) has claimed some differences in the mode of transfer of sugar to the acceptor proteins by dolichol phosphate sugar and retinyl phosphate sugar. Thus it has been claimed that retinyl phosphate acts as a direct donor of mannose to glycoproteins without the build up of oligosaccharides on itself, whereas dolichol builds up the oligosaccharide chain on itself, after which the oligosaccharide is transferred to the acceptor protein. Yet another important difference seems to be that, in the retinol-catalyzed glycosylation, the mannosyl residue incorporated into an oligosaccharide chain (which is bound to a protein) is alkali labile and is probably an O-glycosidic type of linkage. In contrast, in the case of the dolichol-mediated synthesis (probably ovalbumin), the sugar moiety is attached to the asparaginyl residue of the protein by an alkali stable, N-glycosidic bond. However, more definitive information regarding the specificity of the acceptor proteins as well as of the lipid intermediates is needed before such claims can be readily accepted.

Such mechanisms mediated by retinol cannot explain the physiological effects of retinoic acid because as yet it has not been established that retinoic acid can be reduced to retinol in animal systems, nor does it appear possible that retinoic acid can form the phosphate intermediates necessary for such reactions. It should, however, be mentioned in this context that De Luca (1977) has claimed that administration of retinoic acid to vitamin A-depleted rats enhances the incorporation of [^{3}H]mannose into a labeled glycolipic that is chromatographically indistinguishable from authentic mannosyl retinyl phosphate. In addition, by using [^{3}H]retinoic acid in cultured mouse fibroblast system, he isolated a compound that was chromatographically similar to retinyl phosphate. De Luca (1977) has, therefore, suggested that retinoic acid is metabolized to an unidentified derivative containing a hydroxyl group. It must be pointed out, however, that such a compound has not been conclusively identified, nor has its role as an intermediate in such reactions been demonstrated.

Although De Luca (1977) has claimed to have isolated retinyl phosphate from biological membranes the nature of the phosphate donor for retinol leading to the synthesis of retinyl phosphate is still obscure and attempts made by using several nucleotide triphosphates containing labeled phosphate at the γ-position as a potential donor of the phosphate moiety have failed to give labeled retinyl phosphate (Peterson *et al.*, 1974).

Finally, it must not be overlooked that, although retinol is required by higher organisms only, polyprenols take part in sugar-transfer reactions also in bacterial organisms.

V. Transport, Delivery, and Mode of Action of Steroid Hormones

At the time when diverse approaches were being made in many laboratories to the question of systemic mode of action of vitamin A, rapid advances were made in a seemingly unrelated area, the mode of action of steroid hormones; as a result of sustained work of several groups of workers, considerable information is now available regarding the mechanisms of transport of steroid hormones to the nucleus of the target cells.

A. Transport in Blood

While considering transport of hormones in general in blood it should be recognized that there are two distinct chemically defined classes of hormones present. The water-soluble protein and peptide hormones do not appear to bind to other plasma proteins. In sharp contrast, the steroid hormones are mainly associated with some serum proteins, which have been called "carriers" (Westphal, 1970).

B. Delivery and Mode of Action

The steroid hormones are the best-known effectors of gene expression in eukaryotes. The site of action of all steroids in their respective target cells appears to be basically similar, only the resulting effects differ in different target cells, and it is widely believed that the steroid hormones regulate the functions of the target cells by influencing cellular RNA and protein synthesis. Since the cell nucleus is the site of RNA synthesis, there should be a well organized sequence of events leading to the transport of the steroid molecule to the cell nucleus so that it can exert its effects there in a well controlled manner. During the 1970s rapid progress has been made in the elucidation of such sequence of events, and some of the salient features of these findings, especially with respect to the action of estradiol in rat uterus and of estradiol and progesterone in the chick oviduct are summarized below.

1. *Rat Uterus*

Availability of tritium-labeled estradiol was mainly responsible for initiation of the work on the mode of action of the estrogen at the molecular level, and extensive work in this area has been covered in some recent reviews (Jensen *et al.*, 1974; Gorski and Gannon, 1976). It is generally accepted that from the blood plasma the steroid diffuses into the target cells through the plasma membrane, after which it is picked up by a 4 S cytoplasmic binding protein. Available evidence indicates that the ligand-bound 4 S protein is converted to a 5 S form within the cytosol, probably through the addition of a peptide of a molecular weight of about 50,000, which is then translocated to the cell nucleus (Yamamoto and Alberts, 1972).

Binding of the Estrogen–Receptor Complex to the Nucleus and Chromatin, and the Consequent Effect on RNA Synthesis. Several groups of workers have studied the nature of binding of estradiol to the nucleus, after the estradiol–receptor complex is translocated into the nucleus. Thus, Harris (1971) showed that treatment with DNase of the uterine nuclei previously labeled with [³H]estradiol releases the radioactivity into the supernatant, and Musliner and Chader (1972) claimed that pretreatment of the rat uterine nuclei with DNase abolishes the ability of the nuclei to take up the estradiol–receptor complex. On the other hand, Toft (1972) and Clemens and Kleinsmith (1972) reported that native DNA isolated from rat uterus can bind the estradiol–receptor complex.

Although these claims indicated that the estradiol–receptor complex might act through direct binding with DNA, such a mechanism would obviously fail to explain the phenomenon of tissue specificity of the binding of the steroids, which is characteristic of the target cells. But, since the [³H]estradiol–receptor complex of the uterine chromatin is readily extractable with 0.3–0.4 M KCl (Yamamoto and Alberts, 1972; Toft, 1972; Musliner and Chader, 1972), it has been suggested that the nonhistone proteins act as acceptor molecules for the receptor complex on the chromatin, because it is widely recognized that such KCl treatment selectively extracts the nonhistone proteins from the chromatin. Indeed, such an interpretation should explain the phenomenon of tissue specificity of estradiol binding, because the nonhistone proteins are very characteristic of a particular tissue.

There have been some attempts to demonstrate the effect of estradiol on RNA synthesis in the target tissues (Mueller *et al.*, 1958; Gorski and Nicolette, 1963; Hamilton, 1964). It was shown that after estrogen administration RNA polymerases I and II are both activated in rat uterus; this obviously indicates that the estrogen stimulates synthesis of both ribosomal and pre-mRNA (Glasser *et al.*, 1972).

It has already been discussed that the estrogen action is probably mediated by the estradiol–receptor complex through its binding to the chromatin. In fact several investigators have studied the effect of the estradiol–receptor complex on RNA synthesis in the nuclei isolated from target cells. Thus, Raynaud-Jamet and Baulieu (1969) have claimed that addition of a sample of heifer endometrium cytosol, which was previously incubated with estradiol, causes a 2- to 3-fold increase in the RNA polymerase activity of the endometrium nuclei. Later on, Mohla *et al.* (1972) and Jensen *et al.* (1974) reported that such stimulation of the RNA polymerase activity is specific for the nuclei of the hormone-dependent tissue and that such an effect can be seen only with estradiol that is complexed with the transformed 5 S receptor, not with the 4 S receptor. It was even more interesting that such effects could be shown not only with the isolated nuclei, but also with isolated chromatin. Thus, Jensen *et al.* (1974) claimed that, when RNA synthesis was examined with the chromatin isolated from calf endometrium and with partially purified RNA polymerase, the estradiol–receptor complex effected a 2- to 3-fold increase in RNA synthesis.

2. *Chick Oviduct*

Yet another system that has provided very useful information with respect to the mechanism of action of steriod hormones is estrogen-induced development of chick oviduct. The sequence of events that take place during cytodifferentiation of the oviduct of immature chicks under estrogen stimulation has been discussed above, and the information available on the molecular mechanisms involved in the action of steroid hormones in the oviduct is summarized here.

a. Estradiol. One of the earliest effects of an estrogen in the oviduct of immature chicks is activation of the synthesis of rapidly labeled nuclear RNA (O'Malley *et al.*, 1969), which is reflected in a simultaneous increase in the RNA polymerase activity of the isolated nuclei (McGuire and O'Malley, 1968; O'Malley *et al.*, 1969). Since ovalbumin constitutes about 60% of the soluble proteins of the oviduct magnum, ovalbumin synthesis has been used with great advantage as a typical system for the study of estrogen-mediated gene expression. Thus, by measuring translation of mRNA in a heterologous system Means *et al.* (1972) and Rosenfeld *et al.* (1972) found that the estrogen markedly stimulates the synthesis of ovalbumin mRNA in the oviduct. This observation was confirmed by Harris *et al.* (1975), who studied *in vitro* hybridization of total cellular RNA with complementary DNA synthesized against purified ovalbumin mRNA.

No doubt these findings indicated that probably during the process of ovalbumin synthesis the.estrogen acts at the transcriptional level of the chromatin, but more direct evidence in support of such a possibility was provided by Harris *et al.* (1976). By using chromatin isolated from the estrogen-stimulated and unstimulated oviduct these workers showed that transcription of the ovalbumin mRNA sequences, *in vitro,* is readily detected in the chromatin of the estrogen-stimulated oviduct, but not in the unstimulated oviduct. The same workers further showed that withdrawal of estrogen administration for 12 days from the estrogen-primed birds resulted in a 20-fold reduction in the ovalbumin mRNA sequences in the *in vitro* RNA transcripts.

Although these interesting observations indicated the molecular events in the oviduct after estrogen treatment, they did not provide sufficient evidence for direct involvement of an estradiol–receptor complex in these processes. However, using the technique of "exchange assay," M. J. Tsai *et al.* (1975) and Kalimi *et al.* (1976) measured the chromatin-bound estradiol–receptor complex during primary stimulation, withdrawal, and secondary stimulation, and they found that, on discontinuation of the estrogen treatment after 12 days of primary stimulation, the differentiated cells lose their ability to synthesize the cell-specific proteins. The same workers further noticed a concomitant decrease in the levels of the chromatin-bound receptors during the process of withdrawal of the estrogen treatment, and readministration of the estrogen to such chicks resulted in a rapid increase in the chromatin-bound estrogen receptors.

Even though the actual mechanism by which the binding of the estrogen–receptor complex to the chromatin brings about an increase in RNA synthesis is not properly understood, the observations of S. Y. Tsai et al. (1975) and of Schwartz et al. (1975) have indicated that probably the interaction of the estradiol–receptor complex with the chromatin of the target cells leads to an actual increase in the formation of the initiation complex between the RNA polymerase and chromatin. Such a possibility was supported by the observations of Kalimi et al. (1976), who claimed a close relationship between the nucleus-bound estrogen receptor and the number of initiation sites for RNA synthesis during the primary stimulation with estrogen, during withdrawal of estrogen treatment, and during secondary stimulation.

b. Progesterone. In the chick oviduct, progesterone specifically stimulates synthesis of the egg-white protein avidin, which represents about 0.1% of the total egg-white proteins. O'Malley et al. (1969) first showed that the induction of avidin synthesis by progesterone is preceded by an increase in RNA polymerase activity, and in a later report O'Malley et al. (1971) claimed that progesterone administration leads to an increase in the levels of avidin mRNA in the chick oviduct.

At the same time attempts were made to purify the progesterone receptor from the oviduct cytosol. Thus, while Kuhn et al. (1975) were able to purify the progesterone receptor to homogeneity, Schraeder and O'Malley (1972) and Buller et al. (1975) reported that the receptor consists of two subunits, termed A and B. The subunit A has a molecular weight of 110,000, and its ligand-bound form preferentially binds with DNA, whereas the B subunit has a molecular weight of 117,000 and binds to the chromatin in its ligand-bound form. As in the case of the other steroid hormones, the binding of progesterone to the chromatin was shown to require the presence of the receptor and to involve a temperature-dependent translocation process (O'Malley et al., 1971). In their attempts to understand the nature of the interaction of the progesterone receptor with the chromatin, Spelsberg et al. (1972) dissociated the nonhistone proteins and histones of the oviduct chromatin by treatment with 2.0 M NaCl–5.0 M urea at pH 8.3; after this they reconstituted most of the dissociated nonhistone proteins and histones with the DNA back to chromatin by gradient dialysis. In some of these experiments the nonhistone proteins and histones of the chromatin from one tissue were reconstituted with the DNA of another tissue to give hybrid chromatins. The oviduct cytosol containing the [³H]progesterone-receptor complex was then separately incubated with the intact, reconstituted, and hybrid chromatin, when it was found that the homologous reconstituted chromatin binds the progesterone-receptor complex quantitatively like the intact native chromatin, whereas the hybrid chromatin obtained from the reconstitution of the erythrocyte nonhistone protein, oviduct DNA, and histone lost its ability to bind the progesterone-receptor complex. It was thus clear that not only that the nonhistone proteins of the chromatin serve as acceptor molecules for the progesterone-receptor complex but that these proteins are also tissue specific.

Later on, direct evidence for the participation of the progesterone receptor in the modulation of the transcription activity in chick oviduct came from the work of Schwartz *et al.* (1976) and of Buller *et al.* (1976). By using a cell-free system that contained the oviduct chromatin from the estradiol-withdrawn chicks and *E. coli* RNA polymerase, these workers showed that the progesterone-receptor complex increases the initiation sites on the chromatin for RNA synthesis by about 60% of the value obtained with chromatin alone. It was also claimed by the same workers that such stimulatory effects of the purified progesterone receptor are specific for the oviduct chromatin.

VI. TRANSPORT AND DELIVERY OF RETINOL

A. TRANSPORT IN BLOOD

While such advances were being made in the areas of transport, delivery, and mode of action of steroid hormones, similar interesting developments were taking place in the field of vitamin A. There were, however, earlier attempts to understand the manner in which retinol is transported in the blood and stored in the liver. Ganguly *et al.* (1952) demonstrated that ammonium sulfate treatment of chicken plasma precipitates the plasma retinol bound to proteins. Immediately after this work Ganguly and Krinsky (1953) observed that retinol appeared to be transported in rat blood by a specific carrier protein and Krinsky and Ganguly (1953) made similar suggestions regarding storage of retinol in rat liver. Later Krinsky *et al.* (1958) actually showed that in human blood retinol is bound to a protein component that fractionated with the plasma albumin but was different from the plasma albumin. Similarly, by using various protein fractionation and denaturation techniques Krishnamurthy *et al.* (1958a,b) demonstrated that in rat liver supernatant retinol is bound to a protein. Relevant information concerning transport in blood and storage in liver of retinol in association with specific proteins was reviewed by Ganguly (1960).

Later systematic work led to the isolation and characterization of a specific protein that transports retinol in blood. This particular protein has been called RBP (retinol binding protein) and has been isolated from the blood of several mammalian species, e.g., human (Kanai *et al.*, 1968), the rat (Muto and Goodman, 1972), the pig (Huang *et al.*, 1972), the dog (Muto *et al.*, 1973), the monkey (Vahlquist and Peterson, 1972), chickens (Bhat *et al.*, 1977), and the goat (Sreekrishna and Cama, 1978a). The extensive work on the blood RBP has been covered in several recent reviews (Glover, 1973; Glover *et al.*, 1974; Goodman, 1974; Sreekrishna and Cama, 1978b).

The liver is the main storage organ for vitamin A, where it is deposited essentially in the form of its palmitic acid ester (Mahadevan and Ganguly, 1961). The retinyl esters are hydrolyzed in the liver by a hydrolase (Mahadevan *et al.*, 1966), after which the retinol is bound to the apo-RBP in the liver; the holo-RBP thus formed is released into the circulation, where it combines with prealbumin. The interaction of retinol with apo-RBP (a) converts retinol into a water-soluble complex; (b) protects the rather unstable retinol molecule against any degradative processes (Glover, 1973); and (c) prevents the cytolytic effects of retinol, because unbound retinol can attack biomembranes.

The RBP isolated from the blood of several species of animals has been shown to be rather similar in their properties: (a) their molecular weights are in the range of about 21,000; (b) they show α_2-mobility during electrophoresis, and (c), they have similar ultraviolet absorption and fluorescence excitation-emission spectra. It has also been claimed that the binding of all-*trans*-retinol to RBP is not absolutely specific because it can bind *in vitro* with retinyl acetate, retinal, and retinoic acid also, but with varying degrees of affinity.

The holo-RBP circulates in blood in combination with prealbumin having an apparent molecular weight of about 75,000. Here also, such complexing of holo-RBP with prealbumin is of considerable physiological significance, because such combination prevents loss of the small molecular weight RBP through glomerular filtration in the kidney (Kanai, *et al.*, 1968). The findings, however, that large amounts of RBP are excreted through the urine of humans suffering from tubular proteinuria (Peterson and Berggard, 1971) as well as of the Japanese patients with chronic cadmium poisoning and "Itai-Itai" disease (Kanai *et al.*, 1972a,b) are not easily reconcilable with the above concept for the function of prealbumin.

In recent years considerable attention has been focused on the regulation of synthesis of RBP in the liver. Thus, by using the technique of radioimmunoassay, Muto *et al.* (1972) had shown that when rats are depleted of vitamin A their serum RBP levels gradually decline with the progress of depletion. At the same time, however, RBP accumulates in the liver, so that when such rats are given supplements of retinol the serum RBP levels show a steep increase, and the liver RBP contents show a simultaneous decrease. It was further shown by Smith *et al.* (1970) that such rapid increase in the serum RBP levels in the vitamin A-deficient rats given supplements of retinol is not due to enhanced synthesis of RBP in the liver, because such an increase in blood RBP could not be prevented by administration of cycloheximide or puromycin to such rats. Therefore it has been generally accepted that RBP synthesis continues in the liver during vitamin A deprivation and that, without the ligand, secretion of the RBP from the liver into the blood cannot take place.

The work of Glover and associates has further shown that the RBP synthesis in the liver is dependent on the physiological and nutritional status of the animal. Thus it has been reported by Muhilal and Glover (1974) that on low protein intake the plasma RBP levels decline even when the liver contains a sufficient supply of retinol, which suggests that the release of retinol from the liver into the circulation is determined by the extent of RBP synthesis in the liver. This would readily explain the situation frequently encountered in Kwashiorkor children, who may have sufficient vitamin A in their liver, but have blood vitamin A levels that are usually very low. This aspect was thoroughly reviewed by Mahadevan *et al.* (1965).

More recently Glover *et al.* (1978) made the interesting observation that the plasma RBP levels in several species of animals show remarkable seasonal variation that reflects their increased or decreased physiological requirements for vitamin A. Thus, when the holo-RBP concentrations in the plasma of groups of ewes and castrated rams were determined monthly throughout the year, in both groups of animals the plasma RBP concentrations were minimal (20–30 μg/ml) during the summer months, but in late August and early September the values rose to peak levels (80–100 μg/ml), which were about 3-fold higher than the minimum values. It was most significant that such elevated values were maintained during the breeding season but showed a steady decline during November and December, so that by

January the levels were down to 40 μg/ml for the rams and 30 μg/ml for the ewes. These workers pointed out that such seasonal changes in the serum RBP values in both sexes appear to coincide with the development of the gonads in these animals, which starts in the sheep with the shortening of the day length after midsummer. Equally interesting observations were made by these workers with the Japanese quail. In these birds the plasma holo-RBP levels rise steeply in January, reaching a first peak by the end of March, show a slight decline in April, and reach minimum levels by June to July in the males and by July to August in the females. But their most significant observation was that during such seasonal changes the plasma holo-RBP levels rose in the females from 80–100 μg/ml to about 250–280 μg/ml, and it is obvious that so marked an increase in the plasma holo-RBP levels takes place to meet the high demands for egg laying and also for the development of the gonads during this period.

B. Cellular Retinol-Binding Proteins

It is thus clear that animals have evolved highly specialized mechanisms for transport of regulated amounts of retinol in the blood in the form of holo-RBP for delivering the retinol to the tissues. While such work on serum RBP was in progress in some laboratories, Bashor et al. (1973) made the interesting observation that many rat tissues contain yet another type of protein that can bind retinol. By using techniques that have been extensively employed for binding studies for steroids, i.e., [³H]retinol and sucrose density gradient centrifugation, these workers found that the high speed supernatant fractions obtained from the intestinal mucosa, kidney, liver, lung, spleen, testes, etc., of rats can bind [³H]retinol. Bashor et al. further showed that such binding proteins of the tissues are different from the serum binding protein as to their molecular size in that, while the cellular binding proteins sediment at 2 S, the corresponding value for the serum binding protein in combination with prealbumin is 4 S. In order to distinguish the two types of binding proteins, they suggested that the cellular binding protein should be called CRBP. Soon it was reported from the same laboratory (Ong and Chytil, 1975) that various rat tissues, including the brain, eye, ovary, uterus, testes, contain yet another class of proteins, which can bind retinoic acid instead of retinol; such binding proteins were called CRABP. It has been a rather active field in recent years, and the general information on these proteins has been reviewed by Chytil and Ong (1978a,b). Both CRBP and CRABP have been purified to homogeneity, and the reported properties of the purified proteins are summarized in Table VI.

TABLE VI

SOME REPORTED PROPERTIES OF THE CELLULAR RETINOL- AND RETINOIC ACID-BINDING PROTEINS
PURIFIED FROM VARIOUS TISSUES[a]

Source	Molecular weight	Dissociation constants	Reference
CRBP			
Rat liver cytosol	14,600	1.6×10^{-8} M	Chytil and Ong (1978a)
Bovine retina cytosol	16,300	—	Saari et al. (1978)
Rat testis			
Cytosol	14,000	1.5×10^{-10} M (type I)	Shinde et al. (1980)
		2.0×10^{-9} M (type II)	
Nucleosol	14,000	—	Shinde et al. (1980)
Chromatin	14,000	—	Shinde et al. (1980)
Hen oviduct			
Cytosol	13,180	2.7×10^{-8} M (type I)	Das et al. (1978)
		2.5×10^{-7} M (type II)	
Nucleosol	14,500	—	Rao et al. (1979)
Chromatin	14,500	—	Rao et al. (1979)
CRABP			
Rat testis cytosol	14,600	4.2×10^{-9} M	Chytil and Ong (1978b)
Bovine retina cytosol	16,600	—	Saari et al. (1978)

[a] CRBP, cellular retinol-binding protein; CRABP, cellular retinoic acid-binding protein.

The CRBP isolated from different animal tissues appears to be specific for retinol in that, it does not bind retinoic acid. On the other hand, the CRABP also appears to be specific for retinoic acid, because it does not bind retinol. The sedimentation behavior and molecular weights of the two types of proteins are very similar; but they can be separated by DEAE-anion exchange chromatography. It must, however, be pointed out that, in contrast to the rather wide occurrence of CRBP in animal tissues (with the exception of skeletal muscles and heart) distribution of CRABP is rather restricted. Ong and Chytil (1976) have further reported that, although CRBP and CRABP are found extensively in the fetal rat tissues, CRABP disappears from all tissues of the adult rat, excepting the eye, brain, and skin, whereas CRBP persists in the tissues of the rat even after it attains adulthood. They have therefore suggested that such changes might reflect the different and varying requirements for retinol and retinoic acid in the development and maturation of the organs of the particular animal.

In our laboratory Das et al. (1978) have purified a CRBP from the oviduct magnum of laying hens, and Rao et al. (1979) have isolated similar binding proteins for retinol from the cytosol, nucleosol, and chromatin fractions from homogenates of the same source. The three binding proteins isolated in our laboratory have shown similar elution profiles during chromatography through Sephadex G-75 and G-50 columns and during polyacrylamide gel electrophoresis; their molecular weights are also comparable and are in the region of about 14,500. Preliminary immunological tests with antibodies raised in rabbits against the cytosol CRBP have shown that the binding proteins from the chromatin and nucleosol of the oviduct magnum cross-react with such antibodies. These preliminary findings would appear to indicate that all three CRBPs of hen oviduct are probably of common origin. Rao *et al.* (1979) have shown further that, when oviduct minces prepared from vitamin A-depleted and vitamin A-repleted chicks treated with estrogen are incubated with [³H]retinol, nuclear uptake of the radioactivity is severalfold higher in the vitamin A-depleted oviduct, as compared to the vitamin A-repleted ones. These observations confirm the work of others who have previously obtained evidence for the nuclear binding of retinol and retinoic acid in other tissues of animals. Thus Sani (1977) claimed the presence of a CRABP in the chromatin fraction of chick embryo skin, and Wiggert *et al.* (1977) detected CRBP in the nucleosol fraction of human retinoblastoma cell cultures.

C. DELIVERY OF RETINOL

Some information is also available regarding cellular uptake of retinol from the circulating retinol-RBP-prealbumin complex. Here, two groups of workers have used two separate systems. Thus, by incubating the mucosal cells isolated from monkey intestine with [³H]retinol-RBP complex, Peterson and co-workers (1974; Rask and Peterson, 1976) have claimed that the [³H]retinol readily accumulates in the mucosal cells from the [³H]retinol-RBP complex. They have further shown that during this process there is no uptake of the protein part, because uptake of the [³H]retinol took place even when the RBP part of the RBP-retinol complex was linked to Sepharose beads. It has also been claimed by the same workers that such uptake of the [³H]retinol is mediated through a membrane receptor because the retinol uptake displayed saturable kinetics and was competitively inhibited by holo-RBP containing unlabeled retinol. On the other hand, presence of high concentrations of albumin or immunoglobulin G did not affect the uptake of the [³H]retinol by the mucosal cells.

Further evidence in support of participation of a plasma membrane receptor for the binding of RBP was produced by Heller (1975), who used the pigment epithelium of bovine retina. Apparently retinol is transported to the retina from blood via the choroidal surface of these cells. They appear as a single layer next to the outer segment of the photoreceptor cells and contain significant amounts of retinol. An important function of the pigment epithelium is to take up and transport retinol to the photoreceptor cells. Heller (1975), using ^{125}I-labeled RBP, has claimed that the isolated pigment epithelial cells of bovine retina can specifically bind holo-RBP. Heller has further claimed that the binding was at the cell surface and that the process was saturable. Subsequent work of Chen and Heller (1977) has indicated that the uptake of retinol by the pigment epithelium takes place from the retinol–RBP complex. As in the case of the mucosal cells of monkey intestine, here also the apo-RBP was left outside the pigment epithelial cells. Chen and Heller (1977) have further claimed that the retinol taken up by the pigment epithelial cells is found in the cytosol as retinol. About a third of the transported retinol was claimed to be bound to a high molecular weight protein ($> 1.5 \times 10^6$), and the rest appeared as free retinol. The nature of this high molecular weight protein is not clear. But it would be interesting to point out that Heller (1976) could detect some radioactivity of the retinol in the region of 15,000 molecular weight. On the other hand, Wiggert and Chader (1975) have demonstrated in the pigment epithelial cells of chicks a binding protein for retinol having a molecular weight of 17,000. At about the same time, by incubating a bovine pigment epithelium preparation with [^{3}H]retinol-RBP followed by extraction of the isolated plasma membranes with sodium dodecyl sulfate and electrophoresis on polyacrylamide gels, Mariani *et al.* (1977) have shown that the radioactivity could be found in the region of MW 14,500.

It would therefore appear that the initial step during the entry of retinol into these cells consists of interaction of the holo-RBP with a specific receptor on the plasma membrane, after which the retinol is delivered to the cell. It remains, however, to be seen whether such receptors for holo-RBP are present also on the surface of other epithelial cells.

VII. An Overview of the Similarities between the Mode of Action of Retinol and Steroid Hormones

The wealth of information that has been rapidly accumulating in recent years reveals a considerable degree of resemblance between the mode of action of steroid hormones in their functional cells on the one hand and that of retinol in epithelial cells on the other. Steroid hormones are synthesized in the endocrine tissues of higher animals and are transported attached to binding globulins through the blood stream to their target cells. The intracellular receptor proteins for the steroids, which are very characteristic of the target cells, concentrate the steroids from the circulating blood. Although it is not clear how the steroid hormones are transported across the plasma membranes of the target cells, it is generally assumed that they cross the plasma membranes by a process of diffusion. The entry of the steroids into the target cells is followed by a whole series of events that ultimately lead to an activation of the chromatin function in terms of specific gene expression.

Retinol, however, is received by the animal body in the diet as either the vitamin or the provitamin and is stored in the liver. It is then transported through blood to the tissues by the serum RBP in a well regulated manner. Moreover, as in the case of the steroids, cellular binding proteins for retinol have been isolated from several animal tissues, and all have a molecular weight of around 14,000. It has also been claimed that they are present in higher amounts in those cells that regenerate rapidly, but are absent in the tissues like the heart and skeletal muscles, where regeneration of the cells is minimal. The analogy of the cellular binding proteins can be drawn further in that, very recently we have isolated binding proteins for retinol from the cytosol, nucleosol, and chromatin of the oviduct magnum of laying hens, and our preliminary results indicate that these three binding proteins are antigenically similar. Here also, like the cellular receptors for steroids, it is likely that these proteins are of cytoplasmic origin.

It is also generally recognized that the primary action of the steroid hormones in the target cells is activation of RNA polymerases leading to the synthesis of specific mRNAs. Similarly, previous studies have consistently shown that vitamin A deprivation markedly affects the synthesis of RNA in those tissue cells that undergo rapid regeneration, i.e., intestinal mucosa of rats (Zile and De Luca, 1970), tracheal epithelium of hamsters (Kaufman et al., 1972), regenerating rat liver (Jayaram et al., 1975), and testes of rats (Jayaram and Ganguly, 1977). Finally, Tsai and Chytil (1978a,b) have claimed that the RNA synthetic activity is perceptibly less in the nuclei isolated from the livers of vitamin A-deficient rats compared to that from normal controls.

On the other hand, there are some differences in the mode of transport and delivery of the estrogens and retinol. Thus, while retinol is transported in blood by a highly specific protein (RBP), which is apparently dependent upon the physiological and nutritional conditions of the animal, the sex hormone-binding globulin for estrogen is less specific (Murphy, 1969). Similarly, while the estrogens are believed to be transported by simple diffusion across the plasma membrane of the target cells, in the case of retinol it is known that holo-RBP binds to specific receptor sites on the cell surface, where it delivers the retinol for transfer inside the cell. Nevertheless, it is interesting that retinol, like the steroid hormones, is derived from a polyisoprenoid hydrocarbon and appears to function at the nuclear level.

VIII. STATUS OF RETINOIC ACID

How does retinoic acid fit into the picture? This compound was first synthesized by Arens and van Dorp (1946), who showed that it supports growth of vitamin A-deficient rats. Later on, Dowling and Wald (1960) demonstrated that rats raised on a vitamin A-deficient diet supplemented with retinoic acid, although outwardly they appear normal, are actually blind, and Juneja et al. (1964) and Thompson et al. (1964) reported that such rats fail to reproduce. These aspects have been discussed earlier. It has also been discussed that retinoate supplementation is not fully effective in reversing the effects of retinol deprivation in regeneration of rat liver after partial hepatectomy as also in supporting the estrogen-induced growth of the oviduct of immature chicks. It has also been mentioned earlier that according to Takahashi et al. (1975) the rates of cell division of both placenta and fetus of retinoate-fed pregnant rats are markedly less around day 14 of pregnancy. Therefore, it is possible to make a general assumption from all these observations that retinoic acid cannot fully replace retinol in those systems where very rapid division and differentiation of cells take place.

Retinoic acid is rapidly absorbed through the portal route (Fidge et al., 1968) and is quickly excreted through the bile as a glucuronide derivative (Dunagin et al., 1965). Although it can be formed in the liver from the stored retinyl esters and retinol (Ganguly, 1967, 1969), unlike retinol and its esters the liver does not have any machinery to store it. Similarly, unlike retinol there is no special carrier for its transport in blood and, like the long-chain free fatty acids, it is transported in the blood by the serum albumin (Smith et al., 1973). It is thus obvious that immediately after a dose of the acid it is rapidly transported to the tissues, but at the same time it is also constantly eliminated through the bile, so that in course of time, unlike retinol, very little of it is available to the tissues. Yet another important point to be considered here is its transport across the plasma membrane. It has been well recognized that free fatty acids cannot cross biological membranes, nor has it been demonstrated that retinoic acid can do so effectively, like retinol. Therefore it follows that, owing to a sudden flush after a large dose of the acid, small amounts of it can probably enter the cells, but after some time, very little of it would be available to the cells. It is also possible that, once it enters the cell, it is as effective as retinol in growth process because retinoic acid-binding proteins have been isolated from many tissues (Chytil and Ong, 1978a,b). It appears to us that such an interpretation should readily explain the rather anomalous situation that, although a retinoic acid-binding protein has been demonstrated in rat testes, the testes of the retinoate-supplemented rats appear more like those of the vitamin A-deficient rats. It is conceivable that owing to the several limitations discussed above sufficient retinoic acid can never reach the target receptor in the testes.

IX. Summary

The information available on the effect of deprivation of vitamin A in animals, as reviewed here, would indicate that the effect is rather extensive in a variety of tissues of the animal. But it is also evident that the most pronounced and characteristic effects are invariably on the epithelial cells. At the same time it is also well recognized that one of the typical properties of the epithelial cells is that they undergo constant *in situ* regeneration. Therefore it follows that vitamin A is required for their controlled division and differentiation. Indeed, histological and electron microscopic examination of the estrogen-induced growth and development of the oviduct magnum of immature chicks has revealed that ordered division and differentiation of the epithelial cells of the oviduct are markedly affected by deprivation of vitamin A.

Recent work has shown that the steroid hormones circulate in blood bound to proteins, from which they are removed by specific receptor proteins present in the target cells. The steroid–receptor complex in the target cells is translocated into the cell nucleus, where it binds to the chromatin and induces characteristic gene expression. Similarly, retinol is carried in blood by a specific binding protein, which transports it from the site of its storage and presumably delivers it to the cell surface. A cytoplasmic specific binding protein picks up the retinol thus delivered and takes it to the cell nucleus. Preliminary evidence indicates that retinol also ultimately binds to the chromatin, where it is probably required for modulation of gene expression.

ACKNOWLEDGMENTS

Our work was supported by generous grants from the Department of Science and Technology, Government of India, and the University Grants Commission, New Delhi. Dr. M. R. S. Rao is a Senior Research Fellow of this Institute and Dr. K. Sarada was a Senior Research Fellow of the Council of Scientific and Industrial Research, New Delhi. We wish to thank Professor T. C. Anand Kumar and Dr. G. F. X. David of the Department of Anatomy, All-India Institute of Medical Sciences, New Delhi for generous help in the light and electron microscopy work.

REFERENCES

Arens, J. F., and van Dorp, D. A. (1946). *Nature (London)* **157**, 190.

Bashor, M. M., Toft, D. O., and Chytil, F. (1973). *Proc. Natl. Acad. Sci. U.S.A.* **70**, 3483.

Behrens, N. H., Parodi, A. J., Le Loir, L. F., and Krisman, C. R. (1971). *Arch Biochem. Biophys.* **143**, 375.

Behrens, N. H., Carminatti, H., Staneloni, R. J., Le Loir, L. F., and Cantarella, H. I. (1973). *Proc. Natl. Acad. Sci. U.S.A.* **70**, 3390.

Bieri, J. G. (1969). *Am. J. Clin. Nutr.* **22**, 1086.

Bhat, M. K., Sreekrishna, K., and Cama, H. R. (1977). *Indian J. Biochem. & Biophys.* **14**, 125.

Bonnani, F., Levinson, S. S., Wolf, G., and De Luca, L. (1973). *Arch. Biochem. Biophys.* **297**, 441.

Boren, H. G., Pauley, J., Wrigert, E. C., Kaufman, D. G., Smith, J. M., and Harris, C. C. (1974). *Int. J. Vitam. Nutr. Res.* **44**, 382.

Brammer, J. D., and White, R. H. (1969). *Science* **163**, 821.

Buller, R. E., Toft, D. O., Schraeder, W. T., and O'Malley, B. W. (1975). *J. Biol. Chem.* **250**, 801.

Buller, R. E., Schwartz, R. J., Schraeder, W. T., and O'Malley, B. W. (1976). *J. Biol. Chem.* **251**, 5178.

Cacaam, J. F., Jackson, J. J., and Eylar, E. H. (1969). *Biochem. Biophys. Res. Commun.* **35**, 505.

Chen, C. C., and Heller, J. (1977). *J. Biol. Chem.* **252**, 5216.

Chytil, F., and Ong, D. E. (1978a). *In* "Receptors and Hormone Action" (B. W. O'Malley and L. Birnbaumer, eds.), Vol. 2, p. 573. Academic Press, New York.

Chytil, F., and Ong, D. E. (1978b). *Vitam. Horm. (N.Y.)* **36**, 1.

Clemens, L. E., and Kleinsmith, L. J. (1972). *Nature (London), New Biol.* **237**, 204.

Das, R. C., Sarada, K., Murthy, S. K., and Ganguly, J. (1978). *Indian J. Biochem. & Biophys.* **15**, 251.

Das, R. C., Sarada, K., Murthy, S. K., Ganguly, J., and Anand Kumar, T. C. (1979). *Indian J. Exp. Biol.* **17**, 336.

De Luca, L. (1977). *Vitam. Horm. (N.Y.)* **35**, 1.

De Luca, L., and Wolf, G. (1969). *Am. J. Clin. Nutr.* **22**, 1059.

De Luca, L., Little, E. P., and Wolf, G. (1969). *J. Biol. Chem.* **244**, 701.

De Luca, L., Rosso, G., and Wolf, G. (1970a). *Biochem. Biophys. Res. Commun.* **41**, 615.

De Luca, L., Schumacher, M., and Wolf, G. (1970b). *J. Biol. Chem.* **245**, 4551.

De Luca, L., Kleinman, H. K., Little, E. P., and Wolf, G. (1971). *Arch. Biochem. Biophys.* **145**, 332.

De Luca, L., Maestri, N., Rosso, G., and Wolf, G. (1973). *J. Biol. Chem.* **248,** 641.

De Luca, L., Silverman-Jones, C. S., and Barr, R. (1975). *Biochim. Biophys. Acta* **409,** 342.

Dowling, J. E., and Wald, G. (1960). *Vitam. Horm. (N.Y.)* **18,** 515.

Dunagin, P. E., Jr., Meadows, E. H., Jr., and Olson, J. A. (1965). *Science* **148,** 80.

Dunphy, P. J., Kerr, J. D., Pennock, J. F., and Whittle, K. J. (1966). *Chem. Ind. (London)* p. 1549.

Dunphy, P. J., Kerr, J. D., Pennock, J. F., and Whittle, K. J. (1967). *Biochim. Biophys. Acta* **136,** 251.

Fell, H. B., and Mellanby, E. (1953). *J. Physiol.* **119,** 470.

Fidge, N. H., Shiratori, T., Ganguly, J., and Goodman, D. S. (1968). *J. Lipid Res.* **9,** 103.

Friedenwald, J. S., Buschke, W., and Morris, M. E. (1945). *J. Nutr.* **29,** 229.

Ganguly, J. (1960). *Vitam. Horm. (N.Y.)* **18,** 387.

Ganguly, J. (1967). *J. Sci. Ind. Res.* **26,** 110.

Ganguly, J. (1969). *Am. J. Clin. Nutr.* **22,** 923.

Ganguly, J. (1974). *Medikon* **6/7,** 23.

Ganguly, J., and Krinsky, N. I. (1953). *Biochem. J.* **54,** 177.

Ganguly, J., Krinsky, N. I., Mehl, J. W., and Deuel, H. J., Jr. (1952). *Arch. Biochem. Biophys.* **38,** 275.

Ganguly, J., Pope, G. S., Thompson, S. Y., Toothhill, J., Edwards-Webb, J. D., and Waynforth, H. B. (1971a). *Biochem. J.* **122,** 235.

Ganguly, J., Pope, G. S., Thompson, S. Y., Toothhill, J., Edwards-Webb, J. D., and Waynforth, H. B. (1971b). *Biochem. J.* **123,** 669.

Ganguly, J., Sarada, K., Jayaram, M., Joshi, P. S., Das, R. C., Murthy, S. K., Thomas, J. A., and Bhargava, M. K. (1978a). *World Rev. Nutr. Diet.* **31,** 59.

Ganguly, J., Sarada, K., Murthy, S. K., and Anand Kumar, T. C. (1978b). *Curr. Sci.* **47,** 292.

Glasser, S. R., Chytil, F., and Spelsberg, T. C. (1972). *Biochem. J.* **130,** 947.

Glover, J. (1973). *Vitam. Horm. (N.Y.)* **31,** 1.

Glover, J., Jay, C., and White, G. H. (1974). *Vitam. Horm. (N.Y.)* **32,** 215.

Glover, J., Kersham, R. C., and Large, S. (1978). *World Rev. Nutr. Diet.* **31,** 21.

Goodman, D. S. (1974). *Vitam. Horm. (N.Y.)* **32,** 167.

Gorski, J., and Gannon, F. (1976). *Annu. Rev. Physiol.* **38,** 425.

Gorski, J., and Nicolette, J. A. (1963). *Arch. Biochem. Biophys.* **103,** 418.

Gough, D. P., and Hemming, F. W. (1970). *Biochem. J.* **118,** 163.

Hamilton, T. H. (1964). *Proc. Natl. Acad. Sci. U.S.A.* **61,** 83.

Harris, G. S. (1971). *Nature (London), New Biol.* **231,** 246.

Harris, S. E., Rosen, J. M., Means, A. R., and O'Malley, B. W. (1975). *Biochemistry* **14,** 2072.

Harris, S. E., Schwartz, R. J., Roy, A. K., Tsai, M. J., and O'Malley, B. W. (1976). *J. Biol. Chem.* **251,** 524.

Hassell, J. R., Silverman-Jones, C. S., and De Luca, L. M. (1978). *J. Biol. Chem.* **253,** 1627.

Heller, J. (1975). *J. Biol. Chem.* **250,** 3613.

Heller, J. (1976). *J. Biol. Chem.* **251,** 2952.

Helting, T., and Peterson, P. A. (1972). *Biochem. Biophys. Res. Commun.* **46,** 429.

Huang, C. C., Howarth, R. E., and Owen, B. D. (1972). *Comp. Biochem. Physiol. B* **42,** 57.

Jayaram, M., and Ganguly, J. (1977). *Biochem. J.* **166,** 339.

Jayaram, M., Murthy, S. K., and Ganguly, J. (1973). *Biochem. J.* **136,** 221.

Jayaram, M., Sarada, K., and Ganguly, J. (1975). *Biochem. J.* **146,** 501.

Jensen, E. V., Mohla, S., Gorell, T. A., and DeSombre, E. R. (1974). *Vitam. Horm. (N.Y.)* **32**, 89.

Johnson, B. C., Kennedy, M., and Chiba, N. (1969). *Am. J. Clin. Nutr.* **22**, 1048.

Joshi, P. S., Mathur, S. N., Murthy, S. K., and Ganguly, J. (1973). *Biochem. J.* **136**, 757.

Joshi, P. S., Murthy, S. K., and Ganguly, J. (1976). *Biochem. J.* **154**, 249.

Juneja, H. S., Murthy, S. K., and Ganguly, J. (1964). *Indian J. Exp. Biol.* **2**, 153.

Juneja, H. S., Moudgal, N. R., and Ganguly, J. (1969). *Biochem. J.* **111**, 97.

Kahn, R. H. (1954). *Nature (London)* **174**, 317.

Kalimi, M., Tsai, S. Y., Tsai, M. J., Clark, J. H., and O'Malley, B. W. (1976). *J. Biol. Chem.* **251**, 576.

Kanai, M., Raz, A., and Goodman, D. S. (1968). *J. Clin. Invest.* **47**, 2025.

Kanai, M., Monoto, S., Sasaoka, S., and Muto, Y. (1972a). *Proc. Symp. Chem. Physiol. Pathol.* **12**, 319.

Kanai, M., Sasaoka, S., and Naiki, M. (1972b). *Proc. Symp. Chem. Physiol. Pathol.* **12**, 325.

Kaufman, D. G., Baker, M. S., Smith, J. M., Henderson, W. R., Harris, C. C., Sporn, M. B., and Saffioti, U. (1972). *Science* **177**, 1105.

Kim, Y. C., and Wolf, G. (1975). *J. Nutr.* **104**, 710.

Kleinman, H. N., and Wolf, G. (1974). *Biochim. Biophys. Acta* **359**, 90.

Kohler, P. O., Grimley, P. M., and O'Malley, B. W. (1969). *J. Cell Biol.* **40**, 9.

Krause, R. F., Beamer, K. E., McCormick, A. M., Canterbery, R. J., and Trifiates, G. P. (1975). *Br. J. Nutr.* **33**, 73.

Krinsky, N. I., and Ganguly, J. (1953). *J. Biol. Chem.* **202**, 227.

Krinsky, N. I., Cornwell, D. G., and Oncley, J. L. (1958). *Arch. Biochem. Biophys.* **73**, 233.

Krishnamurthy, S., Mahadevan, S., and Ganguly, J. (1958a). *J. Biol. Chem.* **233**, 32.

Krishnamurthy, S., Seshadri Sastry, P., and Ganguly, J. (1958b). *Arch. Biochem. Biophys.* **75**, 6.

Kuhn, R. W., Schraeder, W. T., Smith, R. G., and O'Malley, B. W. (1975). *J. Biol. Chem.* **250**, 4220.

Lasnitzki, I. (1961). *Exp. Cell Res.* **24**, 37.

McGuire, W. L., and O'Malley, B. W. (1968). *Biochim. Biophys. Acta* **157**, 187.

Mahadevan, S., and Ganguly, J. (1961). *Biochem. J.* **81**, 53.

Mahadevan, S., Malathi, P., and Ganguly, J. (1965). *World Rev. Nutr. Diet.* **5**, 209.

Mahadevan, S., Ayyoub, N. I., and Roels, O. A. (1966). *J. Biol. Chem.* **241**, 57.

Mariani, G., Otto Nello, S., Gozzoli, F., and Merli, A. (1977). *Nature (London)* **265**, 681.

Mason, K. E. (1935). *Am. J. Anat.* **57**, 303.

Mason, K. E., and Ellison, E. T. (1935a). *J. Nutr.* **9**, 75.

Mason, K. E., and Ellison, E. T. (1935b). *J. Nutr.* **10**, 1.

Means, A. R., Comstock, J. P., Rosenfeld, G. C., and O'Malley, B. W. (1972). *Proc. Natl. Acad. Sci. U.S.A.* **69**, 1146.

Mohla, S., DeSombre, E. R., and Jensen, E. V. (1972). *Biochem. Biophys. Res. Commun.* **46**, 661.

Moore, T. (1957). *In* "Vitamin A." Elsevier, Amsterdam.

Mori, S. (1922). *Bull. Johns Hopkins Hosp.* **33**, 357.

Mueller, G. C., Herranen, A. M., and Jevrell, K. J. (1958). *Recent Prog. Horm. Res.* **14**, 95.

Muhilal, H., and Glover, J. (1974). *Br. J. Nutr.* **32**, 549.

Murphy, B. P. (1969). *Recent Prog. Hormone Res.* **25**, 563.

Musliner, T. A., and Chader, G. J. (1972). *Biochim. Biophys. Acta* **262**, 256.

Muto, Y., and Goodman, D. S. (1972). *J. Biol. Chem.* **247**, 2533.

Muto, Y., Smith, J. E., Milch, P. O., and Goodman, D. S. (1972). *J. Biol. Chem.* **247**, 2542.

Muto, Y., Smith, F. R., and Goodman, D. S. (1973). *J. Lipid Res.* **14**, 525.

Oka, T., and Schimke, R. T. (1969a). *J. Cell. Biol.* **41**, 816.

Oka, T., and Schimke, R. T. (1969b). *J. Cell. Biol.* **43**, 123.

O'Malley, B. W., McGuire, W. L., Kohler, P. O., and Korenman, S. G. (1969). *Recent Prog. Horm. Res.* **25**, 105.

O'Malley, B. W., Toft, D. O., and Sherman, M. R. (1971). *J. Biol. Chem.* **246**, 1117.

Ong, D. E., and Chytil, F. (1975). *J. Biol. Chem.* **250**, 6113.

Ong, D. E., and Chytil, F. (1976). *Proc. Natl. Acad. Sci. U.S.A.* **73**, 3976.

Palmiter, R. D., and Wrenn, J. T. (1971). *J. Cell Biol.* **50**, 598.

Parnell, J. P., and Sherman, B. S. (1962). *In* "Fundamentals of Keratinization" (E. D. Bucher and R. F. Signaes, eds.), Publ. No. 70, p. 113. Am. Assoc. Adv. Sci., Washington, D.C.

Peterson, P. A., and Berggard, I. (1971). *J. Biol. Chem.* **132**, 585.

Peterson, P. A., Nielson, S. F., Ostberg, L., Rask, L., and Vahlquist, A. (1974). *Vitam. Horm. (N.Y.)* **32**, 181.

Pitt, G. A. J. (1971). *In* "Carotenoids" (O. Isler, ed.), p. 717. Birkhaeuser, Basel.

Rao, M. R. S., Prasad, V. R., Padmanaban, G., and Ganguly, J. (1979). *Biochem. J.* **183**, 501.

Rask, L., and Peterson, P. A. (1976). *J. Biol. Chem.* **251**, 6360.

Raynaud-Jammet, C., and Baulieu, E. E. (1969). *C. R. Acad. Sci. Ser. D* **268**, 3211.

Rosenfeld, G. C., Comstock, J. P., Means, A. R., and O'Malley, B. W. (1972). *Biochem. Biophys. Res. Commun.* **47**, 387.

Rossa, R., Nicolan, J., Fernandes, L. R., and Vacilla, M. (1971). *Int. J. Vitam. Nutr. Res.* **41**, 17.

Rowland, R. L., Letimer, P. H., and Goles, J. A. (1956). *J. Am. Chem. Soc.* **78**, 4680.

Saari, J. C., Futterman, S., and Bredberg, L. (1978). *J. Biol. Chem.* **253**, 6432.

Sani, B. P. (1977). *Biochem. Biophys. Res. Commun.* **75**, 7.

Sarada, K., Ganguly, J., and Lipner, H. (1977). *Indian J. Exp. Biol.* **15**, 1139.

Schraeder, W. T., and O'Malley, B. W. (1972). *J. Biol. Chem.* **247**, 51.

Schwartz, R. J., Tsai, M. J., Tsai, S. Y., and O'Malley, B. W. (1975). *J. Biol. Chem.* **250**, 5175.

Schwartz, R. J., Kuhn, R. W., Buller, R. E., Schraeder, W. T., and O'Malley, B. W. (1976). *J. Biol. Chem.* **251**, 5166.

Sherman, B. S. (1961). *J. Invest. Dermatol.* **37**, 469.

Shinde, R., Das, R. C., Sarada, K., and Ganguly, J. (1980). *Indian J. Biochem-Biophys.* **17**, 135.

Smith, F. R., Raz, A., and Goodman, D. S. (1970). *J. Clin. Invest.* **49**, 1754.

Smith, J. E., Milch, P. O., Muto, Y., and Goodman, D. S. (1973). *Biochem. J.* **132**, 821.

Spelsberg, T. C., Steggles, A. W., Chytil, F., and O'Malley, B. W. (1972). *J. Biol. Chem.* **247**, 1368.

Spencer, B. (1969). *Am. J. Clin. Nutr.* **22**, 1019.

Sreekrishna, K., and Cama, H. R. (1978a). *Proc. Indian Acad. Sci. Sect. B* **87**, 205.

Sreekrishna, K., and Cama, H. R. (1978b). *Biochem. Rev.* **49**, 40.

Takahashi, Y. I., Smith, J. E., Winick, M., and Goodman, D. S. (1975). *J. Nutr.* **105**, 1299.

Thompson, J. N. (1969). *Am. J. Clin. Nutr.* **22**, 1063.

Thompson, J. N., Howell, J. M., and Pitt, G. A. J. (1964). *Proc. R. Soc. London, Ser. B* **159**, 510.

Toft, D. (1972). *J. Steroid Biochem.* **3**, 515.

Tsai, C. H., and Chytil, F. (1978a). *Fed. proc., Fed. Am. Soc. Biol. Chem.* **37**, 2602.

Tsai, C. H., and Chytil, F. (1978b). *Life Sci.* **23**, 1461.

Tsai, M. J., Schwartz, R. J., Tsai, S. Y., and O'Malley, B. W. (1975). *J. Biol. Chem.* **250**, 5164.

Tsai, S. Y., Tsai, M. J., Schwartz, R. J., Kalimi, M., Clark, J. R., and O'Malley, B. W. (1975). *Proc. Natl. Acad. Sci. U.S.A.* **72**, 4228.

Vahlquist, A., and Peterson, P. A. (1972). *Biochemistry* **11**, 4526.

Waechter, C. J., and Lennarz, W. J. (1976). *Annu. Rev. Biochem.* **45**, 95.

Weiss, P., and James, R. (1955). *Exp. Cell Res., Suppl.* **3**, 381.

Wellburn, A. R., Stevenson, J., Hemming, F. W., and Morton, R. A. (1967). *Biochem. J.* **102**, 313.

Westphal, V. (1970). *In* "Biochemical Actions of Hormones" (G. Litwack, ed.), Vol. 1, p. 209. Academic Press, New York.

Wiggert, B. O., and Chader, G. J. (1975). *Exp. Eye Res.* **21**, 143.

Wiggert, B. O., Russel, P., Lewis, M., and Chader, G. (1977). *Biochem. Biophys. Res. Commun.* **79**, 218.

Wolbach, S. B., and Howe, P. R. (1925). *J. Exp. Med.* **42**, 753.

Wolbach, S. B., and Howe, P. R. (1933). *J. Exp. Med.* **57**, 511.

Wong, Y. C., and Buck, R. C. (1971). *Lab. Invest.* **24**, 55.

Yamamoto, K. R., and Alberts, B. M. (1972). *Proc. Natl. Acad. Sci. U.S.A.* **69**, 2109.

Yonemoto, J., and Johnson, B. C. (1967). *Fed. Proc., Fed. Am. Soc. Biol. Chem.* **26**, 635.

Zachman, R. D. (1967). *Life Sci.* **6**, 2207.

Zile, M., and De Luca, H. F. (1970). *Arch. Biochem. Biophys.* **140**, 210.

Zile, M., Bunge, R. C., and De Luca, H. F. (1977). *J. Nutr.* **107**, 552.

VITAMINS AND HORMONES, VOL. 38

Aldosterone Action in Target Epithelia

DIANA MARVER

*Departments of Internal Medicine and Biochemistry, University of Texas
Health Science Center at Dallas, Dallas, Texas*

Aldosterone biosynthesis by the zona glomerulosa of the adrenal cortex is controlled by a number of factors including the renin-angiotensin system, plasma potassium, and, to a lesser degree, ACTH (Bravo, 1977). Renin release increases at times of hyponatremia, hypovolemia, and sympathetic nervous system activity. Therefore, when sodium intake in man is low (25 meq or less), daily aldosterone production may rise to 1000 μg; if sodium intake is high (50–200 meq/day), production decreases to 50–250 μg/day (Knochel and White, 1973). In cases of unrelenting release of aldosterone or administration of mineralocorticoids, a renal compensatory mechanism known as "escape" ensues. Although the exact controlling elements have not been determined, it is generally believed that escape involves recruitment of those factors that are responsible for volume-related natriuresis (Paillard, 1977; Wright *et al.*, 1969; Knox *et al.*, 1980). Addisonian patients, on the other hand, are hyponatremic, hypovolemic, hyperkalemic, and acidotic, indicating a role of cortical steroids in Na^+, K^+, H^+, and volume homeostasis.

A diagram, illustrating a mineralocorticoid-responsive cell, is given in Fig. 1. Na^+ passively enters across the luminal membrane, moving down an electrochemical gradient. It is then pumped out the basolateral cell boundary via sodium–potassium activated adenosinetriphosphatase (Na^+K^+-ATPase) against both concentration and electrical gradients. Because these are "tight" epithelia (backleak and passive permeabilities to ions are low) and the stoichiometry of the pump is the movement of 3 Na^+ ions out for 2 K^+ ions in per molecule of ATP hydrolyzed, the net transport of Na^+ from urine to blood usually results in a lumen ($-$) potential difference (PD) with respect to blood (Skou, 1977). Since the transepithelial PD reflects the movement of anions and cations toward both the blood and urine space, a convenient model to study the action of aldosterone is the toad bladder, in which one can easily determine the amount of current necessary to null the potential across the bladder. Under these circumstances, this short-circuit current (SCC) is essentially equivalent to that produced by the active transport of Na^+ (Ussing and Zerahn, 1951; Crabbé, 1963a). Therefore, as a measure of the influence of aldosterone upon net Na^+ transport, SCC is monitored. In tissues where measurement of SCC is not feasible, investigators evaluate the effect of aldosterone on Na^+ reabsorp-

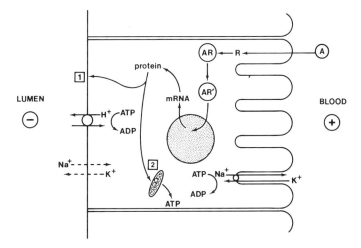

FIG. 1. A schematic representation of a mineralocorticoid target cell. In this model, aldosterone (A) enters the cell and binds to a cytoplasmic receptor (R). This AR-AR' complex attaches to chromatin, initiating a cascade of events including mRNA and protein synthesis. The newly synthesized proteins are thought both to alter the Na^+ permeability across the apical boundary (1) and to enhance the formation of ATP (2) for support of active Na^+ transport and perhaps also H^+ transport.

tion by recording the change in PD, supported by bidirectional flux data obtained with ^{22}Na and ^{24}Na.

I. Historical Introduction

In the 1930s, scientists realized that surgical adrenalectomy resulted in an inability to conserve body sodium and that this lethal process could be reversed by the administration of adrenal extracts (Loeb *et al.*, 1933; Harrop *et al.*, 1936). Indeed, the adrenal was found to be the source of substances that have profound effects on both electrolyte and carbohydrate homeostasis. Even though soldiers were being treated with semipurified preparations of cortisone several years later during World War II, physicians were still not sure whether the mineralocorticoid activity of such preparations was due to a compound with both mineralo- and glucocorticoid activity or to a separate entity. With the emergence of the Bush system of chromatographic separation of steroids and more sensitive bioassays for Na^+-retaining activity, aldosterone was finally purified and assigned the role of physiological mineralocorticoid (Simpson and Tait, 1953; Simpson *et al.*, 1954; Luetscher, 1956; Tait and Tait, 1978).

Two other technical advances laid the groundwork for studies published over the next 10 years. One was the development of the SCC apparatus by Ussing and Zerahn (1951), and the second was the production of radiolabeled steroids of such high specific activity that they could be used as biological tracers. Using such tools, several groups headed by Crabbé, Edelman, Kirsten and Kirsten, and Sharp and Leaf, were the source of much of the evidence for the very early models of aldosterone action. The following paragraphs discuss some of these initial findings and how the models evolved.

The story perhaps began about 1958 when Leaf *et al.* proposed that the toad bladder actively transports Na^+ and that this process is enhanced by vasopressin (antidiuretic hormone, ADH). Crabbé then demonstrated that aldosterone also increased Na^+ transport in this tissue, an effect that was additive to that elicited by ADH (Crabbé, 1961a, 1963a). He also noted a latent period between addition of steroid and the SCC response that was independent of steroid concentration. Two classic papers by Edelman and co-workers contributed to an explanation of this latent period. They indicated (*a*) that actinomycin D and puromycin blocked the aldosterone-mediated rise in SCC if added to bladders before steroid, and (*b*) that the incorporation of [^3H]uridine into RNA was increased with a time course that just preceded the rise in current (Edelman *et al.*, 1963; Porter *et al.*, 1964). Since the presence of an oxidizable substrate such as glucose or pyruvate was necessary for the rise in Na^+ transport to occur, the authors proposed that aldosterone increased RNA and protein synthesis in order to support ATP production. The ATP, generated by substrate flux through the tricarboxylic acid cycle, was deemed in critical supply for maintainence of Na^+ transport via membrane-bound Na^+,K^+-ATPase.

Crabbé, on the other hand, suggested that aldosterone enhanced net Na^+ transport by increasing the permeability of Na^+ at the apical cell membrane, thereby allowing greater access of Na^+ to pump sites (Crabbé, 1963b, 1964). This proposal was supported by Sharp and Leaf, who agreed that aldosterone enhanced utilization of substrates such as glucose, pyruvate, or acetoacetate, but argued that this was tantamount to a cellular adaptation to enhanced Na^+ entry at the apical boundary of target cells (Sharp and Leaf, 1965; Sharp *et al.*, 1966a). In support of this hypothesis, they showed that amphotericin B, an antibiotic that enhances apical Na^+ entry into cells, also increased the SCC, and that the rise in SCC was greater in substrate-replete versus substrate depleted bladders. Therefore, they were able to mimic the action of aldosterone save for the fact that the amphotericin response could not be blocked by puromycin. By analogy, they concluded that aldosterone induced an apical cell membrane protein that behaved in the same way as amphotericin and that the rise in substrate utilization through the tricarboxylic acid cycle was, for both amphotericin and aldosterone, secondary to a rise in intracellular Na^+. Furthermore, to rule out the possibility that aldosterone action was directly linked to net synthesis of ATP, they measured ATP in toad bladder cells isolated from hormone-stimulated and nonstimulated bladders 5–14 hours after incubation and found no difference in steady-state levels. Finally, in support of this hypothesis, Crabbé and Ehrlich (1968) reported that aldosterone reduced the amiloride sensitivity of toad bladder cells, which suggested to these authors that this was as a result of a net increase in the density of luminal Na^+-transporting sites with steroid.

Continuing studies on the energy hypothesis, Edelman and co-workers found that aldosterone-mediated changes in Na^+ transport depended on the provision of a precursor to acetyl-CoA and concluded that one or more of the enzymes in the tricarboxylic acid cycle were directly stimulated by this steroid (Fimognari *et al.*, 1967). In agreement with this concept, the activity of several mitochondrial enzymes (citrate synthase, isocitrate dehydrogenase, and glutamate dehydrogenase) were shown to be increased with administration of aldosterone (Kinne and Kirsten, 1968; E. Kirsten *et al.*, 1968, 1970). Cytochrome oxidase, an intermediate in the electron transport chain, also was elevated (Feldman *et al.,* 1961; R. Kirsten *et al.,* 1970). By 1970, therefore, it was generally agreed that the action of aldosterone on Na^+ transport was dependent on RNA and protein synthesis, but it was still unclear whether the protein products enhanced luminal entry of Na^+ or stimulated ATP synthesis. What follows in this review is a detailed interpretation of some of the earlier reports as well as recent developments. The subdivisions of the review take up in turn the following questions related to aldosterone action: (*a*) the nature and role of the cytoplasmic receptor; (*b*) documentation of increases in RNA and total protein synthesis; (*c*) how aldosterone may enhance the physiological response to ADH; (*d*) the relationship between aldosterone and secretion of H^+ and K^+; (*e*) what is known about the induction of specific proteins; (*f*) the current evidence on the permease and ATP hypotheses; (*g*) what is known about the localization of mineralocorticoid target cells within the kidney and toad bladder; and (*h*) how substances such as spirolactone may antagonize Na^+ transport.

For recent reviews dealing with the physiology and biochemistry of mineralocorticoids, I would direct the reader to the following: Edelman and Fanestil, 1970 (120 references); Porter, 1972 (190 references); Knochel and White, 1973 (106 references); Sharp and Leaf, 1973 (168 references); Crabbé, 1977 (230 references); and Paillard, 1977 (53 references).

II. The Mineralocorticoid Receptor

In 1966, Sharp *et al.* (1966a) described a low and high affinity intracellular binding site for [³H]aldosterone in toad bladder cells, as was inferred from earlier autoradiographic analyses (Edelman *et al.,* 1963). Sharp and Leaf found that displacement of [³H]aldosterone from these sites could be achieved by mineralocorticoid agonists and antagonists (SC 14266), but not by inactive steroids such as cholesterol. These binding sites, or receptors, appeared to be proteins, since they were digested by proteases but not by nucleases, lipases, or neuraminidase (Herman *et al.,* 1968). They have been found in all target tissues thus far examined and are characteristically absent from nontarget tissues, such as liver (Swaneck *et al.,* 1969; Funder *et al.,* 1972; Duval and Funder, 1974; Kusch *et al.,* 1978). Suggested mammalian target organs include kidney, salivary and sweat glands, and colon (Edmonds, 1972; Funder *et al.,* 1972; Frizzel and Schultz, 1978). A recent paper, however, has called into question the previous proposal that the colon is a mineralocorticoid target organ, since both Na^+ and K^+ transport appear to be more sensitive to dexamethasone than to aldosterone in this tissue (Bastl *et al.*, 1980). Table I lists the equilibrium dissociation constants (K_d's) determined for aldosterone–receptor interactions in a variety of species and target tissues. Except for toad bladder ($K_d = 10^{-8}$ M), the K_d's range from 5×10^{-10} M to 4×10^{-9} M, with some variation due to temperature.

The overwhelming evidence suggests that the ability to affect the distribution of the receptor pool determines the physiological response to a given amount of hormone. The relevancy of the mineralocorticoid receptor is emphasized by the close correlation between the kinetics of saturation of the receptor and the kinetics of saturation of the physiological response. At 37°C, the K_d for aldosterone–receptor interaction is 5×10^{-10} M in the rat (Table I). At a concentration of 5×10^{-9} M aldosterone, $> 90\%$ maximal binding of the receptor would be attained.

$$\% \text{ bound} = \frac{100 \text{ (steroid conc.)}}{\text{(steroid conc.)} + K_d}$$

If the receptor is physiologically relevant, one would expect that this concentration of aldosterone would produce a near-maximal increase

TABLE I

Equilibrium Dissociation Constants (K_d's) for Aldosterone–Receptor Interactions

Species	Plasma concentration aldosterone (M)[a]	Tissue[b]	Temperature (°C)	K_d (M)	References[c]
Human	0.8 to 8×10^{-10}	Kidney	37	5×10^{-10}	1, 2
		Kidney	25	2×10^{-9}	3
Sheep	<0.3 to 9×10^{-10}	Kidney	37	5×10^{-10}	4, 5
		Parotid	37	5×10^{-10}	5
Rabbit	3×10^{-10}	Kidney cortex	37	4×10^{-9}	6, 7
		Kidney red medulla	37	4×10^{-9}	7
Rat	1.4×10^{-10}	Kidney	37	5×10^{-10}	8, 9
		Kidney	37	6×10^{-10}	10
		Kidney	25	2×10^{-9}	11
		Parotid	25	2×10^{-9}	11
		Kidney	20	4×10^{-9}	12
Toad	2 to 3×10^{-8}	Bladder	25	1×10^{-8}	13, 14

[a] Concentrations listed reflect either the range of values found in normal animals or a mean value.

[b] The equilibrium dissociation constants listed were determined in slices of tissue (kidney or parotid) or whole bladder rather than in cell-free tissue fractions.

[c] (1) Gottfried *et al.*, 1975; (2) Matulich *et al.*, 1976; (3) Fuller and Funder, 1976; (4) Coghlan and Scoggins, 1967; (5) Butkus *et al.*, 1976; (6) Schwartz and Burg, 1978; (7) Marver, 1980; (8) Bojesen, 1966; (9) Funder *et al.*, 1973a; (10) Baxter *et al.*, 1976; (11) Funder *et al.*, 1972; (12) Rafestin-Olin *et al.*, 1977; (13) Crabbé, 1961b; (14) Kusch *et al.*, 1978.

in Na^+ transport. Indeed, Fanestil and Edelman (1966) estimated that the maximal antinatriuretic effect of aldosterone in rats is obtained at a plasma concentration of approximately 5×10^{-9} M. When a series of steroids were tested for their relative affinity for the receptor versus their relative stimulation of Na^+ transport, there was a close correlation (Fimognori *et al.*, 1967; Herman *et al.*, 1968). Finally, both 17α-isoaldosterone, a stereoisomer of aldosterone, and 17β-estradiol lack demonstrable affinity for the mineralocorticoid receptor and have no effect on Na^+ transport in target epithelia (Fimognari *et al.*, 1967; Herman *et al.*, 1968). In the case of aldosterone antagonists, the relative antagonism of certain steroids such as progesterone or spirolactone also reflect their capacity to bind to this receptor (Sharp *et al.*, 1966a; Herman *et al.*, 1968; Marver *et al.*, 1974; Wambach and Higgins, 1978).

Since all steroid hormones have in common a cytoplasmic steroid-specific receptor, the importance of these receptors has been generally accepted based on evidence from work with either mineralocorticoids, glucocorticoids, or the sex steroids. Therefore, mutants of a lymphoma cell-line that lost cellular response to glucocorticoids, were found to be "receptorless," indicating the crucial role of the receptor (Sibley and Tomkins, 1974). An even more interesting variation on the theme of receptor-mediated hormone action was the observation that an estrogen-insensitive human breast cancer cell line, MCF-7, contained estrogen receptor bound to nuclei in the absence of steroid. Although the cells appeared to be independent of estrogen addition to the media, they could still be inhibited by certain estrogen antagonists. The implication was that whatever modification steroid induces in receptor molecules to allow nuclear binding had already occurred to these altered receptors, thereby eliminating the need for estrogen (Zava *et al.*, 1977).

Perhaps the strongest evidence for the role of receptors in the mechanism of action of aldosterone and other steroid hormones is their association with nuclear sites (Fanestil and Edelman, 1966; Swaneck *et al.*, 1970). When trace quantities of [^{3}H]aldosterone were given i.v. to adrenalectomized rats, there was immediate attachment of labeled aldosterone to a cytoplasmic receptor, followed by a rise in nucleus-associated [^{3}H]aldosterone:receptor complexes with a peak binding occurring about 10 minutes after injection (Marver *et al.*, 1972). Thereafter, the fall in nucleus-associated complexes mimicked the fall in the cytoplasmic and plasma compartments. The inference gaining acceptance over the years, although not proved as yet, is that nuclear association of receptor:steroid complexes activates or derepresses a portion of the genome that codes for the synthesis of mRNAs specific for proteins necessary for the physiological response. There is no doubt that steroid:receptor complexes have a high affinity for chromatin, since steroid-labeled receptor binds rapidly to nuclear chromatin sites *in vitro* at 25° or 37°C (Marver *et al.*, 1972, 1974). Based on such experiments, it has been postulated that the second key event in the mechanism of action of aldosterone is the attachment of steroid-bound mineralocorticoid complexes to specific sites on chromatin.

Control of hormone expression at the nuclear level has been demonstrated in both normal and transformed cells in a number of steroid systems. Variants of both the HTC and lymphoma cell lines contain glucocorticoid receptors but are steroid-unresponsive. In the case of some lymphoma mutants, it appeared that the receptor was "normal" with respect to a steroid binding site, but was deficient in another site on the receptor that was required for nuclear attachment (Gehring and Tomkins, 1974). This study established the concept of a receptor with at least two physiologically important domains. More recently, a hormone-unresponsive HTC cell mutant was described that had normal glucocorticoid receptors but lacked normal binding sites on chromatin (Thompson *et al.*, 1977). Studies with mutants have therefore provided evidence that hormone response requires competent receptors and intact nuclear attachment sites. Further indirect evidence suggests control of hormone action at the genome level. Feldman *et al.* (1978) reported that, by a number of criteria, the glucocorticoid receptor in normal tissue was identical whether it was obtained from rat thymus, kidney, or adipose tissue. Yet when Feldman (1977) compared the ability of glucocorticoids to regulate phosphoenolpyruvate carboxykinase (PEPCK) activity in several tissues, he found that dexamethasone increased PEPCK activity in the kidney, decreased activity in white adipose tissue, and had no effect on activity in brown fat, even though all three tissues contained glucocorticoid receptors. One explanation of these findings is that a level of discrimination is occurring at the nuclear binding site.

The relevance of nuclear association of hormone complexes to Na^+ transport was also shown in experiments by Farman *et al.* (1978) in the toad bladder. In their studies, concentrations of aldosterone that produced a maximal rise in SCC also saturated a specific site on chromatin with a K_d for receptor complexes of 3×10^{-9} *M* and a maximal binding site capacity of 15×10^{-14} mol of [^{3}H]aldosterone bound to macromolecular complexes per milligram of DNA. This is equivalent to approximately 650 nuclear sites per cell. However, the interpretation of simple attachment of receptor to the chromatin matrix is complicated, since 50% of these high-affinity nuclear sites had to be occupied before any rise in SCC occurred. However complicated, if the amount of hormone-bound receptor is a function of plasma steroid level, this dose-response relationship may be translated at the chromatin level by the duration of activation or derepression of key nuclear sites by receptor complexes (Buller and O'Malley, 1976).

Some processing of receptor probably takes place between the initial binding of steroid in the cytoplasm and the subsequent attachment to nuclear sites. The simplest evidence for this appeared some years ago when investigators noted alterations in the sucrose gradient sedimentation profile of receptor complexes pre- and postactivation (Jensen *et al.*, 1972, 1974). For instance, cytoplasmic receptors labeled with steroid *in vitro* at 0°C have a low affinity for nuclear sites. A number of manipulations, including exposure to heat (37°C) or salt, can enhance binding of these receptors to isolated nuclei or chromatin. This process is termed "activation." With this transformation comes a small change in the sedimentation coefficient for the labeled receptor complex (Notides *et al.*, 1976; Puca *et al.*, 1977). It has been proposed that, *in vivo*, some as yet unknown cellular modifier carries out this activation process.

Table II lists the sedimentation coefficients (*s* values) for a number of steroid–hormone receptor complexes. Under low salt conditions, all physiologically active steroids demonstrate an ~ 8 S (± 4 S) complex on sucrose or glycerol density gradients. In the presence of 0.3–0.4 M KCl, a single labeled complex appears, with a sedimentation value of ~ 4 S. The fact that two antagonists of steroid hormone action, spirolactone and cortexolone, do not form the 8 S complex under low-salt conditions will be discussed in a later section on antagonist action.

In conclusion, it appears that receptor occupancy by steroid agonists determines very early in the biochemical pathway the magnitude of the final rise in Na^+ transport. In normal cells, the receptor theory predicts that any steroid that cannot bind to this receptor cannot alter Na^+ transport through the induction pathway. Any steroid that can occupy the receptor *must* either be an agonist, an antagonist, or a partial agonist:antagonist of the induction pathway. One can also predict that once sufficient steroid has been added to occupy the receptor completely, the addition of more steroid cannot further enhance the magnitude of the physiological response. Occupancy of the mineralocorticoid receptor is determined by the affinity of a given steroid for the site and its molar concentration. Therefore, even steroids with a modest affinity for the receptor (such as all glucocorticoids) can bring about enhanced Na^+ transport through the

TABLE II

Sedimentation Coefficients (s Values) of Various [³H]Steroid Labeled
Cytoplasmic Receptors

		s Values (S)		
		---	---	
Steroid	Tissue	Low salt[a]	High salt[a]	References[b]
Agonists				
Aldosterone	Kidney	8.5 4	4.5	1
Triamcinolone	Thymus	7 3.5	4	2
Dexamethasone	Hepatoma	8	4	3
Dihydrotestosterone	Prostate	8 4.5	4.5	4, 5
Estradiol	Uterus	8 4	4.5	6
Progesterone	Oviduct	8 5	4	7
Antagonists				
Spirolactone	Kidney	3	4	8
Cortexolone	Thymus	3.5	3.5	2

[a] The values (in Svedberg units, S) were obtained using glycerol or sucrose density gradients containing either low sale (<0.1 M) or high salt (0.3–0.4 M KCl).

[b] (1) Marver et al., 1972; (2) Kaiser et al., 1972; (3) Baxter and Tomkins, 1971; (4) Baulieu et al., 1971; (5) Mainwaring and Mangan, 1971; (6) Jensen et al., 1972; (7) O'Malley et al., 1971; (8) Marver et al., 1974.

mineralocorticoid-specific pathway if sufficient quantities of those steroids are used. To illustrate this point: if aldosterone has a K_d of 5 × 10⁻¹⁰ M for the mineralocorticoid receptor compared to a K_d of 2.5 × 10⁻⁸ M for dexamethasone for the same site (where the K_d is the concentration of steroid at which 50% of the sites are occupied), then at 5 × 10⁻⁹ M steroid, aldosterone will occupy > 90% of the sites compared to only 17% by dexamethasone. The ultimate rise in Na⁺ transport would reflect these differences in binding. However, if dexamethasone concentration is increased to 2.5 × 10⁻⁷ M, it will also occupy > 90% of the mineralocorticoid sites and have a near-maximal effect on Na⁺ reabsorption.

Experiments in the rat have shown that dexamethasone has about 1/50th the affinity of aldosterone for mineralocorticoid receptors whereas aldosterone has 1/5th the affinity of dexamethasone for glucocorticoid receptors (Feldman et al., 1972). This has practical implications when investigators wish to ascribe changes in a particular biochemical pathway to a mineralocorticoid rather than glucocorticoid domain. To avoid significant occupation of glucocorticoid sites, aldosterone concentrations are kept at moderate levels and the response to equivalent doses of dexamethasone are compared as a control. If glucocorticoids are used that bind appreciably to corticosteroid-binding globulin and are given *in vivo,* then the dose of glucocorticoid must be increased to a point where the plasma "free" concentration is equivalent to "free" concentration of aldosterone (Funder *et al.,* 1973b). Studies that do not address this separation of mineralocorticoid and glucocorticoid responses may be open to criticism.

Little information is available about the nature of the receptor itself. In cell-free form, it is extremely labile but it can be protected to varying degrees by the addition of aldosterone, 15–25% glycerol, 20 mM sodium molybdate, and by maintaining samples at 4°C (Herman *et al.,* 1968; Alberti and Sharp, 1969; Marver *et al.,* 1972; Rafestin-Olin *et al.,* 1977; Marver, 1980). Its propensity to aggregate on column beds and for bound [^{3}H]aldosterone to dissociate irreversibly during chromatographic or electrophoretic procedures has hindered purification attempts. However, using toad bladders, Alberti and Sharp (1969) reported a 100,000 MW cytoplasmic [^{3}H]aldosterone-bound complex on Agarose columns, and Ludens and Fanestil (1971) isolated a 50,000 MW complex from rat kidney in the presence of high salt. These species may coincide with the aggregate 8 S form seen on low salt gradients and the 4 S form seen on high salt gradients (Table II). We have had experience with ion-exchange chromatography for purification of receptors and recently reported a 50- to 200-fold purification of the cytoplasmic receptor from rabbit renal cortex and red medulla, using DE-52 Sephadex and rapid KCl elution (Marver, 1980). Last, in order to study the receptor in pure form, attempts have been made in recent years to label the protein covalently by use of photoactivated diazo- or azidosteroids, and it may be that this approach will ultimately be successful (Wolff *et al.,* 1975; Marver *et al.,* 1976).

III. THE ROLE OF RNA AND PROTEIN SYNTHESIS

Early in the investigation of aldosterone, it was noted that actinomycin D and puromycin blocked the aldosterone-induced increase in Na$^+$ transport in the toad bladder, but had little effect on the similar action of vasopressin (ADH) (Crabbé, 1963a; Porter and Edelman, 1964; Sharp and Leaf, 1964). Actinomycin D also inhibited the stimulation of Na$^+$ transport in adrenalectomized rats given aldosterone (Fimognari *et al.,* 1967). There was also enhanced incorporation of [^{3}H]orotate or [^{3}H]uridine into RNA and [^{3}H]leucine into protein in rat or toad bladders exposed to mineralocorticoid (Fimognari *et al.,* 1967; Rousseau and

Crabbé, 1968; Forte and Landon, 1968; Hutchinson and Porter, 1972). On the basis of such experiments, Porter *et al.* (1964) suggested that the action of aldosterone in target epithelia requires the induction of DNA-dependent RNA synthesis and that the ultimate protein products are responsible for the increased active Na^+ transport. The 60–90 minute latent period between administration of hormone and the initiation of the rise in SCC was considered to be related to the time required for this synthesis and processing of protein (Lahav *et al.*, 1973).

Since then more information has been collected concerning the nature of the RNA products. Studies of Rossier, Wilce, Edelman and co-workers showed a direct correlation between an aldosterone-dependent rise in Na^+ transport and an increase in [^{3}H]uridine labeling of a nonmethylated 9–12 S RNA (Rossier *et al.*, 1974; Wilce *et al.*, 1976a,b). This labeling was rapid, appearing within the first 30 minutes after hormone addition; increases in cytoplasmic 18 S and 28 S RNA were observed about 100 minutes later. On the basis of sucrose density gradient analyses and the polyadenosine [poly(A)] content of the 9–12 S product, the authors concluded that there was synthesis of aldosterone-specific messenger RNA (mRNA) followed by ribosomal RNA (rRNA). The postulated mRNA appeared to be mineralocorticoid-specific, since spirolactone antagonized the increases seen in RNA synthesis with aldosterone, whereas cortisol and 17α-isoaldosterone were ineffective in stimulating RNA synthesis at concentrations equimolar to aldosterone. When rRNA was specifically inhibited with 3'-deoxycytidine, there was little effect on the rise in SCC with aldosterone, which suggested that enhanced synthesis of rRNA played a supportive rather than key role in aldosterone action (Rossier *et al.*, 1977). Rossier *et al.* (1978) continued an analysis of the role of specific RNA products in studies that paired responses to 3'-deoxyadenosine (cordycepin) and actinomycin D. Actinomycin D blocks both poly(A) (+) and poly(A) (−) mRNA, while cordycepin blocks only poly(A) (+) mRNA. Since actinomycin D completely inhibited the SCC response to aldosterone, compared to only a 50% decrease in SCC with cordycepin, it appeared that both poly(A) (+) and poly(A) (−) mRNA are necessary to obtain the full mineralocorticoid response. In addition to enhanced nuclear mRNA and rRNA synthesis with aldosterone, modifications in RNA polymerase I and II activities also have been reported (Mishra *et al.*, 1972; Chu and Edelman, 1972). Finally, it should be noted that actinomycin D does not inhibit the kaliuretic or H^+-secretory stimulation of aldosterone at concentrations of inhibitor that block Na^+ reabsorption, which suggests that these effects are not dependent on the same intermediates as those that stimulate Na^+ transport (William-son, 1963; Fimognari *et al.*, 1967; Lifschitz *et al.*, 1973).

Since both cycloheximide and puromycin are potent inhibitors of aldosterone action on Na^+ transport (Edelman *et al.*, 1963; Crabbé and DeWeer, 1964), several investigators have tried to identify those newly synthesized proteins obtained in the presence of steroid. To this end, Sapirstein and Scott developed procedures to separate isolated cells of the toad bladder into the two major cell types: granular and mito-chondria-rich (Scott *et al.*, 1974; Sapirstein and Scott, 1975). Using [^{3}H]methionine for aldosterone-treated and [^{35}S]methionine for con-trol bladders, there was an increase in the ratio of ^{3}H:^{35}S labeling in the mitochondria-rich cell fraction of some six peaks eluted from Sephadex G-75. No increases in this ratio were noted in the granular cell fraction, which suggested that the mitochondria-rich cell is the sole mineralocorticoid target (Scott and Sapirstein, 1975). Three pro-teins were associated with the plasma membrane fraction (MW = 170,000, 85,000, and 12,000) and three with the cytoplasmic compart-ment (MW = 36,000, 12,000, and 6000) (Scott *et al.*, 1978). When poly(A) (+) containing mRNA was isolated from aldosterone-treated toad bladders and compared in a rabbit reticulocyte cell-free protein synthesis system to mRNA products isolated from control bladders, only two proteins were isolated, one of which had a molecular weight of about 70,000. The exact identification of these proteins has not been achieved.

In the adrenalectomized rat, Law and Edelman (1978) reported a 15–50% increase in [^{3}H]leucine incorporation into total protein in the renal cortex and red medulla, respectively, after injection of aldosterone *in vivo*. When the proteins were fractionated from rat renal medullary mitochondria after double-labeling experiments with [^{3}H]- and [^{35}S]methionine, at least two proteins had enhanced ratios in the presence of aldosterone. With antibody techniques, one of these proteins appeared to be citrate synthase, and the other was not iden-tified. No estimated molecular weight was given for this second pro-tein. It has been felt generally that because the total amount of protein induced is small and because tissue heterogeneity complicates the iso-lation of mRNA coding for mineralocorticoid-specific proteins, this par-ticular approach to the identification of aldosterone-induced proteins has been difficult. Another avenue of investigation is to look for changes in the activity of specific proteins such as Na^+,K^+-ATPase with or without aldosterone; this will be addressed in a following sec-tion.

Since aldosterone may stimulate ADH action and H^+/K^+ secretion

by biochemical pathways other than that proposed for stimulation of
Na^+ reabsorption, the peculiarities of these pathways will be described
first. This is an important consideration in trying to sort out proteins
that may be used as markers of various intracellular sites of action.

IV. ALDOSTERONE INTERACTIONS WITH ANTIDIURETIC HORMONE

In the toad bladder, mineralocorticoids produce a sustained increase
in the SCC after 60–90 minutes of exposure to hormone while ADH
causes an immediate transient rise in the SCC followed by a prolonged
refractory period (Crabbé and De Weer, 1965). However, if bladders
are first exposed to aldosterone for several hours before addition of
ADH, the SCC, the osmotic water flow, and the urea permeability
responses to ADH are enhanced (Fanestil et al., 1967). Similar stimulatory effects of aldosterone are seen when cAMP is added in place of
ADH (Handler et al., 1969a). This has been termed a permissive action
of steroid since aldosterone does not alter osmotic water flow in the
absence of cAMP or ADH. Possible explanations for these findings
follow.

In 1972, Stoff et al. reported that aldosterone markedly increased the
accumulation of cAMP if it was added to ADH-stimulated bladders, but
not when added to unstimulated bladders. When several steroids were
tested for their ability to affect cAMP accumulation, there was no
response to testosterone ($2 \times 10^{-7} M$) in contrast to a 33-fold increase
with dexamethasone and a 30-fold increase with aldosterone (both $2 \times
10^{-7} M$); cycloheximide inhibited the response. Based on an observa-
tion that glucocorticoids decreased phosphodiesterase activity in adrenalectomized rats (Senft et al., 1968), Stoff et al. (1972) proposed that
corticoid steroids have a permissive effect on ADH action by decreasing
the activity of phosphodiesterase, thereby increasing intracellular
cAMP. Subsequently they demonstrated modest (22%) decreases in
toad bladder phosphodiesterase levels after prolonged incubation with
aldosterone (Handler et al., 1973). Other investigators focused on a
second site of corticoid interaction with the ADH pathway, the synthesis
of prostaglandins. Prostoglandin E (PGE) inhibits the osmotic permeability response of toad bladder and renal cortical collecting duct
to ADH, but has no effect on the response to cAMP (Grantham and
Orloff, 1968; Orloff et al., 1965; Urakabe et al., 1975). Zusman and
co-workers (1977, 1978; Zusman and Keiser, 1980) found that steroid
hormones could in turn interfere with PGE production by blocking
the release of arachidonic acid from phospholipid (acylhydrolase/
phospholipase step). This site of action is noted in Fig. 2 and is con-

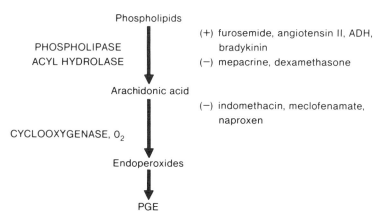

FIG. 2. The biosynthesis of prostaglandins. Positive and negative effectors of the enzymic steps in the synthesis of prostaglandins are given to the right.

trasted to the site of action of other inhibitors, such as indomethacin. Again, when glucocorticoids were compared with aldosterone, both dexamethasone and triamcinolone were more effective in inhibiting PGE biosynthesis than aldosterone, and were more effective in stimulating ADH-responsive water flow. They attributed these changes, therefore, to a glucocorticoid-responsive pathway. Further experiments showed that spirolactone, cycloheximide, and actinomycin D blocked the inhibitory effects of steroids on PGE biosynthesis as well as steroid-stimulated water flow. If this is, as reported, a glucocorticoid-regulated event, then the fact that spirolactone blocked this response suggests either (a) a nonreceptor-mediated inhibitory site for spirolactone, or (b) the addition of such large quantities of spirolactone that they were sufficient to occupy and inhibit glucocorticoid receptor sites. It is interesting to note that this interaction of prostaglandins, steroid hormones, and adenylate cyclase has also been observed in liver, a nontarget tissue for mineralocorticoids (Manganiello and Vaughan, 1972).

The above studies were done with toad bladder, but similar results were obtained in mammals. Schwartz and Kokko (1979) demonstrated that both dexamethasone and aldosterone indistinguishably enhanced osmotic water flow in the presence of ADH in isolated rabbit cortical collecting ducts. Within minutes after addition and at very low concentrations of steroid ($5 \times 10^{-11} M$), there was a 3- to 4-fold increase in the osmotic water permeability coefficient, L_p. Progesterone had no effect. Since 8-bromo-cAMP or a phosphodiesterase inhibitor (1-methyl-3-isobutylxanthine) replaced the steroid requirement, it appeared that

steroids increased accumulation of cAMP by inhibiting phosphodiesterase activity. The results led the authors to conclude that the concentrating defect seen in adrenal insufficiency in man is due to the loss of
the permissive action of corticoids on ADH-induced water flow. While
it is widely appreciated that most patients with adrenal insufficiency
are unable to excrete a free water load normally and therefore have
secondary hyponatremia, these patients also have a concentrating defect whereby they are unable to form a maximally concentrated urine
for any given level of ADH. It is this latter defect that was considered
in the studies by Schwartz and Kokko.

Jard and co-workers have suggested another site of action of steroids
on ADH. They found that adrenalectomy led to a decrease in the efficiency of ADH receptor:adenylate cyclase coupling in rat renal medullary fractions, and that dexamethasone was more potent than aldosterone in repairing this defect (Rajerison *et al.*, 1974; Jard *et al.*, 1977).
Whether this result is related to prostaglandins working as down-
regulators of coupling, or to variations in contaminating phosphodiesterase activity, or to a third site of steroid regulation remains to be
seen. It should be noted that in all the above studies dexamethasone
was either equipotent or more effective than aldosterone.

V. Aldosterone and Cation Secretion

The exact mechanism by which aldosterone stimulates H^+ transport
is still by no means clear, but on the basis of a review of the literature, I
will attempt to present a reasonable working model of mineralocorticoid action on the transport of this ion. From the outset, it is important to remember that the cell that is responsible for mineralocorticoid–sensitive active Na^+ transport may not be the same cell as that
responsible for mineralocorticoid-sensitive H^+ transport, even though
such cells may coexist side by side in target tissues. Secretion of H^+ in
the amphibian bladder (freshwater turtle, toad) requires glucose or
another suitable substrate and is enhanced by the addition of mineralocorticoids (Schwartz and Steinmetz, 1977). Because of the sensitivity
of the transport process to acetazolamide, a carbonic anhydrase inhibitor, it is thought that carbonic anhydrase action is the major
source of protons for secretion (Ziegler *et al.*, 1976; Maren, 1977). The
action of this enzyme results in the production of HCO_3^- as well as H^+
ions, the HCO_3^- being resorbed across the basolateral membrane and
H^+ being secreted into the lumen. Alternatively, carbonic anhydrase
may be necessary to dispose of OH^- generation (Steinmetz, 1974).

These two possibilities are illustrated below:

$$CO_2 + H_2O \xrightarrow{\text{CA}} H_2CO_3 \longrightarrow H^+ + HCO_3^- \tag{1}$$

$$H_2O \longleftrightarrow H^+ + OH^-; OH^- + CO_2 \xrightarrow{\text{CA}} HCO_3^- \tag{2}$$

where CA = carbonic anhydrase.

Secretion of H^+ can be measured either directly with a pH-stat or indirectly by examining the magnitude of the reverse short-circuit current (RSSC). This current (lumen +) is what remains after Na^+ transport is blocked with amiloride or ouabain and may reflect either H^+ secretion into the lumen, HCO_3^- exit into the bath, or a combination of both processes (Ludens and Fanestil, 1974). Aldosterone probably promotes H^+ secretion by at least two processes. One is dependent on Na^+ and one is independent of Na^+. The Na^+-dependent pathway is a secondary response augmented by the establishment of a more negative lumen PD. Previous investigators have found that the extent of H^+ secretion can easily be modulated by altering the transepithelial PD (Ziegler et al., 1976). The primary effect of aldosterone on H^+ secretion is the one best described in the absence of Na^+, and it probably involves alterations in the luminal membrane containing the H^+ transporting site or the H^+ pump itself. One should keep in mind the relative magnitude of these two responses (SCC vs RSCC). In the toad bladder, the Na^+-dependent SCC 3–4 hours after aldosterone administration might be equivalent to 90–400 μamp. In comparison, the RSCC in the absence of Na^+ but in the presence of aldosterone is about 6 μamp (Ludens et al., 1978).

Both Na^+ and H^+ transport require substrate. For Na^+ transport, it makes little difference if the starting substrate is glucose or pyruvate since substrate is channeled into the tricarboxylic acid cycle and is used to enhance ATP synthesis (pathway I, Fig. 3) (Edelman et al., 1963). On the other hand, the magnitude of H^+ transport stimulated by aldosterone, using pyruvate as a substrate, was only 56% of that supported by glucose (Al-Awqati, 1977). The reason given for this finding was that substrate necessary to promote H^+ secretion must be funneled through the pentose phosphate shunt pathway (pathway II, Fig. 3). It now appears that the action of aldosterone on both Na^+ and H^+ transport requires the generation of ATP and is, therefore, antimycin A-sensitive. It also requires the stimulation of NADPH and fatty acid synthesis, and is therefore sensitive to inhibitors of this pathway. We will look at these pathways in more detail.

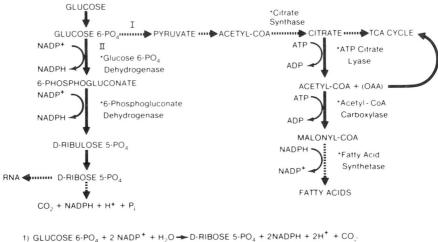

1) $GLUCOSE\ 6\text{-}PO_4 + 2\ NADP^+ + H_2O \rightarrow D\text{-}RIBOSE\ 5\text{-}PO_4 + 2NADPH + 2H^+ + CO_2$

2) $GLUCOSE\ 6\text{-}PO_4 + 12\ NADP^+ \rightarrow 6\ CO_2 + 12\ NADPH + 12H^+ + P_i$

FIG. 3. The hexose monophosphate shunt pathway and the biosynthesis of fatty acids.

Coupling between H^+ transport and the pentose shunt pathway was demonstrated in a number of ways. If H^+ efflux is inhibited by an opposing pH gradient or by acetazolamide, glucose metabolism by the pentose phosphate shunt pathway is reduced (Ziegler *et al.*, 1976; Norby and Schwartz, 1978; Beauwens and Al-Awqati, 1976). Conversely, when H^+ transport is stimulated by imposing either a more favorable pH gradient or by increasing the P_{CO_2}, flux through this pathway increases. As can be seen at the bottom of Fig. 3, glucose 6-phosphate oxidation through the shunt pathway can be driven to ribose 5-phosphate and 2 NADPH or it can be completely oxidized to CO_2, resulting in the generation of 12 NADPH. Norby and Schwartz (1978) suggested that the major end product of this pathway, NADPH, may provide reducing equivalents for fatty acid synthesis or may serve as a source of protons, perhaps coupled at the membrane to a redox transport mechanism.

Dixon and Al-Awqati then asked the question: Is the H^+ pump an ATPase or solely a redox-driven transport system? Their approach was similar to that in the classic study of Garrahan and Glynn (1966, 1967) on the coupling of ATP hydrolysis to Na^+,K^+-ATPase activity in the red blood cell. In the earlier studies, Garrahan and Glynn reversed the chemical potential for membrane-bound Na^+,K^+-ATPase and generated small amounts of ATP in red blood cell ghosts. They could not predict the efficiency of running the Na^+ pump "backward," but they could thermodynamically predict that some ATP would be synthesized if ATP hydrolysis was tightly coupled to ion transport. Similarly, after poisoning endogenous mitochondrial ATP synthetic capacity, Dixon and Al-Awqati (1979) demonstrated ATP accumulation in the presence of adverse transepithelial proton electrochemical gradients across turtle bladders. DCCD (N,N'-dicyclohexylcarbodiimide) abolished both ATP synthesis and H^+ flux. Since this agent had previously been used to inhibit specifically a mitochondrial proton translocating ATPase, the results supported their proposal that luminal H^+ ion translocation in the amphibian bladder is via a H^+-ATPase. There may be another similarity between luminal membrane H^+-ATPase and mitochondrial H^+-ATPase, and that is the presence of an endogenous inhibitor of function, to be discussed a little later.

There have been a number of experiments carried out to see whether aldosterone-mediated changes in H^+ transport as well as Na^+ transport are dependent on intracellular receptors and RNA and protein synthesis. First, if a receptor is involved, as well as an induction mechanism at the nuclear level, one might expect that spirolactone would block the response and that a series of steroids of varying agonist activity on Na^+ transport pathways would have the same relative effect on H^+ secretion. Furthermore, the time course of the responses might be similar. Actually, H^+ transport increases some 60 minutes before Na^+ transport in the turtle bladder (Al-Awqati et al., 1976). Spirolactone SC 14266 prevented the rise in H^+ transport whereas spirolactone SC 9420 promoted H^+ transport (Ludens et al., 1978; Mueller and Steinmetz, 1978). Since SC 9420 appeared to have some agonist activity on the SCC response or net Na^+ flux also, this spirolactone may not be the drug of choice to distinguish clearly between a possible agonist or antagonist action on H^+ secretion. [However, in the adrenalectomized dog, SC 9420 also increased urinary H^+ excretion without a significant change in Na^+ loss (Hulter et al., 1979).] When several hormones were compared for their relative ability to stimulate H^+ secretion, it was found that dexamethasone and aldosterone at 10^{-7} M had similar stimulatory actions, but 17β-estradiol or ADH had no effect as measured by the RSCC (Ludens et al., 1978). Realistically, it may be difficult to rank a large series of potential agonist steroids because the magnitude of the RSCC is so small. Given the differences in time course and the response to spirolactone, the data provided to date neigher clearly implicate nor negate a role for the receptor in mediating enhanced H^+ transport with mineralocorticoids.

When actinomycin D or puromycin was added to unstimulated bladders (i.e., minus hormone), there was a rapid stimulation of H^+ transport. The further addition of steroids did not produce an additive effect (Ludens *et al.*, 1978). This finding has some parallelism in the mammalian system, since Lifschitz *et al.* (1973) found that actinomycin D alone enhanced both K^+ and H^+ secretion in the adrenalectomized dog. The proposed explanation for this increase in H^+ transport goes back to studies on H^+-ATPase in the mitochondrion. It has been long realized that mitochondrial H^+-ATPase has an associated molecule that behaves as a natural inhibitor (Racker, 1976; Pullman and Monroy, 1969). It was postulated, therefore, that luminal membrane H^+-ATPase has a similar molecule attached, with a relatively short half-life. When the synthesis of this inhibitor molecule is blocked with actinomycin D or puromycin, H^+ secretion rises. Thus, one of the possible roles of aldosterone might be to dissociate this inhibitor (Ludens *et al.*, 1978). Until proved otherwise, this would seem a plausible model for the results obtained with RNA and protein synthesis inhibitors. Because of the unusual response to inhibitor alone, one cannot determine at present whether aldosterone increases H^+ secretion by a post-transcriptional or a transcriptional route. The suggestion has been made, however, that aldosterone increases H^+ transport either by increasing the ease with which H^+ moves through the membrane (in keeping with the proposal that an inhibitor "gate" is removed) or by increasing the number of pumps (Al-Awqati *et al.*, 1976; Al-Awqati, 1978). The evaluations were based on experiments in which variable pH gradients were applied across aldosterone-stimulated and unstimulated bladders, and both the slope of H^+ flux versus the applied potential and the potential at which flux = 0 were noted. Under these circumstances, aldosterone increased the slope of H^+ transport per applied gradient, but did not change the maximum electrochemical gradient against which H^+ could be pumped.

If H^+-ATPase relies on ATP for energy and to a large extent on carbonic anhydrase activity for proton generation, why then does glucose oxidation through the pentose shunt pathway vary as a function of proton transport? New data would implicate the necessity of this pathway for the involvement of fatty acid synthesis in the action of aldosterone. As seen in Fig. 3, the conversion of acetyl-CoA to malonyl-CoA, the rate-limiting step in fatty acid synthesis is governed by acetyl-CoA carboxylase activity. Inhibition of this enzyme with 2-methyl- 2- [*p*- (1,2,3,4- tetrahydro- 1- naphthyl)phenoxy]propionic acid (TPIA) in toad bladder resulted in inhibition of the aldosterone-induced increase in Na^+ transport as well as the inhibition of labeled amino acid precursors into several plasma membrane proteins (Lien *et al.*, 1975; Scott *et al.*, 1979). By analogy, it may be that both Na^+ and H^+ fluxes are in some way facilitated by fatty acid synthesis.

Aldosterone may also promote net acid excretion by influencing the metabolism of ammonia. Adrenalectomized rats show a 70% reduction in ammonia production. These losses can be recovered by administration of glucocorticoids or large doses of aldosterone (7 μg/100 gm body weight) (Welbourne, 1974; Welbourne and Francoeur, 1977). In studies by Welbourne and Francoeur (1977), aldosterone increased ammonia production in rats without a significant elevation in K^+ excretion or evidence of hypokalemia. This is an important finding, since previous studies have shown a close correlation between ammonia production and K^+ depletion (Tannen, 1977). The results would suggest, therefore, that aldosterone-stimulated ammonia production is not secondary to steroid effects on K^+ disposition. The exact biochemical locus of steroid-regulated ammoniagenesis is not known, but the rate-limiting steps that have been suggested are (*a*) the entry of glutamine into mitochondria; (*b*) an activation of the mitochondrial enzyme, phosphate-dependent glutaminase; (*c*) an activation of the cytoplasmic enzyme, phosphoenolpyruvate carboxykinase (PEPCK), which alleviates an accumulation of α-ketoglutarate; and perhaps (*d*) the exit of glutamine carbons from mitochondria via the dicarboxylate transporter (Welbourne, 1974; Welbourne and Francoeur, 1977; Welbourne *et al.*, 1976; Snart and Taylor, 1978; Kunin and Tannen, 1979; Cheema-Dhahli and Halperin, 1979). The effects are not peculiar to mineralocorticoids, and further experiments are necessary in order to determine the role of aldosterone in this process (Welbourne *et al.*, 1976; Snart and Taylor, 1978; Tannen, 1978; Frazier and Zachariah, 1979).

Another cation influenced by aldosterone is K^+. Urinary K^+ is a composite of both reabsorptive and secretory processes in various portions of the nephron. In the proximal tubule, some 40–60% of filtered K^+ is reabsorbed, or quantities that reflect the overall reabsorption of water in this segment. At the first accessible portion of the distal convoluted tubule, only 10–15% of filtered K^+ remains, the net K^+ absorption taking place somewhere along the loop of Henle. The distal convoluted and cortical collecting tubules result in net K^+ addition to the urine, while the medullary collecting duct may have the dual capacity both to readsorb and to secret K^+. K^+ excretion is altered by four variables: the K^+ load, the flow rate through the nephron, acid-base balance, and mineralocorticoids (Wright and Giebisch, 1978). Chronic K^+ loading can promote K^+ secretion by producing net addition of sodium pumps to the basolateral membrane of the medullary collecting duct (Hayslett *et al.*, 1979). Also, increasing flow rate to the distal convoluted tubule increases K^+ secretion, while increasing K^+ concentration at a constant flow rate reduces K^+ secretion and can promote reabsorption at high luminal concentrations (Good and Wright, 1979). Both alkalosis and mineralocorticoids increase K^+ excretion, while acidosis and adrenalectomy decrease K^+ loss. Since several parameters govern K^+ transport, changes in load or flow rate can mask mineralocorticoid-sensitive K^+ flux. Therefore, when aldosterone was administered to adrenalectomized rats on normal rat chow (high K^+ content), urinary electrolyte measurements revealed a decrease in Na^+, with no observable change from control values in urinary K^+ levels. When animals were given a low K^+ diet overnight, aldosterone then dramatically increased urinary K^+ loss over control levels (Fimognari *et al.*, 1967).

As with H^+, we would ask whether aldosterone directly stimulates K^+ secretion or whether it does so indirectly by increasing Na^+ transport and thereby creating a more favorable electrical gradient for the movement of K^+ into the lumen. It has been shown in the toad bladder that the influx of K^+ from the serosal surface correlates with the efflux of Na^+ across the same membrane. This process, i.e., K^+ influx, is sensitive to all inhibitors of the Na^+ transport pathway (amiloride, ouabain, puromycin, actinomycin D) (Rodriguez *et al.*, 1975). Since luminal K^+ permeability is low in this species, information is not available concerning the effects of steroids on K^+ efflux across the luminal membrane. In the mammalian cortical collecting duct, however, a target for mineralocorticoid-sensitive Na^+ transport, Schwartz and Burg (1978) found that the net fluxes of both K^+ and Na^+ in the isolated segment were proportional to the plasma aldosterone concentration of the animal (rabbit) *in vivo*. These findings would be in keeping with the proposal that K^+ movement in the presence of aldosterone was dependent on Na^+ moving across Na^+,K^+-ATPase in exchange for K^+, and that K^+ moved down its electrochemical gradient into the lumen. Some questions have been raised about this simple explanation based on *in vivo* studies in rats and dogs. First, spirolactone appears to block K^+ losses when administered in appropriate amounts along with aldosterone. However, as with H^+, the administration of actinomycin D *in vivo* does not block K^+ loss if given before aldosterone. Again actinomycin D has some kaliuretic effect when given alone (Williamson, 1963; Fimognari *et al.*, 1967; Lifschitz *et al.*, 1973; Nicholls *et al.*, 1979). It is this finding that suggests that aldosterone may result in enhanced movement of K^+ and H^+ across the luminal membrane via biochemical pathways activated sooner and in some ways independent of effects on Na$^+$ transport. This question remains to be resolved.

VI. ALDOSTERONE-INDUCED PROTEINS: POSSIBILITIES AND PROBABILITIES

Although aldosterone enhances labeled amino acid uptake into total protein, only a few individual proteins have been extensively studied in connection with the mechanism of action of mineralocorticoids. These are citrate synthase, Na$^+$,K$^+$-ATPase, and, more recently, enzymes involved in flavin metabolism.

A. CITRATE SYNTHASE

Fimognari *et al.* (1967) were the first to suggest that citrate synthase activity (citrate synthetase, condensing enzyme) might be increased by aldosterone. They postulated that the mechanism of action of aldosterone depended on the stimulation of the tricarboxylic acid cycle at some point between citrate synthase and α-ketoglutarate dehydrogenase. The mitochondrial level of this stable enzyme (citrate synthase) is remarkably constant and reflects the oxidative capacity of a given cell type or tissue (Srere, 1971). However, activity is elevated or decreased in concert with several other tricarboxylic acid cycle enzymes in the following few instances: (*a*) muscle enzyme increases after prolonged strenuous exercise (Holloszy *et al.*, 1970); (*b*) liver enzyme increases in vitamin B$_{12}$-deficient animals (Mukerjee *et al.*, 1976); (*c*) enzyme levels increase in several tissues from hyperthyroid rats (Winder, 1979; Tata, 1966; Kadenbach, 1966); and (*d*) rat renal enzyme decreases after adrenalectomy (Kinne and Kirsten, 1968; Law and Edelman, 1978; Kirsten and Kirsten, 1972). In the latter case, modest doses of aldosterone returned renal citrate synthase levels to normal within 3 hours after injection. This effect was inhibitable by spirolactone and could not be reproduced by glucocorticoids. As with prolonged exercise or thyroid hormone, several tricarboxylic acid cycle enzymes were reduced after adrenalectomy and were increased again by acute administration of aldosterone. A coordinate change in tricarboxylic acid enzyme levels is not surprising, since Srere has postulated that complex control of the tricarboxylic acid cycle under any circumstances may require modification of several enzymes, rather than any particular one (Srere, 1969, 1971). In contrast to differences in renal citrate synthase activities with and without aldosterone, liver mitochondria from the same animals had equivalent activities (Law and

Edelman, 1978). Since the liver apparently contains glucocorticoid receptors, but not mineralocorticoid receptors, the differential effects of aldosterone on renal and liver citrate synthase are in keeping with the suggested mineralocorticoid specificity of acute changes in this enzyme (Duval and Funder, 1974). Citrate synthase has also been measured in toad bladders with and without aldosterone addition. In studies by Kirsten et al. (1968), citrate synthase activity increased with the same time course as the rise in aldosterone-stimulated Na^+ transport. Kirsten et al. also found a linear correlation between the percentage incremental in citrate synthase activity and the percentage incremental in Na^+ transport.

Several pieces of evidence rule out the possibility that these findings were secondary to enhanced transepithelial Na^+ transport. First, removal of mucosal Na^+ eliminated the rise in SCC observed with aldosterone, but it did not alter the rise in enzyme activity (Kirsten et al., 1968). Second, the administration of ADH or a combination of cAMP and theophylline, both of which stimulate Na^+ transport in the toad bladder, did not elevate citrate synthase levels (R. Kirsten et al., 1970). These aldosterone-mediated changes in enzyme activity appear to depend on de novo synthesis of citrate synthase, since inhibitors of protein and RNA synthesis block both aldosterone-stimulated Na^+ reabsorption and the rise seen in citrate synthase activity (Kinne and Kirsten, 1968; Kirsten et al., 1968). Furthermore, when Law and Edelman (1978a) examined renal changes in citrate synthase activity in adrenalectomized rats with and without administration of aldosterone (0.8 $\mu g/100$ gm body weight), they found that the rise in activity at 3 hours after injection was consistent with an effect on the kinetic component V_{max} rather than enhanced affinity of either of the substrates, acetyl-CoA or oxaloacetate. Most important, they found that titration of renal fractions with anti-citrate synthase antibodies supported the proposal that increased citrate synthase activity with aldosterone was due to a net increase in enzyme molecules.

All these findings favor a model of aldosterone action in which citrate synthase is a specifically induced protein. Certainly no one has suggested that it is the only induced protein. While it remains to be seen whether this enzyme should be considered a key intermediate in the action of aldosterone on Na^+ transport, one series of experiments would favor this suggestion. Srere (1971) has shown that in comparing several tissues, the ratio of extractable citrate synthase to the oxygen consumption rate varies somewhat. In heart and liver, this ratio is substantially greater than one (i.e. citrate synthase does not appear to be rate-limiting for metabolic activity in these tissues). However,

Kirsten and Kirsten (1972) found that in kidney the ratio of extractable citrate synthase activity to the activity through the tricarboxylic acid cycle was approximately equal to one, which means that in this tissue citrate synthase may be rate-limiting for activity through the cycle and thereby key to the production of energy for aldosterone-mediated Na^+ transport. On the other hand, amphotericin B can stimulate active Na^+ transport without presumably increasing citrate synthase levels (Lichtenstein and Leaf, 1965).

B. NA^+,K^+-ATPASE

The debate that surrounds the question of the association between aldosterone and Na^+,K^+-ATPase activity is complicated by two major problems: (a) how to assay Na^+,K^+-ATPase activity for evaluation of hormonal stimulation; and (b) the need to separate changes produced by glucocorticoid activity from changes to be considered mineralocorticoid-specific.

Since Na^+,K^+-ATPase activity is plasma membrane-bound, assays require homogenization of tissue. During preparation of plasma membrane fractions, vesicularization of membrane fragments probably takes place (Razin, 1972). Apparent cellular Na^+,K^+-ATPase activity is increased by agents used in preparative procedures, such as detergents, which tend to allow better access of substrates (ATP, K^+, Na^+) to substrate-specific sites on the enzyme. However, the rise in activity that is observed with detergents could also be attributed to the mechanical uncovering of latent pumps (i.e., inactive Na^+, K^+-ATPase enzyme molecules). This same criticism appears in much of the literature on aldosterone stimulation of Na^+,K^+-ATPase. If the more usual methods are used to isolate Na^+,K^+-ATPase, (i.e., with detergents) and aldosterone appears to have no effect on enzyme activity, then one may contend that, in isolation of the enzyme, the investigator has inadvertently uncovered latent pumps, thereby obliterating an effect that would naturally belong to the hormone stimulus.

The second question to consider in evaluating experiments on aldosterone and Na^+,K^+ ATPase is whether glucocorticoid controls have been included. It is generally agreed that renal Na^+, K^+-ATPase levels are lower in adrenalectomized than in normal rats. The question that remains is whether this is due to loss of glucocorticoid action, to loss of mineralocorticoid action at particular target sites along the nephron, or to adaptive changes in Na^+ load to various portions of the nephron secondary to a diminished glomerular filtration rate, which is predominantly a glucocorticoid effect.

The available data do not make it possible either to dismiss or accept unequivocally the proposal that aldosterone directly increases the synthesis or activation of Na^+,K^+-ATPase. In Table III, however, I have summarized results of pertinent papers in the field in order to allow the reader to consider the feasibility of direct induction of Na^+,K^+-ATPase by aldosterone. Section A of the table records changes in enzyme activity in toad bladders with and without aldosterone administration. Section B deals with experiments in which 10 μg of aldosterone or less were given to rats or guinea pigs per day per 100 gm body weight. Section C includes studies in which higher doses of aldosterone were used, and Section D compares changes in Na^+,K^+-ATPase activity in experiments where methylprednisolone, a potent glucocorticoid, was given to the animals.

The available data (Table III) indicate that aldosterone does not regulate Na^+,K^+-ATPase activity in the toad bladder (Bonting and Canady, 1964; Hill *et al.*, 1973). Three points should be made about the earlier, oft-quoted study (Bonting and Canady, 1964). Basal Na^+,K^+-ATPase activity was low, and the duration of assay incubation (60 minutes) was longer than has been used in most studies (10–20 minutes), which presents a problem in interpretation because generation of P_i, even in the presence of a continued excess of substrate, tends to be nonlinear beyond 20 or 30 minutes of incubation (Lo *et al.*, 1976). Furthermore, Bonting and Canady, in this study, examined Na^+,K^+-ATPase activity at only one time, 1 hour after hormone addition, whereas initiation of the rise in SCC with aldosterone most commonly occurs between 60 and 90 minutes after hormone addition, with a plateau occurring some 2 hours later (Crabbé, 1977). Depending on the final limiting step in hormone action, a 1-hour time point might, or might not, isolate statistically significant increases in enzyme activity. The second paper, by Hill *et al.* (1973), examined the Na^+,K^+-ATPase response at 2.5 hours and did not find a rise in activity; however, deoxycholate (DOC) was used.

Review of data obtained in the rat and guinea pig (Section B, Table III) showed an inconsistent response to aldosterone under a variety of conditions such as with and without DOC, homogenates versus microsomal preparations, and whole tissue versus subfractionation of kidney into cortex, red medulla, etc. However, it is important to ask if a pattern for mineralocorticoid induction of Na^+,K^+-ATPase can be revealed when specific conditions are examined. Dose of steroid should be considered first, because previous publications showed that 0.3–0.4 μg of aldosterone per 100 gm body weight produced a half-maximal change in both urinary Na^+/K^+ ratios and ^{3}H-labeled precursor incorporation into protein in the rat kidney (Kirsten and Kirsten, 1972; Law and Edelman, 1978a). In Table III, the smallest dose of aldosterone administered, 5 μg/100 gm body weight, should therefore produce > 90% of the maximum possible effect. [Many investigators, including myself, prefer to use ~ 1 μg/100 gm body weight, to avoid occupancy of glucocorticoid receptor sites (Feldman et al., 1972; Marver and Edelman, 1978).] One report showed a 66% rise in cortical Na$^+$, K$^+$-ATPase activity at 1 hour after injection with no changes in medullary activity (−DOC). This is in contrast to a second study (+DOC) in which steroid was administered for 6 days. In this study there was no change in cortical activity, but the activity in red medulla increased 29%. The former experiments used normal rats, and the latter used adrenalectomized rats (Ikeda et al., 1979; Hendler et al., 1972). Using an ultramicro oil-well technique, Schmidt and co-workers (1975) measured Na$^+$,K$^+$-ATPase activity on isolated cortical nephron segments and found that 5 μg of aldosterone per 100 gm body weight resulted in increases of 133–465% in Na$^+$,K$^+$-ATPase in proximal convoluted tubule, distal convoluted tubule, and thick ascending limb of Henle at 1 hour after injection. Deoxycholate was not used in these studies because they had found that it has little effect on activity in this particular system (Schmidt and Horster, 1978). In two other studies, one +DOC and the other −DOC, no rise in Na$^+$,K$^+$-ATPase activity was reported to occur when aldosterone was given to adrenalectomized rats over a 5-day period (10 μg/day) (Chignell and Titus, 1966; Knox and Sen, 1974). In Section B of Table III, therefore, there was no consistent difference in activity between normal and adrenalectomized animals, between (−) and (+) DOC, or between homogenates and microsomal preparations. Section C of Table III, lists experiments in which 20–100 μg of aldosterone per day were used, a dose well above that necessary to produce maximum effects on Na$^+$ reabsorption. One report (Chignell and Titus, 1966) cited 28 or 50% increases in renal Na$^+$,K$^+$-ATPase activities in animals given aldosterone (20 or 100 μg) over a 5-day period. This particular paper, however, reported a very low activity for control adrenalectomized rats, considering that DOC was used. A second group (Charney et al., 1974) found small changes in activity (16 or 17%) if 100 μg of aldosterone was given for 5 days to adrenalectomized rats, but not if the same dose was given to normal rats. Other investigators gave 20 μg/day for 5 days and found a 14% rise in activity (Knox and Sen, 1974). Last, when colon, another mineralocorticoid target tissue, was examined, 60 μg of aldosterone given over a 1-day period to normal animals did not increase Na$^+$,K$^+$-ATPase activity (Frizzell and Schultz, 1978; Thompson and Edmonds, 1974). To this point, there is

TABLE III

Na⁺, K⁺-ATPase Activity (37°C): Response to Aldosterone (A) and Methylprednisolone (MP)[a]

Species and tissue	H/MC[b]	DOC[c] (+) or (−)	Fractionation[d]	Activity[e] Normals	Activity[e] Adz/basal	Dose (A) or (MP) and duration	Response[f] (%)	References[g]
Section A								
1. Toad bladder	H	(−)	—	—	0.3	(A) 5×10^{-5} M; 1 hr	NS	1
2. Toad bladder	H	(+)	—	—	22	(A) 10^{-6} M; 2.5 hr	NS	2
Section B								
1. Rat kidney	H	(−)	PCT	—	0.6	(A) 5 µg; 1 hr	+133	3
			DCT	—	1.7	(A) 5 µg; 1 hr	+465	3
			TALH	—	2.0	(A) 5 µg; 1 hr	+200	3
2. Rat kidney	H	(−)	Cortex	2.9	—	(A) 5 µg; 1 hr	+66	4
			Red Med.	3.4	—	(A) 5 µg; 1 hr	NS	4
			Papilla	1.6	—	(A) 5 µg; 1 hr	NS	4
3. Rat kidney	H	(+)	—	—	1.1	(A) 10 µg × 5 days	NS	5
4. Rat kidney	MC	(−)	—	—	128	(A) 10 µg × 5 days	NS	6
5. Rat kidney	MC	(+)	Cortex	—	53	(A) 5-10 µg × 6 days	NS	7
			Red Med.	—	66	(A) 5-10 µg × 6 days	+29	7
Section C								
1. Rat kidney	H	(+)	—	—	1.1	(A) 20 µg × 5 days	+28	5
			—	—		(A)100 µg × 5 days	+50	5

Tissue	Method		Region			Treatment	Response	Ref.
2. Rat kidney	H	(+)	Cortex	14	—	(A)100 μg × 7 days	NS	8
			Red Med.	31	—	(A)100 μg × 7 days	NS	8
3. Rat kidney	MC	(−)	Cortex	—	11	(A)100 μg × 7 days	+16	8
			Red Med.	—	27	(A)100 μg × 7 days	+17	8
				—	128	(A) 20 μg × 5 days	+14	6
4. Rat colon	H	(+)		6.7[h]	—	(A) 60 μg × 1 day	NS	9
5. Guinea pig heart	H	(−)		2.0	—	(A) 30 μg × 14 days	+42	10
Section D								
1. Rat kidney	H	(+)	Cortex	14	—	(MP) 3 mg × 3 days	+42	8
			Red Med.	31	—	(MP) 3 mg × 3 days	+37	8
2. Rat kidney	MC	(+)		—	31	(MP) 6 mg × 3 days	+77	7
3. Guinea pig heart	H	(−)		—	2	(MP) 8 mg × 24 days	+18	10

[a] Duration of incubation for estimation of Na^+,K^+-ATPase activity ranged from 10 to 20 minutes, except for sample 1 in group A, where incubation was for 60 minutes at 37°C.

[b] MC, microsomes; H, homogenate.

[c] DOC, deoxycholate.

[d] PCT, proximal convoluted tubule; DCT, distal convoluted tubule; TALH, thick ascending limb of Henle; Med., medulla.

[e] Activity: micromoles of P_i per hour per milligram of protein; Adx, adrenalectomized.

[f] Percentage of increase under response is to be compared with appropriate control (either normal or adrenalectomized) for each experiment. If normal activity is reported, steroids were given to normal animals. If Adx values are given, steroids were given to Adx animals. The term basal was added to indicate activities in toad bladders where endogenous mineralocorticoid activity was suppressed but not necessarily totally absent. NS, not significant.

[g] References: (1) Bonting and Canady, 1964; (2) Hill et al., 1973; (3) Schmidt et al., 1975; (4) Ikeda et al., 1979; (5) Chignell and Titus, 1966; (6) Knox and Sen, 1974; (7) Hendler et al., 1972; (8) Charney et al., 1974; (9) Thompson and Edmonds, 1974; (10) Hegyvary, 1977.

[h] Activity in this one experiment is expressed as micromoles of P_i per hour per micromole of K^+.

one consistent finding within the very high-dose aldosterone group. In each case aldosterone given to normal animals was ineffective. However, when given to adrenalectomized rats, there was always an increase in activity both with and without DOC. Guinea pig heart was added to the list because heart is not a mineralocorticoid target organ, but it does respond to glucocorticoids (Duval and Funder, 1974). When 30 μg of aldosterone was given to normal guinea pigs for 14 days, there was a 42% increase in heart Na^+,K^+-ATPase activity (Hegyvary, 1977). This brings us to Section D of Table III, which deals with animals given methylprednisolone. In each case, with or without DOC, in both normal and adrenalectomized rats, methylprednisolone increased Na^+,K^+-ATPase activity.

In summary, maximum doses of aldosterone (5–10 μg/day) do not produce a consistent change in renal Na^+,K^+-ATPase activity even when given over a period of days to normal or adrenalectomized rats. In the case of supramaximal doses, aldosterone increased activity in adrenalectomized, but not in normal, rats. Methylprednisolone increased activity in both. None of the data consistently supports the proposal that deoxycholate obliterates the hormonal response or that aldosterone induces Na^+,K^+-ATPase as part of the receptor-linked pathway that leads within hours to enhanced Na^+ reabsorption. Based on the data in Table III, however, I agree with the model of Jorgensen (1972), who attributed increases in Na^+,K^+-ATPase activity after prolonged cortical steroid administration as an indirect adaptation of chronic changes in Na^+ load to responsive nephron segments. Changes in Na^+ load would be brought about by fluctuations in glomerular filtration rate, a parameter that is hormonally sensitive to glucocorticoids. Indeed, it has recently been reported that manipulations of glomerular filtration rate by adrenalectomy, glucocorticoids, or reduction of renal mass have all resulted in alterations in renal Na^+,K^+-ATPase content per cell (Rodriguez and Klahr, 1980). If future studies support the proposal that Na^+ load can regulate renal Na^+,K^+-ATPase, then one of the most interesting questions to be answered in renal physiology and biochemistry in the future is the molecular mechanism by which Na^+ per se increases the synthesis of or activates this membrane protein.

C. FLAVIN ENZYMES

The general biochemical pathway for flavin metabolism is outlined in Fig. 4. Flavin mononucleotide (FMN) is synthesized from riboflavin by the action of the enzyme flavokinase (enzyme I, Fig. 4), in the presence of Mg^{2+} and ATP. (Flavin adenine dinucleotide (FAD) is de-

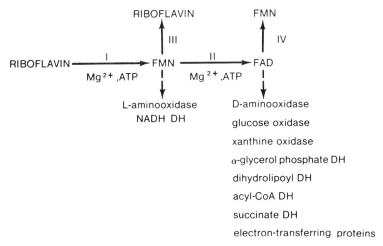

FIG. 4. The biosynthesis of FMN and FAD from riboflavin. The key enzymes are flavokinase (I), pyrophosphorylase (II), and FMN- and FAD-specific phosphatases (III, IV). A number of proteins dependent on either FMN or FAD biosynthesis are also shown.

rived from FMN via the enzyme FAD pyrophosphorylase (enzyme II, Fig. 4), which also requires Mg^{2+} and ATP for action; phosphatases specific for either FMN or FAD dephosphorylate the flavins (enzymes III and IV, Fig. 4). FMN and FAD are in turn bound covalently or noncovalently to a number of enzymes including succinic dehydrogenase and NADH dehydrogenase. Since free flavin is rapidly metabolized by phosphatases, the presence of flavin-binding proteins stabilizes synthesized FMN and FAD. Therefore, tissue concentrations of these flavins depend on the level of riboflavin as substrate, the levels of both synthetic and degradative enzymes, the level of ATP as a second substrate, and the level of flavin-containing apoenzymes. Hormones interacting with this pathway could theoretically interact at any one of these sites. With the administration of ^{14}C-labeled riboflavin in tracer quantities, the accumulation of riboflavin + FMN/FAD is greatest in kidney, followed by liver and heart, which in turn have much higher concentrations than the remaining tissues (Yagi, 1954). The high riboflavin levels in kidney are a consequence of both renal concentration and excretion of this vitamin, since some 20% of [^{14}C]riboflavin is excreted in the urine 1 hour after s.c. injection. However, a significant portion of the riboflavin penetrates renal cells and is used for the synthesis of FAD and FMN (Fazekas and Sandor, 1973). It is believed that, once in the cells, most, if not all, of the flavin biosynthesis takes place in the cytoplasmic compartment, whereas bound

FAD/FMN are concentrated in the mitochondrial and nuclear compartments (Fazekas and Sandor, 1973). The cytoplasmic level of riboflavin, on the other hand, appears to be directly proportional to the plasma concentration, which suggests the lack of major riboflavin cytoplasmic receptors other than the metabolizing enzymes themselves. In the liver, 70% of the total radioactivity is associated with nuclei and mitochondria 90 minutes after injection of [^{14}C]riboflavin, largely bound as FAD.

With these few generalizations about the synthesis of flavins, we will examine what is known about the interaction of aldosterone with this pathway. A suggestion that adrenal corticoids are involved in the pathway came from the early work of Fazekas and Sandor (1971), who found that ACTH (60 IU/day for 2 days) given to normal rats along with [^{14}C]riboflavin increased FMN accumulation by 88% in liver and 57% in kidney at 1 hour, compared to noninjected controls. Riboflavin and FAD levels were invariant with or without ACTH loading. The authors held this to be the result of increased flavokinase activity, probably mediated by glucocorticoids (Fazekas and Sandor, 1971). Tan and Trachewsky (1975) and Trachewsky (1978) subsequently examined the possibility of corticoid control of flavin biosynthesis. In the earlier paper, the levels of accumulated [^{14}C]riboflavin, [^{14}C]FMN, and [^{14}C]FAD at 1 hour after injection of diluent or steroid along with labeled riboflavin were determined. In the second paper the same accumulation pattern was examined 3.5 hours after injection. Dexamethasone (15 μg/100 gm body weight) was given the evening before the experiment to suppress endogenous ACTH. In the earlier study (Tan and Trachewsky, 1975), 75 adrenalectomized controls and 79 adrenalectomized animals given aldosterone (2 μg/100 gm body weight) were examined. At 1 hour after injection of steroid, there was a significant rise in renal FAD levels (range 8 to 28% above controls in 5 series) with no apparent change in labeled tissue riboflavin and FMN. Progesterone (1 mg/100 gm body weight) and corticosterone (0.65 mg/100 gm body weight) were less effective than aldosterone in increasing tissue FAD. Concentrations of actimonycin D that blocked 49% of RNA synthesis, and of cycloheximide that blocked 88% of protein synthesis, were used to examine the mode of action of steroid on FAD accumulation. Cycloheximide blocked the rise in tissue FAD, which implied that the rise in FAD with aldosterone alone was dependent on protein synthesis. However, actinomycin D was ineffective. To interpret lack of a decrease with actinomycin D to mean that the rise in FAD is not mediated through RNA synthesis would still be questionable, since only 49% of RNA synthesis was inhibited. Also, there was no significant change in flavin accumulation in liver samples. Last, spironolactone (6.5 mg/100 gm body weight) given with aldosterone blocked the rise in renal FAD seen with aldosterone alone. One could conclude that at 1 hour after aldosterone there was a significant rise in FAD in kidney, with no change in FMN. It should be noted that at 1 hour the ratio of FMN/riboflavin levels was 0.84 in adrenalectomized rats and FAD/riboflavin was 5.10 (FAD/FMN = 4.26).

In a second paper Trachewsky (1978) examined flavin levels 3.5 hours after administration of aldosterone and [^{14}C]riboflavin. The accumulation of flavins (in particular FMN) relative to riboflavin was higher than in the previous study. The ratio of FMN/riboflavin in adrenalectomized controls was 2.13, while FAD/riboflavin was 5.81 and FAD/FMN was 2.72. With the administration of aldosterone to adrenalectomized rats (1.5 μg/100 gm body weight), there was a 19% increase in [^{14}C]riboflavin deposition [numbers expressed as disintegrations per minute per microgram (dpm/μg) of total flavin], a 27% increase in FMN, and a 14% increase in FAD. Only the increases in FMN and FAD, compared to adrenalectomized controls, were statistically significant (N = 78-80 animals per group). These findings appeared to be compatible with an aldosterone-induced increase in flavokinase and pyrophosphorylase activities at 3.5 hours. However, if one examines the ratio of FMN/riboflavin and FAD/riboflavin in the steroid-treated vs untreated groups, there was only a 5% rise in the ratio of FMN/riboflavin (2.28 vs 2.13 = ratio in aldosterone group vs ratio in controls) with a 4% fall in FAD/riboflavin concentrations (5.58 vs 5.81), resulting in an overall fall in the ratio of FAD/FMN of 10% (2.44 vs. 2.72). Therefore, depending on how the findings at 3.5 hours after aldosterone are evaluated, as seen with ACTH, renal FMN accumulation is increased, and renal FAD accumulation may or may not be. Most important, the changes in renal FAD at 1 hour and renal FMN at 3.5 hours could reflect changes in the enzymes involved in the flavin synthetic–degradative pathway, increases in the level of induced proteins that bind these flavins, or even increases in ATP availability to the flavin pathway. A direct hormonal control of enzymes in the synthesis of flavin nucleotides is not without precedent, however, since thyroid hormone appears to modulate flavokinase activity in target tissues (Rivlin, 1970).

Finally, the question of the importance of flavins to the physiological action of aldosterone has been evaluated by the use of riboflavin analog, known to be competitive antagonists of riboflavin at the level of flavokinase (Trachewsky, 1978). When aldosterone (1.5 μg/100 gm body weight) was given to adrenalectomized rats, the urinary Na$^+$/K$^+$ ratio fell from 4.75 to 1.53 at 3.5 hours later. Riboflavin analogs injected in varying doses along with aldosterone, antagonized the action of aldosterone on Na^+ reabsorption; K^+ excretion was not affected. (Riboflavin analogs, given alone, had no significant effect on Na^+ or K^+ excretion.)

At the present time, it is difficult to determine whether the inhibition of aldosterone-stimulated Na^+ transport by riboflavin analogs reflects a primary or secondary effect due to flavin participation in aldosterone action. For instance, flavin nucleotides, in particular FMN, are in a fairly rapid state of turnover. In normal rat liver, the rate of turnover of FAD per hour is 2%; of FMN, 7%; and of riboflavin, 34% (Fazekas and Sandor, 1973). Therefore, if flavokinase is blocked at the same time that aldosterone is administered, and if free flavin nucleotide is rapidly degraded, the induction of flavin-requiring apoenzymes necessary for enhanced flux through the tricarboxylic acid cycle and through the respiratory chain would be futile; therefore those physiological parameters that depend on these pathways might be retarded whether or not aldosterone specifically increased flavin-nucleotide biosynthetic enzymes, such as flavokinase. The implication of the flavin biosynthetic pathway in the mechanism of action of aldosterone is an exciting new development. Further studies must be completed, however, to determine whether this is tantamount to induction of either flavokinase or pyrophosphorylase. The suggestion by some that riboflavin analogs might ultimately provide a clinical alternative to spirolactone with fewer harmful side effects seems difficult to reconcile at this time with the wide range of enzymes (Fig. 4) that depend on FMN or FAD for function.

VII. The Two Models: Permease vs Energy

It would be impossible to project an updated model of aldosterone action on target epithelia without incorporating portions of both the permease and energy models. However, before discussing the supporting evidence, it should be emphasized that these models may represent the combined action of aldosterone on more than one cell type and through more than one definable pathway.

A. Permease or Plasma Membrane Theory

The permease theory originally considered only luminal membrane permeability changes, but the following discussion will also include the proposal that the lipid environment surrounding basolateral membrane-bound Na^+,K^+-ATPase enzyme molecules is modified so as to increase apparent enzyme activity (i.e., latent pump theory). In the early years, the strongest defense of the permease model by Sharp and Leaf (1964, 1965) was based on two indirect findings. Sharp and Leaf argued that if aldosterone increased ATP synthesis and if this in turn was responsible for the rise in SCC, then toad bladders exposed to aldosterone should have more ATP per cell than controls. When they were unable to detect a rise in intracellular ATP in hormone-stimulated bladders they rejected the energy theory (Sharp et al., 1966a; Handler et al., 1969a). Viewed retrospectively, the findings are not surprising, since ATP is a negative modifier of a number of enzymes in the glycolytic-tricarboxylic acid cycle pathway including phosphofructokinase, pyruvate kinase, citrate synthase, and isocitrate dehydrogenase (Bhagavan, 1978). Because of feedback controls that involve both ATP and ADP, cellular ATP/ADP$\cdot$P$_i$ ratios remain relatively constant (Racker, 1976; Kirsten et al., 1972; Erecińska et al., 1977). Therefore, rather than obtaining a major increase in the steady-state level of ATP, one would expect to find an increased capacity to synthesize and utilize ATP as long as Na^+ was available to drive the pumps and therefore consume ATP, and as long as pyruvate or another suitable substrate was available to produce reducing equivalents for ATP synthesis. Although this proposal seems rational on paper, it has been difficult for investigators to design experiments that clearly show that aldosterone stimulates the energy pathway divorced from its effects on luminal Na^+ entry. This is illustrated by the second argument of Sharp and Leaf against the energy theory.

Amphotericin B, an antibiotic that increases luminal Na^+ permeability, mimics the action of aldosterone on toad bladders. Therefore, both aldosterone and amphotericin independently increased pyruvate utilization, the O_2 consumption rate, and the SCC (Sharp et al., 1966a; Lichtenstein and Leaf, 1965). The absolute magnitude of pyruvate oxidation with amphotericin was less than that stimulated by aldosterone (1.3-fold rise vs 1.5-fold, respectively). However, as amphotericin increases luminal permeability to K^+, H^+, Cl^-, and thiourea as well as to Na^+, one can make only qualitative rather than quantitative statements about the relative stimulation of active Na^+ transport for a given change in luminal Na^+ conductance with amphotericin compared to aldosterone. Based on these findings, Sharp and Leaf proposed that aldosterone, like amphotericin B, (a) enhanced luminal permeability to Na^+; (b) increased intracellular Na^+ concentration and therefore stimulated pump activity and the hydrolysis of ATP; and (c) as a result of increased ATP utilization, there was a secondary stimulation of glycolysis and ATP formation. As further evidence of this secondary effect, Sharp and Leaf reported that removal of mucosal Na^+ blocked the rise in pyruvate oxidation, O_2 consumption, and SCC in bladders treated with either aldosterone or amphotericin. While the results with amphotericin support the permease theory, they are not incompatible with the energy theory. Again, because of feedback controls on ATP synthesis, the fact that Na^+ removal decreased all these parameters with aldosterone or amphotericin was to have been expected, because Na^+ is an obligatory substrate for ATP hydrolysis under the circumstances. The experiments with amphotericin B did yield two very important findings. First, intracellular Na^+ must be a limiting substrate for pump activity in the unstimulated state; and second, enhancement of intracellular Na^+ concentrations can produce a marked stimulation of aerobic metabolism in the absence of aldosterone. That is to say, the rate-limiting enzymes in the tricarboxylic acid cycle and respiratory chain still have a reserve capacity to increase ATP synthesis in the absence of new enzyme production.

In support of an aldosterone action on apical membrane Na^+ permeability, isolated toad bladder cells incubated with aldosterone were found to contain more Na^+ than paired controls (180 ± 10 μeq vs 92 μeq/gm dry weight, $p < 0.001$). Although neither ADP or ATP levels were altered in these experiments, the phosphocreatine:creatine ratio was significantly reduced from 3.7 to 1.7 with addition of aldosterone, indicating to the authors that increases in transport activity had placed a drain on cellular energy reserves (Handler et al., 1969a, 1972). [The latter finding is to be contrasted with work in the adrenalectomized rat kidney, in which aldosterone increased the phosphocreatine:creatine ratio from 0.31 to 0.65 (Kirsten et al., 1972).]

An increase in intracellular Na^+ content brought about by aldosterone has also been inferred from recent experiments with amiloride (Crabbé, 1980). The inhibitory effects of a given dose of amiloride were reduced in aldosterone-treated amphibian skin and bladder. From a series of manipulations including ADH, ouabain, and insulin administration, Crabbé found that agents that decreased intracellular Na^+ increased amiloride sensitivity, and agents that increased intracellular Na^+ decreased amiloride sensitivity. He concluded that intracellular as well as extracellular Na^+ competed with amiloride for Na^+ "pores." Since aldosterone reduced amiloride sensitivity, Crabbé reasoned that aldosterone increased intracellular Na^+ via apical membrane Na^+ permeability changes. Glucose addition, as a final control, both stimulated SCC and tended to increase again the amiloride sensitivity in aldosterone-treated preparations. Here glucose would tend to decrease intracellular Na^+ by providing energy requirements for Na^+, K^+-ATPase.

For some time, changes in resistance (or conductance) across bladders treated with aldosterone also have been noted. Civan and Hoffman (1971) and Siegel and Civan (1976) found a reduction in transepithelial resistance after aldosterone that mirrored the rise in SCC. Both responses were sensitive to inhibitors of RNA and protein synthesis. Two explanations for the rise in SCC were ruled out. First, the E_{Na}, or the maximal electrochemical driving force against which Na^+ could be actively transported, did not change. This precludes a direct effect of aldosterone on increasing the driving force of the sodium pump as a mechanism of enhancing net Na^+ transport. Second, aldosterone might increase net Na^+ transport by decreasing passive backflux of Na^+. However, experiments by Saito and Essig (1973) disproved this hypothesis by showing that passive conductance pathways were unaffected by aldosterone. Since previous studies in the toad bladder had shown a linear relationship between the rise in SCC and the rise in citrate synthase activity, does such a dose-related kinship exist between SCC and changes in resistance (E. Kirsten *et al.*, 1970)? Only one study provides information about this question. Civan and Hoffman (1971) found a 90% increase in SCC matched with an 18% decrease in transepithelial resistance. They then allowed a series of bladders to become slowly substrate-depleted by incubating them over a period of 6 hours. When pyruvate was added, the SCC rose an additional 23%, while resistance decreased a barely preceptible 3%. This suggests a lack of tight coupling between aldosterone-stimulated increases in SCC and decreases in resistance. Indeed, the results with amiloride versus aldosterone obtained by Spooner and Edelman (1975) would support this finding, since at 5 hours after the administration of aldosterone, the energy pathway appeared to dominate the overall stimulation of Na^+ transport. These experiments will be discussed further in Section VII, B.

Spooner and Edelman (1976) also reported that aldosterone could increase SCC anaerobically as had been demonstrated earlier by Handler *et al.* (1969a). In the absence of oxidative phosphorylation, the SCC dropped 90%. Remaining was a small, but statistically significant, difference between steroid-stimulated and unstimulated bladders. Amiloride did not reduce this steroid-dependent anaerobic SCC, and, in fact, tracer analyses showed that this SCC was not equivalent to active transport of Na^+, but to some other ion(s). While the exact ionic nature of the current was not determined, it appeared that aldosterone increased certain permeability properties of the membrane through anaerobic pathways. Again the question arises, how independent are the effects of aldosterone on membrane permeability and energy formation? A recent report briefly discussed experiments in which the investigator looked at the reasons for the drop in resistance across the luminal membrane with aldosterone. He set out to determine whether the response could be attributed to an increase in conductance through individual Na^+ channels or to an increase in the number of transporting sites (Edelman, 1979). In these analyses, aldosterone elevated the luminal membrane Na^+ permeability and SCC to the same degree (161 and 163%). Na^+ conductance of single channels was unaffected but overall channel number increased 123%. This value is, in fact, quite similar to that proposed by Cuthbert and Shum (1975, 1976), who used radiolabeled amiloride to show a 115% rise in [^{14}C]amiloride binding sites (presumably Na^+ channels) in aldosterone-treated hemibladders over controls. However, the above-mentioned studies by Edelman (1979) brought forth what may seem to some in the field a tour de force.

The suggestion was made that metabolic energy is necessary to obtain or maintain the increase in luminal membrane Na^+ conductance. The inference was based on the findings that changes in apical membrane Na^+ permeability and the resultant rise in SCC were equally dependent on glucose metabolism. This could be dissociated from sodium effects in that ouabain blocked the SCC to the same degree as that seen with 2-deoxyglucose treatment, but ouabain had only a minor inhibitory effect on the aldosterone-stimulated increase in luminal Na^+ permeability. Therefore, luminal conductance may be dependent on the energy pathway rather than the energy pathway playing a secondary role serving increased intracellular Na^+ concentrations and increased energy demands. However, one caveat remains. Since 2-deoxyglucose blocks metabolism through the glycolytic and hexose monophosphate shunt pathway, given the available data, we cannot determine whether the glucose-dependence of membrane Na^+ conductivity is via generation of mitochondrial NADH and ATP or via generation of cytoplasmic NADPH and fatty acid synthesis.

Phospholipid analyses provided by Goodman, Rasmussen, and co-workers support the proposal that aldosterone modifies target cell membranes. These investigators considered the turnover of phospholipids in toad bladders (Goodman et al., 1980). Within 20 minutes, aldosterone stimulated glucose oxidation via the hexose monophosphate shunt pathway as evidenced by an increase in labeled CO_2 production from [1-^{14}C]glucose at a time when labeled CO_2 production from [6-^{14}C]glucose was unchanged (Goodman *et al.*, 1971). [These data are in contrast to those of Kirchberger *et al.* (1968), who found a decrease in hexose monophosphate shunt pathway activity in toad bladders in the presence of aldosterone. The disagreement between the two laboratories may in part be due to the fact that Kirchberger *et al.* examined glucose metabolism hours, rather than minutes, after aldosterone.] Using [^{14}C]pyruvate, there was increased incorporation of label into the 2-position of phospholipids during a 60-minute incubation with aldosterone, and after 6 hours, phospholipids from aldosterone-treated bladders showed an increase in the weight percentage and specific activity of several long-chain polyunsaturated fatty acids. Furthermore, the addition of phospholipase A$_2$ reduced the latent period from 93 to 72 minutes. Aldosterone also stimulated the oxidation of [^{14}C]oleate to cytoplasmic acetyl-CoA and the authors suggested that this acetyl-CoA was then utilized for lipid synthesis (Goodman *et al.*, 1975). Cordycepin, cycloheximide, and TPIA, an acetyl-CoA carboxylase inhibitor, but not amiloride, blocked these metabolic changes. TPIA also blocked the rise in SCC (Lien *et al.*, 1975, 1976). If TPIA is specific for acetyl-CoA carboxylase (rather than acting as a general "sink" for acetyl-CoA), the complete lack of an aldosterone-stimulated increase in SCC in the presence of TPIA would place a strong emphasis on a requirement for fatty acid synthesis for the SCC response. [TPIA has been reported to be a competitive inhibitor of acetyl-CoA in this reaction (Maragoudakis, 1969).] Since TPIA also prevented the aldosterone-enhanced incorporation of ^{3}H-labeled amino acid precursors into specific plasma membrane proteins, it may well be that aldosterone action depends on both membrane and membrane-protein turnover (Scott *et al.*, 1978). Last, increases in activity of renal ATP citrate lyase, transaldolase, and transketolase, all key enzymes in lipogenesis, were demonstrated at 3 hours after aldosterone (5 μg/100 gm body weight) injection of adrenalectomized rats. Fatty acid synthetase and 6-phosphogluconate dehydrogenase were unaffected by this treatment (see Fig. 3) (Kirsten *et al.*, 1978).

It has not been determined whether changes in phospholipid environment occur at the luminal or basolateral membrane or at both, and whether they modify H$^+$ as well as Na$^+$ transport. Investigators have suggested that part of the phospholipid alteration may include the environment around Na$^+$,K$^+$-ATPase since they have demonstrated a 10-fold increase in the sensitivity of this enzyme to ouabain in aldosterone-treated bladders (Goodman *et al.*, 1969). Furthermore, both deoxycorticosterone and dexamethasone increase the basolateral cell membrane surface area in particular cells within the renal cortical collecting duct, a target segment for mineralocorticoids (Wade *et al.,* 1979).

In considering possible membrane effects with aldosterone, two other papers should be included. The first, by Liu and Greengard (1974), reported that aldosterone increased a protein phosphatase activity in toad bladder. They demonstrated an increase in the endogenous dephosphorylation of a membrane-bound protein in steroid-treated bladders, an effect that could be reproduced by cAMP. Unfortunately, glucocorticoids were not tested. Since both aldosterone and dexamethasone inhibit phosphodiesterase activity in the toad bladder (see Section IV), the dephosphorylation of the membrane-bound protein in these studies may be related to a corticoid effect on the degradation of cAMP. This remains to be seen. Second, Yorio and Bentley (1978) related that various inhibitors of prostaglandin synthesis, such as indomethacin, produced a 70% inhibition in aldosterone-stimulated SCC in toad bladder and suggested by inference that prostaglandins may play an important role in stimulating steroid-sensitive Na^+ transport. This seems surprising, since prostaglandins have been shown to inhibit, rather than stimulate, both ADH effects in toad bladder and aldosterone-stimulated Na^+ transport in the cortical collecting tubule (Zusman *et al.,* 1977, 1978; Stokes and Kokko, 1977). Some problems arise in interpreting these data, since indomethacin decreased basal as well as aldosterone-stimulated SCC. After correcting for this decrease in basal current with indomethacin, the percentage rise in SCC above the appropriate control values was 122% in the case of aldosterone alone, and 129% in the case of aldosterone + indomethacin. Under these circumstances, indomethacin appears to have no deleterious effect on aldosterone-mediated events but rather on the basal SCC. Therefore, before a final statement can be made concerning a possible (positive) role for prostaglandins or enzymes involved in prostaglandin synthesis on aldosterone action, a more detailed analysis has to be made.

B. ENERGY THEORY

In the preceding section, I mentioned that it is difficult to design experiments that clearly show that aldosterone increases the energy potential of target cells independent of increased energy demands (i.e., independent of increased Na^+ flux). Perhaps the most important and convincing experiment attempting to accomplish this feat was by Spooner and Edelman (1975). They chose to use amiloride rather than amphotericin B to change Na^+ conductance across the luminal membrane, probably because amiloride is more selective for Na^+ conductance pathways than amphotericin. Then they simply asked the question: What is the relationship between the change in SCC (ΔSCC) and in conductance (ΔK) brought about by amiloride, compared to the relationship between the ΔSCC and ΔK in the presence of aldosterone. With varying amiloride concentrations, they found a linear correlation between ΔSCC and ΔK. The linear regression equation, measured over a wide range of SCC and conductances, was $\Delta SCC = 1.02 \, (\Delta K) - 3.17$. In another series of bladders, ΔSCC and ΔK were tabulated at 2, 3, 4, and 5 hours after aldosterone addition. With time, there was an increasing, nonlinear deviation from the regression analysis line determined with amiloride. Aldosterone, compared to amiloride, produced a greater change in ΔSCC for a given ΔK. In fact, at 5 hours, ΔSCC was almost twice that predicted by the amiloride experiments. These results strongly suggest that aldosterone has cellular effects beyond increasing luminal membrane Na^+ permeability, and it would seem appropriate to suggest that the energy pathway provides this additional boost in active transport.

In a similar vein, Weiner (1980) reported that even though ATP synthesis in toad bladders was uncoupled from respiration by dinitrophenol (DNP), aldosterone still increased CO_2 production compared to paired controls (DNP without aldosterone). If, in addition to steroid and DNP, amiloride was added to block Na^+ entry and thereby the permease pathway, there was still a significant increase in CO_2 production ($117 \pm 8\%$, $p < 0.05$) compared to nonsteroid-treated bladders. These results can be easily applied to a model in which aldosterone enhances flux through metabolic pathways, presumably by influencing enzyme intermediates. In these experiments, therefore, CO_2 production was increased despite lack of Na^+ flux and ATP synthesis, which would indicate a primary effect of aldosterone on the metabolic machinery of the cell. No information was given, however, concerning the pathways involved in the generation of this CO_2.

In addition, citrate synthase measurements support this hypothesis. In the toad bladder, the rise in citrate synthase activity has the same time course as the rise in SCC, is prevented by actinomycin D, cycloheximide, or spirolactone, and the incremental rise in activity is a linear function of the incremental rise in SCC, which suggests that these two events are intimately coupled. The removal of mucosal Na^+ does not diminish the enzyme response (Kirsten et al., 1968). Law and Edelman (1978b) determined that the apparent increase in citrate synthase activity in the adrenalectomized rat treated with aldosterone was not related to a change in affinity of either of the substrates, oxaloacetate (OAA) or acetyl-CoA, but rather to a change in the parameter N_{max} or the maximum number of sites. They reaffirmed their proposal of an increased number of enzyme molecules by using an antibody raised against rat citrate synthase. Citrate synthase measured by the antibody or by enzyme activity was similarly increased in rats treated with aldosterone (Law and Edelman, 1978b).

There is some controversy as to the rate-limiting enzyme in the tricarboxylic acid cycle; suggestions have been citrate synthase, isocitrate dehydrogenase, or a coordinate control at multiple sites (Krebs, 1970; Bhagavan, 1978; Srere, 1969). However, Figs. 5 and 6 illustrate the proposed effect of increases in citrate synthase activity, i.e., enhanced production of reducing equivalents in the form of mitochondrial NADH or $FADH_2$ and ultimately ATP synthesis. Kirsten and Kirsten (1972) have been able to demonstrate an elevation in the ratio of rat mitochondrial $NADH/NAD^+$ as well as cytoplasmic $NADPH/NADP^+$ after aldosterone, but not in the ratio of $ATP/ADP \cdot P_i$ (Kirsten et al., 1972). The $NADH/NAD^+$ ratio after adrenalectomy fell from 0.34 to 0.27; this was returned to a ratio of 0.34 at 4 hours after aldosterone administration. Likewise, $NADPH/NADP^+$ fell after adrenalectomy

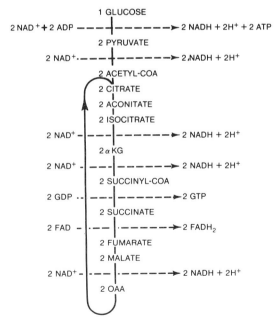

FIG. 5. The reducing equivalents provided by the Emden-Meyerhof and tricarboxylic acid cycle for ATP synthesis.

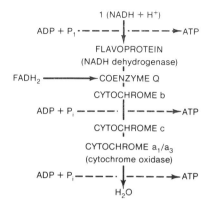

FIG. 6. The electron-transport chain.

from a ratio of 4.35 to 2.94 and returned to a ratio of 4.35 at 4 hours after the administration of aldosterone. The return with aldosterone to a more reduced state in both the cytoplasmic and mitochondrial compartments seems to be an appropriate trend, given the suggestion that aldosterone stimulates the tricarboxylic acid cycle and hexose monophosphate shunt pathway activity.

However, another group of investigators (Ogata *et al.*, 1977) have obtained the opposite response. Using a fluorometer that detects reduced pyridine nucleotides as it is laid against the surface of the kidney *in situ*, they found that within 2 minutes after the administration of aldosterone to normal or adrenalectomized rats, the fluorescence decreased, indicating a shift from reduced to oxidized nucleotides. The smallest detectable change was obtained with a dose of 0.2 μg/100 gm body weight of aldosterone; however, the maximal effect required 20–25 μg/100 gm body weight, a dose well beyond that required to produce a maximal change in urinary Na^+/K^+ in the rat. At these levels, steroid decreased fluorescence 20%. The response was maximal at 10 minutes and could be sustained if large enough doses of steroid were given. Actinomycin D, cycloheximide, and spirolactone prevented the oxidation reaction (Ogata *et al.*, 1977). Some questions arise about the magnitude of this response. Since approximately 90% of the kidney surface tubule population consists of proximal convoluted tubules and, of the remainder, about 5% is distal convoluted tubules and 5% is cortical collecting ducts, and since, of these, aldosterone appears to act solely on the cortical collecting tubule, the finding of a 20% decrease in overall surface NADH + NADPH fluorescence is surprisingly large (Kaissling and Kriz, 1979; Marver and Schwartz, 1980; Schwartz and Burg, 1978; Gross and Kokko, 1977). Furthermore, when rats were partially exsanguinated, aldosterone no longer produced a detectable shift from reduced to oxidized pyridine nucleotides. While these findings are provocative, at the present time it is difficult to place them into an overall model of hormone action. It should be noted, however, that the authors *did* use glucocorticoid controls, and these steroids had the opposite effect or an immediate shift toward a more reduced state. Therefore, aldosterone was not working through a glucocorticoid receptor in this setting.

Beyond changes in citrate synthase activity and an increase in intramitochondrial $NADH/NAD^+$ ratios, ATP synthesis may be additionally supported by an increase in cytochrome oxidase activity and by stimulation of enzymes in the flavin biosynthetic pathway (Feldman *et al.*, 1961; Trachewsky, 1978). Experiments in which aldosterone action on cytochrome oxidase activity was estimated bear repeating, however, since the earlier studies used pharmacologic doses of steroid (100 μg/100 gm body weight).

This section may be summed up as follows: Energy is needed to support active Na^+ and H^+ transport. Any interference with ATP synthesis would be expected to block transport of these ions. Aldosterone, working through a specific protein receptor, stimulates RNA and protein synthesis and alters metabolism through at least two biochemical pathways in target cells. One involves modification of the luminal membrane and specifically increases Na^+ permeability. The present aggregate data would suggest that this is the key step in the action of aldosterone. A second site of action is the mitochondrion, where an increase in enzyme synthesis results in an enhanced capacity to synthesize ATP. This augmentation of energy production adds to the overall capacity to transport Na^+. Whether some cellular response may be obtained without the mediation of receptors or RNA synthesis or if more than one cell type responds to aldosterone remains to be seen. As a final point, Taylor and Windhager (1979) have recently proposed that intracellular Ca^{2+} ion is a controlling element in transepithelial Na^+ transport. While no specific data are now available on cytosolic levels of Ca^{2+} with and without aldosterone treatment, it may well be that one day Ca^{2+} disposition will be added to a list of aldosterone-induced cellular changes.

VIII. Cellular Targets for Aldosterone

In this section are considered those particular segments within the renal nephron and those particular cells within the toad bladder that may represent the mineralocorticoid target sites for Na^+ and H^+ transport. A schematic representation of both superficial (short loops) and juxtamedullary nephrons (long loops of Henle) and their relationship to the cortical and medullary zones of the kidney is given in Fig. 7. Studies in the rat and rabbit kidney suggest that the cortex and outer medulla contain mineralocorticoid-responsive sites, but that the papilla does not. This indirect evidence consists of the presence or the absence of mineralocorticoid-specific cytoplasmic receptors, increases in [^{3}H]leucine incorporation into total protein, and increases in citrate synthase activity in the presence of aldosterone vs controls (Funder *et al.* 1973a; Marver, 1980; Law and Edelman, 1978a,b). Currently we know more about the location of mineralocorticoid-sensitive sites within the renal cortex than in the outer medulla. The renal cortex contains all of the glomeruli, proximal convoluted tubules (PCT), and distal convoluted tubules (DCT) in the kidney, as well as the cortical portions of the proximal straight tubule (PST), thick ascending limb of Henle (cTALH), and collecting tubule (CCT). Of these, the PCT, DCT, and CCT are assessible by *in vivo* micropuncture techniques. It was concluded from early micropuncture studies that the PCT and DCT are targets for aldosterone based on the reabsorptive capacity or trans-

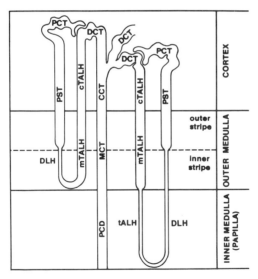

FIG. 7. A schematic representation of superficial and juxtamedullary nephrons. The various segments shown are: proximal convoluted tubule (PCT), proximal straight tubule (PST), descending limb of Henle (DLH), thin ascending limb of Henle (tALH), thick ascending limb of Henle—medullary and cortical (mTALH, cTALH), distal convoluted tubule (DCT), and collecting duct—cortical, medullary, and papillary (CCT, MCT, PCD).

epithelial PD generated in those segments with and without steroid treatment (Wiederholt, 1966; Wiederholt et al., 1972; Hierholzer and Stolte, 1969). Actually, more recent experiments have raised the possibility that neither of these segments represent direct targets for aldosterone. Part of the problem in evaluating micropuncture studies performed some years ago is that investigators were less aware of the pitfalls associated with the use of larger amounts of steroids (i.e., the problems with obtaining glucocorticoid responses) and also, punctures that were thought to be in the DCT, may have actually been in the CCT (remember that the accessible DCT and CCT sites represent only a minor fraction of the surface loops). Keeping these problems in mind, we will examine the more recent data on target sites in the cortex.

Using an enrichment technique for the separation of proximal and distal tubule elements from collagenase-treated preparations of whole rat renal cortex, Scholer and co-workers (Scholer and Edelman, 1979; Scholer et al., 1979) found that tubule populations enriched for distal segments contained about a 10-fold higher concentration of [^{3}H]aldosterone-bound receptor sites compared to fractions enriched in proximal tubule elements. With the rabbit, however, it is possible to dissect out individual tubule segments to gain an even closer look at aldosterone target sites in the cortex. When the potential difference (PD) was measured across isolated single rabbit DCT and CCT segments, it was found that only the CCT appeared to be responsive to the previous administration of deoxycorticosterone acetate in vivo. The PD in the isolated CCT in the absence of deoxycorticosterone acetate was +3.7± 1.9 mV compared to −30.8 ± 3.9 mV in the presence of steroid pretreatment (lumen negative). On the other hand, there was no statistically significant difference between the PDs across DCTs obtained from steroid-replete or steroid-depleted rabbits (−40 ± 2.8 mV without deoxycorticosterone acetate vs −33.8 ± 5.5 mV with deoxycorticosterone acetate treatment) (Gross et al., 1975). The authors concluded that, of these two segments, only ion transporting systems in the CCT responded to mineralocorticoids. [With long-term treatment (11–18 days) deoxycorticosterone acetate can further stimulate transport in this segment (PD > −50 mV) (O'Neil and Helman, 1977; Helman and O'Neil, 1977).] Since then, the effect of steroid on the CCT has been examined in a number of papers. Schwartz and Burg (1978) reported that there was a linear relationship between the in vivo mineralocorticoid status of rabbits and the in vitro PD, net Na$^+$ flux, and net K$^+$ flux across isolated CCTs. Hanley and Kokko (1978) have also demonstrated stimulation of net Cl$^-$ flux in CCTs from deoxycorticosterone acetate-treated rabbits.

Our own work with citrate synthase supports a role for aldosterone in the CCT as opposed to other segments within the cortex (Marver and Schwartz, 1980). Since aldosterone specifically increases the activity and net synthesis of citrate synthase in direct correlation with changes in Na^+ transport, we used this enzyme as a cellular marker of target sites. The studies were carried out on microdissected rabbit nephron segments using an enzymic cycling method perfected by Lowry and co-workers (Lowry and Passonneau, 1972; Lowry *et al.*, 1978). As seen in Fig. 8, citrate synthase activity was unaffected by mineralocorticoid status in PCT, PST, cTALH, and DCT, suggesting that aldosterone does not alter transport in these segments. However, in the CCT, there was a 55% reduction in citrate synthase activity in adrenalectomized rabbits compared to normals. When aldosterone (1 μg/100 gm body weight) was given to adrenalectomized rabbits, citrate synthase activity returned to normal levels at 90 minutes; the same dose of dexamethasone was ineffective. Last, spirolactone (SC 26304) antagonized the rise in activity seen with aldosterone alone. All these findings suggest that the CCT is the primary target for mineralocorticoid-stimulated Na^+ reabsorption within the renal cortex. Since, in previous studies in the toad bladder, a direct correlation between changes in citrate synthase activity and net Na^+ transport was demonstrated, until further data are available, we cannot predict that citrate synthase activity will localize cells in which aldosterone stimulates H^+ secretion.

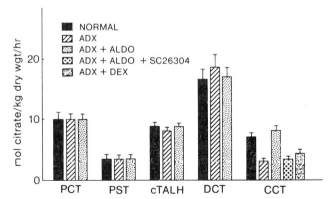

FIG. 8. Citrate synthase activities in various portions of the rabbit cortical nephron at 28° C. The segments assayed were proximal convoluted tubule (PCT), proximal straight tubule (PST), thick ascending limb of Henle (cTALH), distal convoluted tubule (DCT), and cortical collecting tubule (CCT). Both aldosterone (ALDO) and dexamethasone (DEX) were given (1 μg/100 gm body weight) 90 minutes before sacrifice. Spirolactone SC 26304 (150 μg/100 gm body weight) was injected 30 minutes before aldosterone. Results are ± SEM. ADX, adrenalectomized.

This same portion of the collecting duct responds to ADH, as evidenced by analyses of adenylate cyclase activity, osmotic water flux, freeze-fracture, and electron micrograph studies (Imbert-Teboul *et al.*, 1978; Grantham and Burg, 1966; Schwartz and Kokko, 1979; Harmanci *et al.*, 1978; Woodhall and Tisher, 1973). Both aldosterone and dexamethasone have been shown to have a permissive effect on the osmotic water flux response to ADH in this segment (Schwartz and Kokko, 1979). It is of extreme interest, therefore, that the CCT, a prime target for the actions of aldosterone on Na^+, K^+, and Cl^- transport as well as for ADH responses, has a poor capacity to reabsorb HCO_3^- (Lombard *et al.*, 1979; McKinney and Burg, 1977). This would suggest that this segment is not likely to be involved in aldosterone-mediated changes in acid-base balance. Since the medullary collecting duct has both a high capacity to reabsorb HCO_3^- and an abundant supply of carbonic anhydrase, it may well be that steroids will be found to enhance H^+ transport somewhere within the medullary collecting duct system (Lombard *et al.*, 1979; Lonnerholm, 1971; Rosen, 1972). As techniques become more sophisticated, investigators have begun to ask if a particular cell type within the cortical collecting tubule is responsive to ADH and mineralocorticoid-stimulated Na^+ reabsorption. There are two basic cells in this segment: the principal or "light" cell and the intercalated or "dark" cell. The intercalated cell contains many mitochondria and has an electron-dense ground substance, indicating an abundance of ribosomes and filamentous material (Tisher, 1981; Kaissling and Kriz, 1979). Definitive experiments are not available, yet it has been suggested that the "dark" cell is the mineralocorticoid target for Na^+ transport within the renal cortex, but there is no evidence to suggest a differential effect of ADH on either "light" or "dark" cells (Stokes *et al.*, 1978; Burg and Orloff, 1973).

In the toad bladder, there are four main cell types, the granular, mitochondrial-rich, goblet, and basal. Of these, only the first three touch the luminal surface, the granular cells comprising some 85% of this population, followed by 10% mitochondria-rich and 5% goblet cells (Saladino *et al.*, 1969; DiBona *et al.*, 1969). More recently, the basal cell population has been subdivided into a microfilament-rich cell and an undifferentiated population (Rossier *et al.*, 1979; Kraehenbuhl *et al.*, 1979).

What is the evidence concerning the action of aldosterone on these various cell types? First, carbonic anhydrase activity was found associated with the mitochondria-rich cell, which implicates this cell as the possible target for H^+ secretion (Sapirstein and Scott, 1975; Schwartz and Rosen, 1979). This same cell appeared to be most sensitive to amphotericin B. Within minutes after the administration of amphotericin B, the SCC rose and cellular changes were noted in mitochondria-rich cells (Saladino *et al.*, 1969). However, in the presence of ADH and an osmotic gradient, only granular cells became distended (DiBona *et al.*, 1969). Also, Civan and Frazier (1968) found that nearly all the epithelial cells successfully probed by microelectrodes reacted to ADH with an increase in luminal membrane permeability. Based on the fact that the majority of luminal toad bladder cells are granular, this suggests that the granular cell is tantamount to the ADH-responsive cell. Since aldosterone has a favorable effect on ADH responses when it is incubated with bladders for a period of time, Lipton and Edelman (1971) concluded that aldosterone stimulated the granular cell. Another indirect piece of evidence was suggested by citrate synthase activation in the toad bladder. In paired hemibladders, incremental changes in citrate synthase activity with aldosterone compared to controls have been as high as 50% (Kirsten *et al.*, 1968). Unless the granular cell has a very low citrate synthase level, the finding of a 50% increase in the activity of this enzyme might be difficult to reconcile with an effect solely on a population of cells comprising 10% or less of the luminal cells. Yet most of this evidence is highly circumstantial and should be compared with the work of Scott and Sapirstein, who have provided dramatic evidence that the mitochondria-rich cell is both the mineralocorticoid and ADH target cell in the toad bladder. They have used an EDTA-dissociated, Ficoll gradient-enriched preparation of granular and mitochondria-rich cells. In their hands, oxytocin increased cAMP accumulation 3.4-fold per milligram of protein in mitochondria-rich cells and only 1.1-fold in the granular-cell fraction. Carbonic anhydrase activity was three times higher in the mitochondria-rich fraction than in the granular fraction. (Scott *et al.*, 1974).

The results with oxytocin in the mitochondria-rich cell conflict with those of DiBona *et al.* (1969), who found morphological changes in the granular cell with ADH. As Scott and Sapirstein (1975) have pointed out, however, there may be some kind of cellular communication between mitochondria-rich and granular cells that determine the final hormonal response, and such a mechanism would explain both findings. Sapirstein and Scott (1975) also quantitated mineralocorticoid receptors in these two cell populations and again found that the mitochondria-rich as opposed to the granular cell contained the great majority of the receptor pool. When ^{3}H-labeled amino acid precursors were added to the cell fractions, aldosterone enhanced the labeled amino acid content of several proteins in the supernatent of the mitochondria-rich cell fraction, but not in the granular cell. On the other hand, corticosterone enhanced amino acid incorporation into proteins within the soluble fraction of the granular cell (Scott and Sapir-stein, 1975). Membrane fractions were not examined. When poly(A) (+) mRNA was isolated over oligo(dT) columns and used as a template in a rabbit reticulocyte protein-synthetic assay, the synthesis of several proteins was increased in aldosterone-treated preparations of mitochondria-rich cells, but not of granular cells. Poly(A) (−) mRNA was not characterized. Certainly all this information would suggest that aldosterone enhances some biochemical pathway in the mitochondria-rich cell, but it remains to be determined if all transport effects of aldosterone are mediated through this one cell type.

IX. Aldosterone Antagonists

Spirolactone blocks aldosterone-stimulated Na^+ and K^+ transport, and may either block or stimulate H^+ secretion (Marver et al., 1974; Ludens et al., 1978, Mueller and Steinmetz, 1978). Spirolactones and progesterone compete with aldosterone for cytoplasmic receptors in both kidney and toad bladders and the concentrations necessary to occupy receptors effectively reflects their antagonist–agonist prop-erties (Marver et al., 1974; Funder et al., 1974; Warnock and Edelman, 1978; Ausiello and Sharp, 1968; Wambach and Higgins, 1978; Sakauye and Feldman, 1976; Claire et al., 1979). It has been recognized for some time that spirolactones may have some agonist activity (i.e., they may stimulate Na^+ reabsorption to some degree), and the degree of agonism-antagonism may vary from species to species (Sakauye and Feldman, 1976). Several years ago, we attempted to determine the mechanism of spirolactone inhibition of Na^+ transport. Figure 9 shows that when increasing doses of spirolactone SC 26304 were injected along with a tracer dose of [³H]aldosterone into adrenalectomized rats, spirolactone progressively reduced [³H]aldosterone binding to both renal cytoplasmic and nuclear proteins. As spirolactone displaced al-dosterone, the urinary K^+/Na^+ ratios dropped. The question was then asked: If spirolactone was displacing aldosterone by binding to the receptor itself, why did it block the physiological response? To answer this question, rat renal slices were incubated for various periods of time at 25°C with either [³H]aldosterone or [³H]SC 26304 (Fig. 10). Both steroids bound to the cytoplasmic receptors but, unlike [³H]aldo-sterone, [³H]SC 26304 receptor complexes could not be recovered from nuclei extracted with either Tris or 0.3–0.4 M KCl. It appeared as though the affinity of [³H]SC 26304-labeled cytoplasmic complexes for chromatin was far less than that for [³H]aldosterone-labeled complexes

(Marver *et al.*, 1974). The lack of nuclear binding was not related to an inability to cross the nuclear membrane, since in cell-free incubations of ^{3}H-labeled receptors and isolated renal chromatin, [^{3}H]aldosterone-labeled receptors rapidly bound to chromatin whereas [^{3}H]SC 26304-labeled receptors did not. Therefore, spirolactone seemed to prevent the physiological response to aldosterone by displacing aldosterone

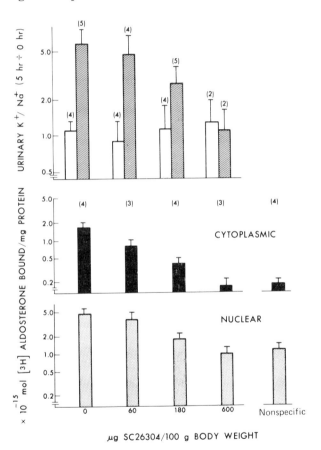

μg SC26304/100 g BODY WEIGHT

Fig. 9. Effects of spirolactone (SC 26304) on the physiological response to aldosterone and on the renal cytoplasmic and nuclear binding of [^{3}H]aldosterone in adrenalectomized rats. The upper panel shows the urinary K$^+$/Na$^+$ ratios after the injection of aldosterone (0.3 μg/100 gm body weight) and 0–600 μg of SC 26304. The two lower panels give the amount of [^{3}H]aldosterone bound to renal cytoplasmic and nuclear proteins from kidneys obtained 20 minutes after the injection of [^{3}H]aldosterone ± various concentrations of SC 26304. Nonspecific binding was estimated in rats given [^{3}H]aldosterone plus a 1000-fold excess of unlabeled aldosterone. The number of animals is given in parentheses, and results are ± SEM. □, Control; ▨, + aldosterone. From Marver *et al.*, 1974.

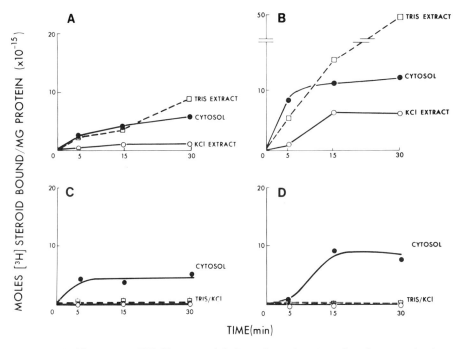

FIG. 10. The *in vitro* [³H]aldosterone labeling of cytoplasmic and nuclear proteins in rat renal slices. Adrenalectomized rat kidney slices were incubated for various periods of time at 25°C with either (A) 1.3×10^{-9} M [³H]aldosterone, (B) 1.3×10^{-8} M [³H]aldosterone, (C) 5.2×10^{-9} M [³H]spirolactone (SC 26304), or (D) 5.2×10^{-8} M [³H]spirolactone. The values given represent the moles of [³H]steroid bound/per milligram of protein in both cytoplasmic and nuclear (KCl and Tris-soluble) fractions isolated from the renal slices. Samples have been corrected for nonspecific binding, estimated in parallel incubations containing 1000-fold excess aldosterone. From Marver *et al.*, 1974.

from cytoplasmic receptor sites and preventing the next step in the pathway, attachment to chromatin. A similar distinction was found by Claire *et al.* (1979), who examined [³H]aldosterone vs [³H]prorenone (SC 23233) binding to rat renal cytoplasmic and nuclear sites.

Density gradient sedimentation analyses indicated that there may be some conformational differences between receptor–steroid complexes containing either agonists or antagonists. In Table II, the sedimentation values of a number of ³H-labeled steroid agonists bound to their respective receptors have been tabulated. In low salt, gradients contained an 8 S complex as well as a 4–5 S complex. This is in contrast to high-salt gradients (0.3 to 0.4 M KCl), which contain only a 4–5 S complex. In the case of the two antagonists, SC 26304 and cortexolone, the 8 S complex was absent in low salt with some shift in s value under high-salt conditions (4.5 S to 4 S for spirolactone and 4 S to 3.5 S for cortexolone). Since the 8 S complex probably represents an aggregate of receptor, the results suggest that the surface charge or hydrophobic properties differ between the agonist and antagonist complexes. Spirolactone may block the physiological response because it is incapable of inducing or maintaining a stable receptor conformation necessary either to (a) expose the nuclear attachment site on the receptor; or (b) allow another molecule/subunit to interact with or dissociate from the receptor; which in turn is necessary for nuclear interaction. In a recent paper it has in fact been suggested that small molecular weight substances that bind to receptors may act as inhibitors and regulate activation *in vivo* (Sato *et al.*, 1980). It is conceivable that spirolactone could stabilize a conformation that would enhance the affinity of such inhibitors for the receptor and disallow activation. Figure 11 schematically presents this model. Depending on the affinity for one of two conformations of the receptor, steroids can be classed as inactive, agonists, antagonists, or mixed agonists–antagonists (suboptimal inducers). In the kidney, cytoplasmic receptors are in vast excess to those bound to chromatin. Therefore, the number of chromatin-bound steroid complexes is a function of the number of activated receptors found in the cytoplasm. With naturally occurring steroids, there appears to be only one mineralocorticoid antagonist, and that is progesterone (Wambach and Higgins, 1978). The only naturally occurring steroid that has been demonstrated to be a suboptimal inducer of the

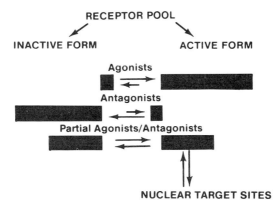

FIG. 11. A schematic representation of the inhibitory role of steroid antagonists on the physiological action of aldosterone. In this model, antagonists and partial antagonists compete with aldosterone for cytoplasmic receptor binding sites. Based on their inability to stabilize a particular conformation of the receptor, which is necessary for subsequent attachment to chromatin, they inhibit the promulgation of the response.

mineralocorticoid pathway is 11-deoxycortisol. The remainder of the
hormonal steroids either are inactive (testosterone, estradiol) or have
diverse agonist activities. Among the spirolactones, however, agonist
and antagonist properties vary greatly (Sakauye and Feldman, 1976).

Until recently, this version of the mechanism of action of spirolactone seemed to suffice. However, the studies outlined in Fig. 12 require
a reconsideration of this simple proposal. Generally, spirolactone is
added just before or along with aldosterone in toad bladder experiments. Under these conditions, spirolactone can prevent the entire rise
in SCC obtained with aldosterone alone. If spirolactone were to be
added after the peak response to aldosterone had developed, the decrease in SCC should reflect a combination of the half-lives of the in-

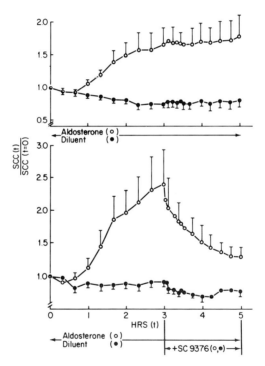

FIG. 12. The short-circuit current (SCC) response to the addition of spirolactone (SC
9376) after preincubation with aldosterone or diluent. In the upper and lower panels,
aldosterone ($5 \times 10^{-8}\,M$) (○) or diluent (●) was added to both sides of *Bufo marinus* toad
bladders mounted as Bentley bags. In the lower panel, spirolactone SC 9376 ($2 \times 10^{-5}\,M$)
was added 3 hours later. For purposes of comparison, nothing was added to experiments
shown in the upper panel. The number of bladders per group was 10, and the values
represent the ratio of the SCC at any time (t) divided by the SCC at time $0 \pm$ SEM.

duced mRNA and the induced proteins. The $t_{\frac{1}{2}}$ for citrate synthase in rat liver is 3.9 days (Mukherjee *et al.*, 1976). One might suspect that the actual $t_{\frac{1}{2}}$ of the decay of the SCC would be a time shorter than this and would be the result of a more rapidly turning over induced protein. What in fact happens is an immediate and very rapid ($t_{\frac{1}{2}} \sim 40$ minutes) decay of the SCC after the addition of spirolactone (SC 9376) to a value of about 50-60% of the total aldosterone-stimulated level (Fig. 12, lower panel). Thereafter the SCC decays with a much slower rate of fall.

These results support the observations of Rossier and Claire (1978), who demonstrated both a rapid and a slow decay of the SCC after the addition of SC 9420 to aldosterone-stimulated bladders. The rapid component can be compared to the 15-minute $t_{\frac{1}{2}}$ of the decay of the SCC after the addition of ouabin to aldosterone-stimulated bladders (Handler *et al.*, 1969b). In the case of ouabain, the decay curve is monophasic and the SCC continues to fall until it meets the control values in about 70 min. We can also compare the $t_{\frac{1}{2}}$ of spirolactone to that of puromycin and actinomycin D. When puromycin was added to bladders 150 minutes after aldosterone, there was an immediate fall in SCC with a $t_{\frac{1}{2}}$ of 90 min. With actinomycin D, SCC fell only after 15 minutes and then decayed with a 150-minute half-life (DeWeer and Crabbé, 1968). The fact that SC 9376 decreased the SCC at a rate faster than actinomycin D or puromycin indicates that it may inhibit a pathway beyond or independent of these steps. Although Rossier and Claire (1978) did not estimate the $t_{\frac{1}{2}}$ of the rapid decrease in SCC, they stated that it took some 13 hours for the SCC in the spirolactone-treated bladders to fall finally to control values. Furthermore, in their experiments, the addition of an excess of aldosterone in addition to spirolactone reversed the rapidly declining SCC into a rapidly rising SCC, after a 30-minute delay. These findings imply that the net SCC obtained after 3 or more hours of aldosterone incubation is the composite of two processes. Spirolactone can inhibit both; however, one process can be inhibited immediately, which suggests a direct effect on a membrane component or an effect on a very rapidly turning over component of the transport system. These results with SC 9376 and SC 9420 are in contrast to the earlier studies of Porter (1968), using SC 14266. Porter found that if SC 14266 was added after aldosterone, there was a delay of 2-3 hours before spirolactone produced a reversal of the SCC. As SC 14266 is a weak antagonist in the toad bladder (Sakauye and Feldman, 1976), this might explain the varied responses.

Certainly results such as those obtained with SC 9420 and SC 9376 will require a reexamination of the model of aldosterone/spirolactone action.

X. Comments

I hope that this review has raised as many interesting questions about aldosterone action as it has answered. I feel confident in saying that aldosterone increases Na^+ transport because it results in both increased ATP synthesis and increased luminal Na^+ permeability. Its role in H^+ and even K^+ secretion is less clear. I would like to stress several points that are unresolved and important to a better understanding of the mechanism of action of aldosterone. First, do all responses to aldosterone require the receptor as an intervening factor? Second, which responses require the induction of RNA and protein synthesis, and which do not? Furthermore, what is the role of the receptor at the chromatin level? Is the proposed model of agonist vs antagonist affinity for active:inactive receptor conformations correct? What are the key enzymes regulated by aldosterone in the cytoplasmic, nuclear, and mitochondrial compartments? Does aldosterone modify Na^+,K^+-ATPase activity in any way other than by increasing intracellular Na^+ and ATP availability? What are the renal medullary target sites for aldosterone? Does aldosterone stimulate H^+ secretion and Na^+ reabsorption in the same cell? If it does, is there a common biochemical pathway involved? Why does H^+ transport depend on hexose monophosphate shunt activity, and how does K^+ interact with H^+ ions at the luminal membrane? Does aldosterone have a steroid-specific effect on NH_3 production? There are many more questions.

Finally, I would like to close with a quotation from G. B. Shaw's *Advice to a Young Critic,* which I found in one of the delightful passages in E. Racker's book (1976), "A New Look at Mechanisms in Bioenergetics":

> You say you are scarcely competent to write books just yet. That is just why I recommend you to learn. If I advised you to learn to skate, you would reply that your balance was scarcely good enough yet. A man learns to skate by staggering about making a fool of himself. Indeed he progresses in all things by resolutely making a fool of himself.

So, we continue, I hope a little less foolish and a little more learned about aldosterone action than before.

Acknowledgments

This chapter is respectfully dedicated to each and every member of the San Francisco team who so diligently worked over the years on various aspects of hormone action. The work cited from the author's laboratory was supported by Grant AM 21576 from the National Institutes of Health. D. M. is an Established Investigator of the American Heart Association.

REFERENCES

Al-Awqati, Q. (1977). *J. Clin. Invest.* **60**, 1240-1247.

Al-Awqati, Q. (1978). *Am. J. Physiol.* **235**, F77-F88.

Al-Awqati, Q., Norby, L., Mueller, A., and Steinmetz, P. R. (1976). *J. Clin. Invest.* **58**, 351-358.

Alberti, K. G. M. M., and Sharp, G. W. G. (1969). *Biochim. Biophys. Acta* **192**, 335-346.

Ausiello, D. A., and Sharp, G. W. G. (1968). *Endocrinology* **82**, 1163-1169.

Bastl, C. P., Binder, H. J., and Hayslett, J. P. (1980). *Am. J. Physiol.* **238**, F181-F186.

Baulieu, E. E., Jung, I., Blondeau, J. P., and Robel, R. (1971). *Adv. Biosci.* **7**, 179-191.

Baxter, J. D., and Tomkins, G. M. (1971). *Adv. Biosci.* **7**, 331-347.

Baxter, J. D., Schambelan, M., Matulich, D. T., Spindler, B. J., Taylor, A. A., and Bartter, F. C. (1976). *J. Clin. Invest.* **58**, 579-589.

Beauwens, R., and Al-Awqati, Q. (1976). *J. Gen. Physiol.* **68**, 421-439.

Bhagavan, N. V. (1978). *In* "Biochemistry," pp. 230-231. Lippincott, Philadelphia, Pennsylvania.

Bojesen, E. (1966). *Eur. J. Steroids* **1**, 145-150.

Bonting, S. L., and Canady, M. R. (1964). *Am.' J. Physiol.* **207**, 1005-1009.

Bravo, E. L. (1977). *Adv. Nephrol.* **7**, 105-120.

Buller, R. E., and O'Malley, B. W. (1976). *Biochem. Pharmacol.* **25**, 1-12.

Burg, M. B., and Orloff, J. (1973). *In* "Handbook of Physiology" (J. Orloff and R. W. Berliner, eds.), Sect. 8, pp. 156-157. Am. Physiol. Soc., Washington, D.C.

Butkus, A., Coghlan, J. P., Paterson, R., Scoggins, B. A., Robinson, J. A., and Funder, J. W. (1976). *Clin. Exp. Pharmacol.* **3**, 557-565.

Charney, A. N., Silva, P., Besarab, A., and Epstein, F. H. (1974). *Am. J. Physiol.* **227**, 345-350.

Cheema-Dhadli, S., and Halperin, M. L. (1979). *Eur. J. Biochem.* **99**, 483-489.

Chignell, C. F., and Titus, E. (1966). *J. Biol. Chem.* **241**, 5083-5089.

Chu, L. L. H., and Edelman, I. S. (1972). *J. Membr. Biol.* **10**, 291-310.

Civan, M. M., and Frazier, H. S. (1968). *J. Gen. Physiol.* **51**, 589-605.

Civan, M. M., and Hoffman, R. E. (1971). *Am. J. Physiol.* **220**, 324-332.

Claire, M., Rafestin-Olin, M. E., Michaud, A., Roth-Meyer, C., and Corvol, P. (1979). *Endocrinology* **104**, 1194-1200.

Coghlan, J. P., and Scoggins, B. A. (1967) *J. Clin. Endocrinol. Metab.* **27**, 1470-1486.

Crabbé, J. (1961a). *J. Clin. Invest.* **40**, 2103-2110.

Crabbé, J. (1961b). *Endocrinolgy* **69**, 673-682.

Crabbé, J. (1963a). "The Sodium-Retaining Action of Aldosterone." Editions Arscia, Brussels.

Crabbé, J. (1963b). *Nature (London)* **200**, 787-788.

Crabbé, J. (1964). *West-Eur. Symp. Clin. Chem.* Vol. 3, pp. 59-79.

Crabbé, J. (1977). *In* "Receptors and Mechanism of Action of Steroid Hormones" (J. R. Pasqualini, ed.), pp. 513-568. Dekker, New York.

Crabbé, J. (1980). *Pfluegers Arch.* **383**, 151-158.

Crabbé, J., and DeWeer, P. (1964). *Nature (London)* **202**, 298-299.

Crabbé, J., and DeWeer, P. (1965). *J. Physiol. (London)* **180**, 560-568.

Crabbé, J., and Ehrlich, E. N. (1968). *Pfluegers Arch.* **304**, 284-296.

Cuthbert, A. W., and Shum, W. K. (1975). *Proc. R. Soc. London* **189**, 543-575.

Cuthbert, A. W., and Shum, W. K. (1976). *J. Physiol. (London)* **260**, 213-235.

DeWeer, P., and Crabbé, J. (1968). *Biochim. Biophys. Acta* **155**, 280-289.

DiBona, D. R., Civan, M. M., and Leaf, A. (1969). *J. Membr. Biol.* **1**, 79-91.

Dixon, T. E., and Al-Awqati, Q. (1979). *Proc. Natl. Acad. Sci. U.S.A.* **76**, 3135-3138.

112   DIANA MARVER

Duval, D., and Funder, J. W. (1974). *Endocrinology* **94**, 575-579.
Edelman, I. S. (1979). *J. Endocrinol.* **81**, 49P-53P.
Edelman, I. S., and Fanestil, D. D. (1970). In "Biochemical Action of Hormones" (G. Litwack, ed.), Vol. 1, pp. 321-364. Academic Press, New York.
Edelman, I. S., Bogoroch, R., and Porter, G. A. (1963). *Proc. Natl. Acad. Sci. U.S.A.* **50**, 1169-1177.
Edmonds, C. J. (1972). *J. Steroid Biochem.* **3**, 143-149.
Erecińska, M., Stubbs, M., Miyata, Y., Ditre, C. M., and Wilson, D. F. (1977). *Biochim. Biophys. Acta* **462**, 20-35.
Fanestil, D. D., and Edelman, I. S. (1966). *Proc. Natl. Acad. Sci. U.S.A.* **56**, 872-879.
Fanestil, D. D., Porter, G. A., and Edelman, I. S. (1967). *Biochim. Biophys. Acta* **135**, 74-88.
Farman, N., Kusch, M., and Edelman, I. S. (1978). *Am. J. Physiol.* **235**, C90-C96.
Fazekas, A. G., and Sandor, T. (1971). *Can. J. Biochem.* **49**, 987-989.
Fazekas, A. G., and Sandor, T. (1973). *Can. J. Biochem.* **51**, 772-782.
Feldman, D. (1977). *Am. J. Physiol.* **233**, E147-E151.
Feldman, D., Vander Wende, C., and Kessler, E. (1961). *Biochim. Biophys. Acta* **51**, 401-403.
Feldman, D., Funder, J. W., and Edelman, I. S. (1972). *Am. J. Med.* **53**, 545-560.
Feldman, D., Funder, J. W., and Loose, D. (1978). *J. Steroid Biochem.* **9**, 141-145.
Fimognari, G. M., Porter, G. A., and Edelman, I. S. (1967). *Biochim. Biophys. Acta* **135**, 89-99.
Forte, L., and Landon, E. J. (1968). *Biochim. Biophys. Acta* **157**, 303-309.
Frazier, L. W., and Zachariah, N. Y. (1979). *J. Membr. Biol.* **49**, 297-308.
Frizzell, R. A., and Schultz, S. G. (1978). *J. Membr. Biol.* **39**, 1-26.
Fuller, P. J., and Funder, J. W. (1976). *Kidney Int.* **10**, 154-157.
Funder, J. W., Feldman, D., and Edelman, I. S. (1972). *J. Steroid Biochem.* **3**, 209-218.
Funder, J. W., Feldman, D., and Edelman, I. S. (1973a). *Endocrinology* **92**, 994-1004.
Funder, J. W., Feldman, D., and Edelman, I. S. (1973b). *Endocrinology* **92**, 1005-1013.
Funder, J. W., Feldman, D., Highland, E., and Edelman, I. S. (1974). *Biochem. Pharmacol.* **23**, 1493-1501.
Garrahan, P. J., and Glynn, I. M. (1966). *Nature (London)* **211**, 1414-1415.
Garrahan, P. J., and Glynn, I. M. (1967). *J. Physiol. (London)* **192**, 237-256.
Gehring, U., and Tomkins, G. M. (1974). *Cell* **3**, 301-306.
Good, D. W., and Wright, F. S. (1979). *Am. J. Physiol.* **236**, F192-F205.
Goodman, D. B. P., Allen, J. E., and Rasmussen, H. (1969). *Proc. Natl. Acad. Sci. U.S.A.* **64**, 330-337.
Goodman, D. B. P., Allen, J. E., and Rasmussen, H. (1971). *Biochemistry* **10**, 3825-3831.
Goodman, D. B. P., Wong, M., and Rasmussen, H. (1975). *Biochemistry* **14**, 2803-2809.
Goodman, D. B. P., Davis, W. L., and Jones, R. G. (1980). *Proc. Natl. Acad. Sci. U.S.A.* **77**, 1521-1525.
Gottfried, H., Gottfried, P. E., and Mamikunian, G. (1975) In "Steroid Hormones" (R. I. Dorfman, ed.), pp. 241-272. Am. Elsevier. New York.
Grantham, J. J., and Burg, M. B. (1966). *Am. J. Physiol.* **211**, 255-259.
Grantham, J. J., and Orloff, J. (1968). *J. Clin. Invest.* **47**, 1154-1161.
Gross, J. B., and Kokko, J. P. (1977). *J. Clin. Invest.* **59**, 82-89.
Gross, J. B., Imai, M., and Kokko, J. P. (1975). *J. Clin. Invest.* **55**, 1284-1294.
Handler, J. S., Preston, A. S., and Orloff, J. (1969a). *J. Clin. Invest.* **48**, 823-833.
Handler, J. S., Preston, A. S., and Orloff, J. (1969b) *J. Biol. Chem.* **244**, 3194-3199.
Handler, J. S., Preston, A. S., and Orloff, J. (1972) *Am. J. Physiol.* **222**, 1071-1074.
Handler, J. S., Stoff, J. S., and Orloff, J. (1973). *Exp. Eye Res.* **16**, 235-240.

Hanley, M. J., and Kokko, J. P. (1978). *J. Clin. Invest.* **62**, 39-44.

Harmanci, M. C., Kachadorian, W. A., Valtin, H., and DiScala, V. A. (1978). *Am. J. Physiol.* **235**, F440-F443.

Harrop, G. A., Nicholson, W. M., and Strauss, M. (1936). *J. Exp. Med.* **64**, 233-251.

Hayslett, J. P., Kastegar, A., and Kashgarian, M. (1979). *Clin. Res.* **27**, 497A (abstr.).

Hegyvary, C. (1977). *Experientia* **33**, 1280-1281.

Helman, S. I., and O'Neil, R. G. (1977). *Am. J. Physiol.* **233**, F559-F571.

Hendler, E. D., Torretti, J., Kupor, L., and Epstein, F. H. (1972). *Am. J. Physiol.* **222**, 754-760.

Herman, T. S., Fimognari, G. M., and Edelman, I. S. (1968). *J. Biol. Chem.* **243**, 3849-3856.

Hierholzer, K., and Stolte, H. (1969). *Nephron* **6**, 188-204.

Hill, J. H., Cortas, N., and Walser, M. (1973). *J. Clin. Invest.* **52**, 185-189.

Holloszy, J. O., Oscai, L. B., Don, I. J., and Mole, P. A. (1970). *Biochem. Biophys. Res. Commun.* **40**, 1368-1373.

Hulter, H. N., Glynn, R. D., and Sebastian, A. (1979). *Kidney Int.* **16**, 821 (abstr.).

Hutchinson, J. H., and Porter, G. A. (1972). *Biochim. Biophys. Acta* **281**, 55-68.

Ikeda, F., Ikeda, Y., Inagaki, C., and Takaori, S. (1979). *Jpn. J. Pharmacol.* **29**, 138-140.

Imbert-Teboul, M., Charbardes, D., Montegut, M., Clique, A., and Morel, F. (1978). *Endocrinology* **102**, 1254-1261.

Jard, S., Roy, C., Ragerison, R., Butlen, D., and Guillon, G. (1977). *In* "Structural and Kinetic Approaches to Plasma Membrane Functions" (C. Nicolau and A. Paraf, eds.), pp. 173-187. Springer-Verlag, Berlin and New York.

Jensen, E. V., Mohla, S., Gorell, T., Tanaka, S., and DeSombre, E. R. (1972). *J. Steroid Biochem.* **3**, 445-458.

Jensen, E. V., Brecher, P. I., Mohla, S., and DeSombre, E. R. (1974). *Acta Endocrinol.* (Copenhagen), *Suppl.* **191**, 159-172.

Jorgensen, P. L. (1972). *J. Steroid Biochem.* **3**, 181-191.

Kadenbach, B. (1966). *In* "Regulation of Metabolic Processes in Mitochondria" (J. M. Tager, S. Pappa, E. Quagliariello, and E. C. Slater, eds.), pp. 508-517. Elsevier, Amsterdam.

Kaiser, N., Milholland, R. J., Turnell, R. W., and Rosen, F. (1972). *Biochem. Biophys. Res. Commun.* **49**, 516-521.

Kaissling, B., and Kriz, W. (1979). *Adv. Anat., Embryol. Cell Biol.* **56**, 1 123.

Kinne, R., and Kirsten, E. (1968). *Pfluegers Arch. Gesamte Physiol. Menschen Tiere* **300**, 244-254.

Kirchberger, M. A., Martin, D. G., Leaf, A., and Sharp, G. W. G. (1968). *Biochim. Biophys. Acta* **165**, 22-31.

Kirsten, E., Kirsten, R., Leaf, A., and Sharp, G. W. G. (1968). *Pfluegers Arch. Gesamte Physiol. Menschen Tiere* **300**, 213-225.

Kirsten, E., Kirsten, R., and Sharp, G. W. G. (1970). *Pfluegers Arch.* **316**, 26-33.

Kirsten, E., Kirsten, R., and Salibian, A. (1972). *J. Steroid Biochem.* **3**, 173-179.

Kirsten, R., and Kirsten, E. (1972). *Am. J. Physiol.* **223**, 229-235.

Kirsten, R., Brinkhoff, B., and Kirsten, E. (1970). *Pfluegers Arch.* **314**, 231-239.

Kirsten, R., Nelson, K., Rabah, E., Ruschendorf, U., Scholz, T., Stuve, J., and Ulbricht, R. (1978). *In* "Biochemical Nephrology" (W. G. Guder and U. Schmidt, eds.), pp. 389-396. Huber, Bern.

Knochel, J. P., and White, M. G. (1973). *Arch. Intern. Med.* **131**, 876-884.

Knox, F. G., Burnett, J. C., Kohan, D. E., Spielman, W. S., and Strand, J. C. (1980). *Kidney Int.* **17**, 263-276.

Knox, W. H., and Sen, A. K. (1974). *Ann. N. Y. Acad. Sci.* **242,** 471-488.
Kraehenbuhl, J. P., Pfeiffer, J., Rossier, M., and Rossier, B. C. (1979). *J. Membr. Biol.* **48,** 167-180.
Krebs, H. A. (1970). *Adv. Enzyme Regul.* **8,** 335-353.
Kunin, A. S., and Tannen, R. L. (1979). *Am. J. Physiol.* **237,** F55-F62.
Kusch, M., Farman, N., and Edelman, I. S. (1978). *Am. J. Physiol.* **235,** C82-C89.
Lahav, M., Dietz, T., and Edelman, I. S. (1973). *Endocrinology* **92,** 1685-1699.
Law, P. Y., and Edelman, I. S. (1978a). *J. Membr. Biol.* **41,** 15-40.
Law, P. Y., and Edelman, I. S. (1978b). *J. Membr. Biol.* **41,** 41-64.
Leaf, A., Anderson, J., and Page, L. B. (1958). *J. Gen. Physiol.* **41,** 657-668.
Lichtenstein, N. S., and Leaf, A. (1965). *J. Clin. Invest.* **44,** 1328-1342.
Lien, E. L., Goodman, D. B. P., and Rasmussen, H. (1975). *Biochemistry* **14,** 2749-2754.
Lien, E. L., Goodman, D. B. P., and Rasmussen, H. (1976). *Biochim. Biophys. Acta* **421,** 210-217.
Lifschitz, M. D., Schrier, R. W., and Edelman, I. S. (1973). *Am. J. Physiol.* **224,** 376-380.
Lipton, P., and Edelman, I. S. (1971). *Am. J. Physiol.* **221,** 733-741.
Liu, A. Y.-C., and Greengard, P. (1974). *Proc. Natl. Acad. Sci. U.S.A.* **71,** 3869-3873.
Lo, C.-S., August, T. R., Liberman, U. A., and Edelman, I. S. (1976). *J. Biol. Chem.* **251,** 7826-7833.
Loeb, R. F., Atchley, D. W., Benedict, E. M., and Leland, L. (1933). *J. Exp. Med.* **57,** 775-792.
Lombard, W. E., Jacobson, H. R., and Kokko, J. P. (1979). *Kidney Int.* **16,** 827 (abstr.).
Lonnerholm, G. (1971). *Acta Physiol. Scand.* **81,** 433-439.
Lowry, C. V., Kimmey, J. S., Felder, S., Chi, M. M.-Y., Kaiser, K. K., Passonneau, P. N., Kirk, K. A., and Lowry, O. H. (1978). *J. Biol. Chem.* **253,** 8269-8277.
Lowry, O. H., and Passonneau, J. V. (1972). "A Flexible System of Enzymatic Analysis," pp. 43-60 and 223-260. Academic Press, New York.
Ludens, J. H., and Fanestil, D. D. (1971). *Biochim. Biophys. Acta* **244,** 360-371.
Ludens, J. H., and Fanestil, D. D. (1974). *Am. J. Physiol.* **226,** 1321-1326.
Ludens, J. H., Vaughn, D. A., and Fanestil, D. D. (1978). *J. Membr. Biol.* **40,** Spec. 191-211.
Luetscher, J. A. (1956). *Recent Prog. Horm. Res.* **12,** 175-198.
McKinney, T. D., and Burg, M. B. (1977). *J. Clin. Invest.* **60,** 766-768.
Mainwaring, W. I. P., and Mangan, F. R. (1971). *Adv. Biosci.* **7,** 165-177.
Manganiello, V., and Vaughan, M. (1972). *J. Clin. Invest.* **51,** 2763-2767.
Maragoudakis, M. E. (1969). *J. Biol. Chem.* **244,** 5005-5013.
Maren, T. H. (1977). *Am. J. Physiol.* **232,** F291-F297.
Marver, D. (1980). *Endocrinology* **106,** 611-618.
Marver, D., and Edelman, I. S. (1978). *J. Steroid Biochem.* **9,** 1-7.
Marver, D., and Schwartz, M. J. (1980). *Proc. Natl. Acad. Sci. U.S.A.* **77,** 3672-3676.
Marver, D., Goodman, D., and Edelman, I. S. (1972). *Kidney Int.* **1,** 210-223.
Marver, D., Stewart, J. W., Funder, J. W., Feldman, D., and Edelman, I. S. (1974). *Proc. Natl. Acad. Sci. U.S.A.* **71,** 1431-1435.
Marver, D., Chiu, W.-H., Wolff, M. E., and Edelman, I. S. (1976). *Proc. Natl. Acad. Sci. U.S.A.* **73,** 4462-4466.
Matulich, D. T., Spindler, B. J., Schambelan, M., and Baxter, J. D. (1976). *J. Clin. Endocrinol. Metab.* **43,** 1170-1174.
Mishra, R. K., Wheldrake, J. F., and Feltham, L. A. W. (1972). *FEBS Lett.* **24,** 106-108.
Mueller, A., and Steinmetz, P. R. (1978). *J. Clin. Invest.* **61,** 1666-1670.
Mukherjee, A., Srere, P. A., and Frenkel, E. P. (1976). *J. Biol. Chem.* **251,** 2155-2160.
Nicholls, M. G., Ramsay, L. E., Boddy, K., Fraser, R., Morton, J. J., and Robertson, J. I. S. (1979). *Metab., Clin. Exp.* **28,** 584-593.

Norby, L. H., and Schwartz, J. H. (1978). *J. Clin. Invest.* **62**, 532-538.

Notides, A. C., Hamilton, D. E., and Muechler, E. K. (1976). *J. Steroid Biochem.* **7**, 1025-1030.

Ogata, E., Nishiki, K., Kugai, N., and Kishikawa, T. (1977). *Am. J. Physiol.* **232**, E401-E407.

O'Malley, B. W., Sherman, M. R., Toft, D. O., Spelsberg, T. C., Schrader, W. T., and Steggles, A. W. (1971). *Adv. Biosci.* **7**, 213-234.

O'Neil, R. G., and Helman, S. I. (1977). *Am. J. Physiol.* **233**, F544-F558.

Orloff, J., Handler, J. S., and Bergström, S. (1965). *Nature (London)* **205**, 397-398.

Paillard, M. (1977). *Adv. Nephrol.* **7**, 83-104.

Porter, G. A. (1968). *Mol. Pharmacol.* **4**, 224-237.

Porter, G. A. (1972). *In* "Enzyme Induction" (D. V. Parke, ed.), pp. 105-141. Plenum, New York.

Porter, G. A., and Edelman, I. S. (1964). *J. Clin. Invest.* **43**, 611-620.

Porter, G. A., Bogoroch, R., and Edelman, I. S. (1964). *Proc. Natl. Acad. Sci. U.S.A.* **52**, 1326-1333.

Puca, G. A., Nola, E., Sica, V., and Bresciani, F. (1977). *J. Biol. Chem.* **252**, 1358-1366.

Pullman, M. E., and Monroy, G. C. (1969). *J. Biol. Chem.* **238**, 3762-3769.

Racker, E. (1976). "A New Look at Mechanisms in Bioenergetics." Academic Press, New York.

Rafestin-Olin, M. E., Michaud, A., Claire, M., and Corvol, P. (1977). *J. Steroid Biochem.* **8**, 19-23.

Rajerison, R., Marchetti, J., Roy, C., Bockaert, J., and Jard, S. (1974). *J. Biol. Chem.* **249**, 6390-6400.

Razin, S. (1972). *Biochim. Biophys. Acta* **265**, 241-296.

Rivlin, R. (1970). *Adv. Enzyme Regul.* **8**, 239-252.

Rodriguez, H. J., and Klahr, S. (1980). *Clin. Res.* **28**, 460A (abstr.).

Rodriguez, H. J., Wiesmann, W. P., and Klahr, S. (1975). *Am. J. Physiol.* **229**, 99-106.

Rosen, S. (1972). *Histochem. J.* **4**, 35-48.

Rossier, B. C., and Claire, M. (1978). *In* "Aldosterone Antagonists in Clinical Medicine, Proceedings of the Searle Symposium" (N. W. Asmussen *et al.*, eds.), pp. 10-16. Excerpta Med. Found., Amsterdam.

Rossier, B. C., Wilce, P. A., and Edelman, I. S. (1974). *Proc. Natl. Acad. Sci. U.S.A.* **71**, 3101-3105.

Rossier, B. C., Wilce, P. A., Inciardi, J. F., Yoshimura, F. K., and Edelman, I. S. (1977). *Am. J. Physiol.* **232**, C174-C179.

Rossier, B. C., Gaggeler, H. P., and Rossier, M. (1978). *J. Membr. Biol.* **41**, 149-166.

Rossier, M., Rossier, B. C., Pfeiffer, J., and Kraehenbuhl, J. P. (1979). *J. Membr. Biol.* **48**, 141-166.

Rousseau, G., and Crabbé, J. (1968). *Biochim. Biophys. Acta* **157**, 25-32.

Saito, T., and Essig, A. (1973). *J. Membr. Biol.* **13**, 1-18.

Sakauye, C., and Feldman, D. (1976). *Am. J. Physiol.* **231**, 93-97.

Saladino, A. J., Bentley, P. J., and Trump, B. F. (1969). *Am. J. Pathol.* **54**, 421-466.

Sapirstein, V. S., and Scott, W. N. (1975). *Nature (London)* **257**, 241-243.

Sato, B., Noma, K., Nishizawa, Y., Nakao, K., Matsumoto, K., and Yamamura, Y. (1980). *Endocrinology* **106**, 1142-1148.

Schmidt, U., and Horster, M. (1978). *Methods Pharmacol.* **4B**, 259-296.

Schmidt, U., Schmid, J., Schmid, H., and Dubach, U. C. (1975). *J. Clin. Invest.* **55**, 655-660.

Scholer, D. W., and Edelman, I. S. (1979). *Am. J. Physiol.* **237**, F350-F359.

Scholer, D. W., Mishina, T., and Edelman, I. S. (1979). *Am. J. Physiol.* **237**, F360-F366.

Schwartz, G. J., and Burg, M. B. (1978). *Am. J. Physiol.* **235**, F576-F585.

Schwartz, J. H., and Rosen, S. (1979). *Kidney Int.* **16**, 837 (abstr.).

Schwartz, J. H., and Steinmetz, P. R. (1977). *Am. J. Physiol.* **2**, F145–F149.

Schwartz, M. J., and Kokko, J. P. (1979). *Kidney Int.* **16**, 874 (abstr.).

Scott, W. N., and Sapirstein, V. S. (1975). *Proc. Natl. Acad. Sci. U.S.A.* **72**, 4056–4060.

Scott, W. N., Sapirstein, V. S., and Yoder, M. J. (1974). *Science* **184**, 797–800.

Scott, W. N., Reich, I. M., Brown, J. A., and Yang, C.-P. H. (1978). *J. Membr. Biol.* **40**, Spec. 213–220.

Scott, W. N., Reich, I. M., and Goodman, D. B. P. (1979). *J. Biol. Chem.* **254**, 4957–4959.

Senft, G., Schultz, G., Munske, K., and Hoffman, M. (1968). *Diabetologia* **4**, 330–335.

Sharp, G. W. G., and Leaf, A. (1964). *Proc. Natl. Acad. Sci. U.S.A.* **52**, 1114–1121.

Sharp, G. W. G., and Leaf, A. (1965). *J. Biol. Chem.* **240**, 4816–4821.

Sharp, G. W. G., and Leaf, A. (1973). *In* "Handbook of Physiology" (J. Orloff and R. W. Berliner, eds.), Sect. 8, pp. 815–830. Am. Physiol. Soc., Washington, D.C.

Sharp, G. W. G., Komack, C. L., and Leaf, A. (1966a). *J. Clin. Invest.* **45**, 450–459.

Sharp, G. W. G., Coggins, C. H., Lichtenstein, N. S., and Leaf, A. (1966b). *J. Clin. Invest.* **45**, 1640–1647.

Sibley, C. H., and Tomkins, G. M. (1974). *Cell* **2**, 221–227.

Siegel, B., and Civan, M. M. (1976). *Am. J. Physiol.* **230**, 1603–1608.

Simpson, S. A., and Tait, J. F. (1953). *Mem. Soc. Endocrinol.* **2**, 9–24.

Simpson, S. A., Tait, J. F., Wettstein, A., Neher, R., von Euw, J., Schindler, O., and Reichstein, T. (1954). *Experientia* **10**, 132–133.

Skou, J. C. (1977). *In* "Structural and Kinetic Approach to Plasma Membrane Functions" (C. Nicolau and A. Paraf, eds.), pp. 145–151. Springer-Verlag, Berlin and New York.

Snart, R. S., and Taylor, E. (1978). *J. Physiol. (London)* **274**, 447–454.

Spooner, P. M., and Edelman, I. S. (1976). *Biochim. Biophys. Acta* **444**, 663–673.

Srere, P. A. (1969). *Biochem. Med.* **3**, 61–72.

Srere, P. A. (1971). *Adv. Enzyme Regul.* **9**, 221–233.

Steinmetz, P. R. (1974). *Physiol. Rev.* **54**, 890–956.

Stoff, J. S., Handler, J. S., and Orloff, J. (1972). *Proc. Natl. Acad. Sci. U.S.A.* **69**, 805–808.

Stokes, J. B., and Kokko, J. P. (1977). *J. Clin. Invest.* **59**, 1099–1104.

Stokes, J. B., Tisher, C. C., and Kokko, J. P. (1978). *Kidney Int.* **14**, 585–593.

Swaneck, G. E., Highland, E., and Edelman, I. S. (1969). *Nephron* **6**, 297–316.

Swaneck, G. E., Chu, L. L. H., and Edelman, I. S. (1970). *J. Biol. Chem.* **245**, 5382–5389.

Tait, J. F., and Tait, S. A. S. (1978). *Trends Biochem. Sci.* **3**, N273–N275.

Tan, E. L., and Trachewsky, D. (1975). *J. Steroid Biochem.* **6**, 1471–1475.

Tannen, R. L. (1977). *Kidney Int.* **11**, 453–465.

Tannen, R. L. (1978). *Am. J. Physiol.* **235**, F265–F277.

Tata, J. R. (1966). *In* "Regulation of Metabolic Processes in Mitochondria" (J. M. Tager, S. Pappa, E. Quagliariello, and E. C. Slater, eds.), pp. 489–507. Elsevier, Amsterdam.

Taylor, A., and Windhager, E. E. (1979). *Am. J. Physiol.* **236**, F505–F512.

Thompson, B. D., and Edmonds, C. J. (1974). *J. Endocrinol.* **62**, 489–496.

Thompson, E. B., Aviv, D., and Lippman, M. E. (1977). *Endocrinology* **100**, 406–419.

Tisher, C. C. (1981). *In* "The Kidney" (B. M. Brenner and F. C. Rector, eds.), pp. 47–52. Saunders, Philadelphia, Pennsylvania.

Trachewsky, D. (1978). *J. Clin. Invest.* **62**, 1325–1333.

Urakabe, S., Takamitsu, Y., Shirai, D., Yuasa, S., Kimura, G., Orita, Y., and Abe, H. (1975). *Comp. Biochem. Physiol.* **52**, 1-4.

Ussing, H. H., and Zerahn, K. (1951). *Acta Physiol. Scand.* **23**, 110-127.

Wade, J. B., O'Neil, R. G., Pryor, J. L., and Boulpaep, E. L. (1979). *J. Cell Biol.* **81**, 439-445.

Wambach, G., and Higgins, J. R. (1978). *Endocrinology* **102**, 1686-1693.

Warnock, D. G., and Edelman, I. S. (1978). *Mol. Cell. Endocrinol.* **12**, 221-233.

Weiner, M. W. (1980). *Clin. Res.* **28**, 65A (abstr.).

Welbourne, T. C. (1974). *Am. J. Physiol.* **226**, 555-559.

Welbourne, T. C., and Francoeur, D. (1977). *Am. J. Physiol.* **233**, E56-E60.

Welbourne, T. C., Phenix, P., Thornley-Brown, C., and Welbourne, C. J. (1976). *Proc. Soc. Exp. Biol. Med.* **153**, 539-542.

Wiederholt, M. (1966). *Pfluegers Arch. Gesamte Physiol. Menschen Tiere* **292**, 334-342.

Wiederholt, M., Behn, C., Schoormans, W., and Hansen, L. (1972). *J. Steroid Biochem.* **3**, 151-159.

Wilce, P. A., Rossier, B. C., and Edelman, I. S. (1976a). *Biochemistry* **15**, 4279-4285.

Wilce, P. A., Rossier, B. C., and Edelman, I. S. (1976b). *Biochemistry* **15**, 4286-4291.

Williamson, H. E. (1963). *Biochem. Pharmacol.* **12**, 1449-1450.

Winder, W. W. (1979). *Am. J. Physiol.* **236**, C132-C138.

Wolff, M. E., Feldman, D., Catsoulacos, P., Funder, J. W., Hancock, C., Amano, Y., and Edelman, I. S. (1975). *Biochemistry* **14**, 1750-1759.

Woodhall, P. B., and Tisher, C. C. (1973). *J. Clin. Invest.* **52**, 3095-3108.

Wright, F. S., and Giebisch, G. (1978). *Am. J. Physiol.* **235**, F515-F527.

Wright, F. S., Knox, F. S., Howards, S. J., and Berliner, R. W. (1969). *Am. J. Physiol.* **216**, 869-875.

Yagi, K. (1954). *J. Biochem. (Tokyo)* **41**, 757-762.

Yorio, T., and Bentley, P. J. (1978). *Nature (London)* **271**, 79-81.

Zava, D. T., Chamness, G. C., Horwitz, K. B., and McGuire, W. L. (1977). *Science* **196**, 663-664.

Ziegler, T. W., Fanestil, D. D., and Ludens, J. H. (1976). *Kidney Int.* **10**, 279-286.

Zusman, R. M., and Keiser, H. R. (1980). *Kidney Int.* **17**, 277-283.

Zusman, R. M., Keiser, H. R., and Handler, J. S. (1977). *J. Clin. Invest.* **60**, 1339-1347.

Zusman, R. M., Keiser, H. R., and Handler, J. S. (1978). *Am. J. Physiol.* **234**, F532-F540.

Thyroid-Stimulating Autoantibodies

D. D. ADAMS

Autoimmunity Research Unit, Medical Research Council of New Zealand, University of Otago Medical School, Dunedin, New Zealand

I. Introduction

A. Fruits of the Germ Theory of Disease

Two pathways trace back from modern understanding of the thyroid-stimulating autoantibodies, over 100 years, to one of the greatest conceptual advances ever to be made in medicine. This was the introduction by Louis Pasteur of the germ theory of disease (Dubos, 1951), today so taken for granted that it is difficult to imagine medicine without it. Our first pathway leads through the work of Joseph Lister, whose introduction of antisepsis, to be followed by asepsis, enabled the development of surgery, now freed from inevitable wound infection (Cameron, 1948). Swiss surgeons were encouraged to attempt the surgical removal of large goiters, which were common in their iodine-deficient country. Initial satisfaction at the success of such operations turned to dismay, some months later, as the patients developed the horrifying picture of myxedema (Harington, 1933). However, it was soon discovered that dried extracts of thyroid tissue, fed by mouth, would effect a cure. In this way, the essential endocrine function of the thyroid gland was established.

Our second pathway leads through the discovery that defense against germs is mediated by the immunity system, with antibodies of myriad specificities capable of identifying foreign invaders and destroying them through the agency of powerful, nonspecific, executive systems, such as complement. Observing how readily a foreign red blood corpuscle could be lysed by antibody and complement, Paul Ehrlich and others wondered if the system ever malfunctioned and attacked the host, to cause disease? This story will be taken up again later in this review.

B. GRAVES' DISEASE

The clinicians, Parry, Graves (1838), and von Basedow all independently recognized the syndrome that came to be called Graves' disease in English-speaking countries. The cardinal features noted were tachycardia, intense nervousness, tremor, enlargement of the thyroid, and, more or less, exophthalmos. Möbius (1886) suggested that a pathological alteration in the thyroid gland was the basis of the condition, a view that received strong support from observation of the similarity of the features of Graves' disease to the effects of overtreatment of myxedema with dried thyroid. Histological study showed that the thyroid gland was hyperplastic in Graves' disease. Moreover, it was found that extracts of thyroid tissue administered to animals would elicit features of Graves' disease, and, most significantly, that far from being more potent than a normal thyroid, the Graves' disease gland was less so, indicating that it did not contain any toxic principle not present in a normal thyroid. Thus, by the turn of the century, Graves' disease was well established as including a state of thyroid gland overactivity, a state of hyperthyroidism. The cause of this hyperthyroidism was to remain a mystery for over 50 years.

C. THE BEGINNING OF THE SEARCH FOR THE CAUSE OF GRAVES' DISEASE

Early in this century it was observed that deficiency of iodine would cause thyroid hyperplasia and that administration of iodine would correct this (Marine and Lenhart, 1909). The iodine-deficient gland took up extra iodine and retained it, the active secretion continuing to be released at the normal rate. The hyperplastic thyroid of Graves' disease, on the other hand, while taking up extra iodine and undergoing morphological involution, did not cease to pour out its active secretion at an increased rate, although iodine treatment had a useful effect in mitigating this, temporarily. Kocher (1910) used the expressive term *"thyroid diarrhoea"* to describe this outpouring of the Graves' thyroid gland. What caused it?

A candidate appeared in the 1920s when Smith and Smith (1922) showed that injection of extracts of bovine pituitary glands would stimulate thyroid secretion in hypophysectomized tadpoles. That thyroid secretion occurred was evident from the occurrence of metamorphosis, which was known from the work of Gudernatsch (1914) to be dependent on thyroid activity. Subsequently, after developing a technique for hypophysectomizing rats, Phillip Smith was successful in demonstrating the action of thyroid-stimulating hormone (TSH) in the mammal (Smith, 1926). Was excessive secretion of TSH from the pituitary the cause of the hyperthyroidism of Graves' disease? Many clinicians assumed so, but Charles Harington (1933), writing a brilliantly clear analysis of thyroid chemistry, physiology, and pathology, was sceptical in the absence of any supportive evidence. Harington's major achievement is the discovery of the chemical structure of thyroxine but, additionally, with his powerful scientific mind, he opposed Plummer's aberrant theory that Graves' disease was a dysthyroidism based on a qualitatively abnormal thyroid secretion and he was unimpressed by Marine's theory that Graves' disease is based on adrenal lesions that free the thyroid from a postulated adrenal inhibitory influence. Harington considered the etiology of Graves' disease to be the outstanding remaining thyroid problem of his day.

D. Toxic Adenoma

In people living in regions where the soil is deficient in iodine, goiters occur. One such region surrounds Rochester, Minnesota, where Henry Plummer worked at the Mayo Clinic. Having a flair for the recording and analysis of meaningful data, Plummer (1913) was able to substantiate an impression that a proportion of cases of endemic goiter developed constitutional symptoms resembling those of mild Graves' disease. On average, 14.5 years elapsed between the first appearance of the goiter and the insidious onset of the constitutional symptoms. With notable perspicacity, Plummer concluded that a second form of hyperthyroidism exists, distinct from Graves' disease, based on the development of hyperfunctioning adenomas in endemic goiters. The term thyrotoxicosis was then coming into use as an apt synonym for hyperthyroidism, and for the newly recognized disorder Plummer coined the commendably precise name "toxic adenoma."

Years later, when radioactive iodine became available, Plummer's concept of toxic adenoma (Plummer's disease) was validated by autoradiography. One or more biochemically hyperactive adenomas were found in such goiters, together with inactive normal tissue (Cope et al., 1947; Dobyns and Lennon, 1948). It was concluded that when autonomously active tissue of an adenoma caused mild hyperthyroidism, it also caused inhibition of TSH secretion by negative feedback, which in turn caused regression of normal thyroid tissue.

The pathogenesis of toxic adenoma is discussed in the light of modern knowledge in Section V,E.

E. From Horror Autotoxicus to Autoimmune Thyroiditis

It is ironical that Paul Ehrlich has been misquoted as stating that autoimmunity does not occur. With Morgenroth, he was able to cause goats to produce antibodies by injecting them with red blood cells of other goats, but attempts to immunize goats against their own red cells did not succeed (Ehrlich and Morgenroth, 1901). The general finding that animals will not normally make antibodies against their own tissues was described by Ehrlich as *"horror autotoxicus"* and is accepted today as immunological tolerance to self components, an obvious necessity for health. What has often been overlooked is that Ehrlich correctly postulated that "possible failure of the internal regulation" of immune processes might be "the explanation of many disease-phenomena" (Ehrlich and Morgenroth, 1900). My colleague W. E. Griesbach recalled that search for autoimmunity as a cause of disease was a common activity in Germany before World War I. However, after this great disruption of academic life, a generation grew up that carelessly misquoted Ehrlich and taught their pupils that he had proved autoimmunity to be impossible. This intellectual sloth delayed the discovery of autoimmune disease by decades. When Dameshek and Schwartz (1938) found autoantibodies against red blood corpuscles in cases of hemolytic anemia, the general phenomenon was still not accepted, being described as "so-called" autoimmunity, or "autoallergy" (see Dameshek, 1965). The turn of the tide came when Doniach and Roitt (1957) looked for and found thyroid autoantibodies in Hashimoto's disease and Witebsky *et al.* (1957) produced experimental autoimmune thyroiditis in rabbits by applying the discovery by Freund *et al.* (1948) of agents that act as mutagenic adjuvants to immunization.

II. Long-Acting Thyroid Stimulator (LATS)

A. Attempts to Determine Blood TSH Levels in Graves' Disease

After the discovery of TSH, it was repeatedly noted that the histological changes that could be induced in the thyroids of laboratory animals by injections of pituitary extracts closely resembled the hyperplasia occurring in Graves' disease (Loeb and Bassett, 1930; Schockaert, 1931). With a view to determining whether or not excessive TSH secretion caused the hyperthyroidism of Graves' disease, attempts began to be made to measure TSH levels in human blood and urine by bioassay in laboratory animals. One of the pioneers was Aron (1931), who used histological change in guinea pig thyroids as his index and noted more TSH activity in myxedema sera than in sera from cases of Graves' disease, but like many subsequent investigators, he mistook nonspecific effects for TSH activity in sera from normal people. Gradually the technology improved. Rawson and Starr (1938) made histological evaluation more objective by taking actual measurements of thyroid cell height. The early work of Hertz and Oastler (1936) is a landmark. Using hypophysectomy to increase the sensitivity of rats to injected TSH, they assayed human urine extracts and blood and found undetectable TSH levels in eight normal people and in eight cases of Graves' disease, but raised levels in nine cases of myxedema. They concluded that hypersecretion of TSH was not the cause of Graves' disease.

The next decade saw little progress, but then two improved methods, using guinea pigs, provided puzzling data. De Robertis (1948) found that the counting of microdroplets of colloid in thyroid cells provided a particularly sensitive measure of thyroid stimulation. Applying this, he observed raised levels of TSH in myxedema and, additionally, in several cases of Graves' disease, but only in those with exophthalmos. Purves and Griesbach (1949) used strict statistical treatment of cell height measurements in thyroxine-treated guinea pigs to obtain data that today can be seen as accurate. Activity was absent in sera from cases of untreated thyrotoxicosis, but it was present in myxedema and in antithyroid drug-treated thyrotoxicosis, which suggested normal pituitary function in thyrotoxicosis. However, two cases of malignant exophthalmos showed very high activity, eliciting mean cell heights of 9.2 and 9.7 μm (controls 3.58 $\pm$ 0.07). Of the remaining 25 cases of malignant exophthalmos studied, most elicited cell heights in the myxedema range (4.5–8 μm), but 11 cases showed no activity. It was 1971 before these observations became explicable. Purves and Griesbach speculated that malignant exophthalmos might be the result of a lesion in the brainstem affecting the orbit and the pituitary by neural pathways.

B. AN ABNORMAL THYROID-STIMULATING HORMONE IN GRAVES' DISEASE

The advent of radioactive iodine provided a powerful new tool for thyroid research. Several groups of investigators developed new bioassays for TSH, using [131]I (see Crigler, 1960). Most methods were based on measurement of thyroid uptake of carrier-free ^{131}I iodide in thyroid-hormone-treated animals. However, Adams and Purves (1955), drawing on the previous bioassay experience of Purves, developed a method that utilized measurement of secretion of ^{131}I from the thyroids of thyroxine-treated, weanling guinea pigs. Tests showed that measurement of the decrease in thyroid ^{131}I was a less sensitive index than measurement of the increase in plasma ^{131}I level (Adams, 1975). Striving for sensitivity, the investigators adopted a technique that enabled test materials to be injected intravenously, via a dilated ear vein, the gain being a factor of 5 over the intraperitoneal route. Maximal responses occurred 3 hours after injection of a large (12.5 mU) dose of TSH, earlier for smaller doses (Fig. 1). The magnitude of the response was remarkably sensitive to change in dosage (Adams and Purves, 1957), an indication that the parameter being measured (increased secretion of thyroid hormone) was a primary effect of TSH, in contrast to increase in thyroid weight or cell height. At low TSH dosage the change in response exceeded direct proportionality to the change in dosage, which suggested the existence of an intracellular amplification mechanism.

Purves was aware that the major variation in bioassays is due to variation in the responsiveness of individual animals. To correct this,

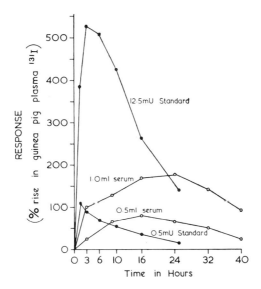

FIG. 1. The prolonged time course of the responses elicited by two doses of serum from a case of thyrotoxicosis with exophthalmos (LATS) compared to the responses elicited by two doses of USP Standard TSH. Reproduced, with permission, from Adams (1958).

he proposed using the same animals repeatedly on successive days. This proved practicable and enabled the development of an accurate assay method in which a group of six prepared guinea pigs were used on up to six successive days, each animal receiving all the test materials in a balanced order (Adams and Purves, 1957). Gaddum's (1953) index of precision, λ, which is s/b, was about 0.1. The sensitivity was such that, in a single assay, a dose of 0.1 mU/ml could be significantly distinguished from injections of saline.

When the method was applied to the examination of human serum samples, normal subjects showed no activity, but four untreated, congenitally hypothyroid children showed TSH levels ranging from 1.0 to 2.5 mU/ml, the activity disappearing with thyroxine treatment of the patients (Adams, 1958). Several untreated thyrotoxic patients showed no activity. However, we then encountered a Mrs. MC, with recurrent thyrotoxicosis and exophthalmos after subtotal thyroidectomy. Her serum elicited only a modest effect at 3 hours, but then the system of using the animals repeatedly paid an unexpected dividend. The guinea pig blood sample taken next day as a baseline for measurement of the next response showed that, instead of falling overnight in the usual manner, the ^{131}I level had risen strikingly. Exploration of the effect showed it to be consistent, indicating that Mrs. MC had in her blood a thyroid stimulator that differed from ordinary TSH in having a markedly longer time course of action after a single intravenous injection (Adams and Purves, 1956).

In a detailed study it was found that MC serum, in a dosage of 0.5 ml, elicited a maximal response at 16 hours, and in 1.0 ml dosage at 24 hours, whereas 0.5 mU of standard TSH (bovine) had a maximal effect at 1.5 hours, and 12.5 mU at 3 hours (Fig. 1) (Adams, 1958). A mixture of MC serum and standard TSH had an additive effect. To test whether the abnormal response was due to a blockage of the inhibitory effect of thyroxine in the assay animals, with thyroid stimulation by TSH secreted from the animals' own pituitaries, a massive dose (1 mg) of thyroxine was injected before a 1.0 ml dose of MC serum. The response was unabated.

For study of materials from various sources, 3 hours and 16 hours were chosen as times that would differentiate between normal (TSH standard-like) and abnormal (MC serum-like) responses. Extracts of human, rat, and mouse pituitary glands all elicited normal-type responses, as did plasma from thyroidectomized rats, from congenitally hypothyroid children, and from two thyrotoxic patients who had been rendered hypothyroid by overtreatment with methylthiouracil. Of six untreated thyrotoxic patients, three showed no activity, but serum from three others elicited small but significant abnormal-type responses. It was concluded that a thyroid-stimulating hormone distinct from TSH occurs in thyrotoxicosis and might play the causative role (Adams, 1958).

C. The McKenzie Mouse Bioassay

1. *An Improved Method*

Meanwhile, E. B. Astwood, in Boston, had realized the virtues of the mouse as a bioassay animal. Its small size enables the use of large numbers and minimizes the quantity of test material needed. Furthermore, like the guinea pig and unlike the rat, the mouse was known to be relatively sensitive to TSH (bovine). J. M. McKenzie, working in Astwood's laboratory, was developing a mouse bioassay for TSH based on measurement of thyroid uptake of ^{131}I, when the abnormal TSH was reported. McKenzie (1958b) succeeded in adapting the Adams and Purves guinea pig assay to the mouse, utilizing tail veins for bleeding and for intravenous injection of the test materials. Because of the advantages mentioned above, I changed to McKenzie's mouse method, which also came into general use.

2. *Confirmation of the Existence of LATS*

McKenzie (1958a) confirmed the existence of the abnormal TSH, as did Munro (1959), using McKenzie's assay. In the mouse, TSH produced its peak effect between 2 and 3 hours after intravenous injection, according to dosage, the abnormal TSH at about 12 hours, given in what is now seen as low dosage.

After establishment of the properties described in the next section, the names "abnormal TSH," "abnormal thyroid stimulator," and "thyroid activator of hyperthyroidism" (McKenzie, 1959) became replaced by "long-acting thyroid stimulator" (LATS) (Adams, 1961), which will be used henceforth in this review.

3. *Confusion from Nonspecific Effects*

In the guinea pig method, a maximum dosage of 1.0 ml of test serum is injected into animals weighing 200 gm or more. Serum from euthyroid people appeared to be inactive (Adams, 1958), but was not tested exhaustively against saline injections. In the mouse method, 0.5 ml is injected into 25 gm animals. An occasional human serum is toxic to both guinea pigs and mice, an effect that weakens with storage of the serum in the frozen state and may be due to antibodies with chance specificity for cellular antigens in the test animals. Separate from this effect is the general capacity of human sera to elicit small but significant responses in the mouse assay when compared to saline injections (Adams *et al.*, 1966). The magnitude of the effect at 2 hours is up to 300% of the initial blood ^{131}I level, with a similar value at 10 hours. Frozen serum shows less effect than fresh. The albumin fraction of the serum proteins elicits the effect as well as the globulin fraction (Adams *et al.*, 1966).

Before it was recognized as such, the nonspecific effect caused confusion. It was thought that LATS was demonstrable in normal people (Major and Munro, 1962), that TSH was demonstrable in unfractionated serum from normal people (Yamazaki *et al.*, 1961), that LATS was distributed throughout all the serum proteins (McKenzie, 1961), and that a shorter-acting variant of LATS existed (Adams *et al.*, 1962b).

The specificity of responses to small doses of TSH can be established by demonstrating significant loss of activity after incubation with antiserum to TSH. For LATS, specificity can be established by a similar neutralization test with antiserum to immunoglobulin or by demonstration of a significantly more prolonged time course (Adams *et al.*, 1966).

D. BIOLOGICAL PROPERTIES OF LATS

1. *Evidence of Thyroid Stimulation*

Release of ^{131}I from thyroid hormone-treated guinea pigs and mice can be caused by thyroid cell damage, as well as by thyroid cell stimulation. McKenzie (1959, 1960) obtained important evidence by injecting LATS into mice twice daily for 4 days, then measuring several indices of thyroid stimulation. He found plasma protein-bound ^{127}I levels to be increased 2- to 3-fold over values in control animals. Histologically, the thyroid glands showed activation with reduction of acinar colloid and increase in the epithelial cell height, in accord with previously observed effects of sera from certain cases of Graves' disease (Purves and Griesbach, 1949). Finally, using thyroid hormone-treated mice, McKenzie (1959, 1960) showed that single injections of LATS sera significantly increased thyroid ^{131}I uptake over that in saline-injected controls. Powerful effects on thyroid histology and thyroid ^{131}I uptake were demonstrated by Major and Munro (1960) with an exceptionally potent LATS serum obtained from a Mrs. C who, like Mrs. MC, had persistent exophthalmos after subtotal thyroidectomy for thyrotoxicosis.

2. *Action in Hypophysectomized Mice*

The pituitary gland was an obvious possibility for the site of action of LATS, but Munro (1959) excluded this by obtaining unabated responses in hypophysectomized mice. This finding, which was confirmed by Adams *et al.* (1961), made it clear that LATS acts directly on the thyroid gland.

3. *Prolonged Stay in the Circulation*

The occurrence of very high LATS levels in occasional patients, such as Mrs. MC, provided material of sufficient potency to enable measurement of its rate of disappearance from circulating blood after an intravenous injection (Adams, 1960). The rat was chosen as the test animal because its size is sufficient to provide multiple blood samples for assay in the mouse. The results were striking (Fig. 2). One hour after injection, the level of human and bovine TSH had fallen to less than 5% of the 2-minute level, whereas the LATS had a half-life of 7.4 hours (confidence limits at $p = 0.05$, 23.3, and 4.4). Despite the greater

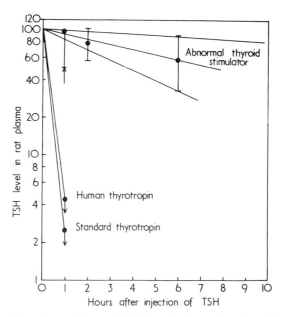

FIG. 2. Markedly prolonged stay of LATS in the circulating blood of the rat, after intravenous injection, compared to human TSH and USP Standard TSH (bovine). Each point represents a mean value from 8–14 assay mice. Limits of error are at $p=0.05$. Reproduced, with permission, from Adams (1960).

technical difficulties, McKenzie (1959, 1961) succeeded in obtaining similar data on the length of stay of LATS in the circulation of the mouse.

4. *The Dose-Response Relationship*

A quite remarkable property of LATS is its dose-response relationship (Fig. 3), which shows it to be a more effective thyroid stimulator than TSH itself (Adams, 1961). The dose-response line is steeper than that for TSH, and the maximal response attainable is much higher. Kriss *et al.* (1964) found the LATS response to plateau when dosage was sufficient to cause approximately 30-fold increases in the mouse blood ^{131}I level (Fig. 4). In contrast, we observed responses to TSH to plateau when the ^{131}I level was about 5 times the initial value (400% increase*) (Fig. 3). Moreover, the prolonged action of LATS after a single injection additionally increases the total thyroid secretion compared to that caused by a TSH injection.

The prolonged stay of LATS in the circulation (Fig. 2) offers an explanation for its superiority to TSH as a circulating thyroid stimulator. Whether or not this is the whole explanation is discussed in Section VI.

5. *Site of Production*

The source of LATS is the blood of patients with Graves' disease, but its site of production was a complete mystery for several years.

a. Not the Pituitary Gland. Exclusion of the pituitary gland came when McKenzie (1962a) demonstrated the presence of TSH, not LATS, in pituitary tissue obtained at biopsy or necropsy from patients with demonstrable LATS in their blood. Major and Munro (1962) confirmed this finding using necropsy tissue from four cases of Graves' disease, additionally noting low content of TSH in two of their four cases, suggestive of inhibition of TSH production by negative feedback from raised thyroid hormone levels (see Section III).

b. Evidence for an Origin in Forbidden Clones of Immunocytes. The indivisibility of LATS from serum immunoglobulins (see Section II,E) first suggested its autoantibody nature. The concept of autoimmunity had been blocked for decades (see Section I,E), but Doniach and Roitt (1957) had recently broken the inhibition by demonstrating the exis-

---

*At the time of the study shown in Fig. 3, the assay mice were receiving excessive dosage of T_4, which reduced sensitivity through an effect of the contained iodine (see Section III,D,1). With optimal preparation, responses to TSH plateau at about 900 (percentage of increase in mouse blood ^{125}I level) and responses to LATS at 4000 to 5000 (Knight, 1977).

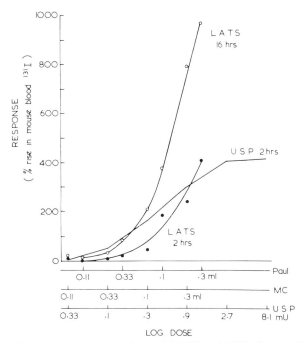

FIG. 3. The dose-response relationships of LATS and USP Standard TSH in the McKenzie mouse bioassay. Reproduced, with permission, from Adams (1961).

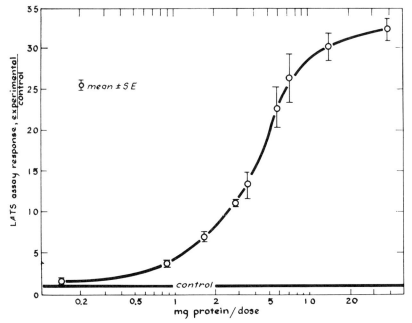

FIG. 4. The full range of the LATS dose-response curve. Reproduced, with permission, from Kriss *et al.* (1964).

tence of autoantibodies to thyroglobulin. At the Second Asia and Oceanic Congress of Endocrinology in Sydney in 1963, I suggested that LATS was an autoantibody against a thyroid protein with which TSH reacts. However, it was Meek *et al.* (1964) and Kriss *et al.* (1964) who played the leading role in establishing the concept, with reports showing the presence of LATS activity in highly purified 7 S γ-globulin and a neutralizing reaction with antiserum to 7 S γ-globulin. Additionally, Kriss *et al.* demonstrated a neutralizing reaction with thyroid tissue (see Section II,E,2,d).

After Nowell (1960) had discovered the powerful effect of the plant lectin phytohemagglutinin on lymphocytes cultured *in vitro*, it was possible to demonstrate LATS production from peripheral blood lymphocytes obtained from cases of Graves' disease (McKenzie and Gordon, 1965; Miyai *et al.*, 1967; Wall *et al.*, 1973). Phytohemagglutinin appears to act via T lymphocytes through a "helper" effect presumably involving production of a lymphokine (Knox *et al.*, 1976a). The acme of evidence from lymphocyte culture came from Knox *et al.* (1976b), who showed that an antigenic stimulus provided by a component of normal human thyroid tissue can replace the effect of phytohemagglutinin in causing detectable secretion of thyroid-stimulating autoantibody by lymphocytes from patients with Graves' disease.

As LATS is not present in normal people and as the unit of immunological specificity is the *clone,* it can be stated that LATS is produced by forbidden clones (Burnet, 1959) of immunocytes peculiar to patients with Graves' disease.

6. *Incidence*

a. In Untreated Thyrotoxicosis. The first large-scale study showed LATS to be present in 54% (38 of 71) cases of thyrotoxicosis (Major and Munro, 1962). However, this was before awareness of nonspecific responses (see Section II,C,3). Significant responses were found in 29% (17 of 60) of normal people studied concurrently. This figure can be used to correct the figure for the thyrotoxic patients, which reduces the incidence to 25%, in close agreement with the 26% (10 of 38) found by Kriss *et al.* (1967) and the 26% (16 of 61) found by Pinchera *et al.* (1969). A consecutive, unselected series of 50 cases of untreated diffuse toxic goiter was studied by Adams *et al.* (1974a), who assayed sixfold immunoglobulin concentrates of negative or doubtful sera to increase sensitivity and to distinguish LATS activity from the nonspecific effect. The use of the concentration procedure increased the incidence of LATS only marginally, to 30% (15 of 50).

b. In Exophthalmos and Pretibial Myxedema. From the time of the discovery of LATS in a patient with exophthalmos, it has been found to be more closely associated with this condition than with thyrotoxicosis. McKenzie and McCullagh (1968) found LATS in 46% (30 of 65) of a series of cases of exophthalmos, an incidence in close agreement with the 45% (10 of 22) observed in the series of Adams *et al.* (1974a). Severe exophthalmos is often associated with pretibial myxedema, where LATS shows its highest incidence, being found in all of 7 cases studied by Kriss *et al.* (1964).

c. After Treatment of Thyrotoxicosis. All of the 7 cases with pretibial myxedema in which Kriss *et al.* (1964) found LATS had been treated by radioiodine or surgery. Subsequent studies (Pinchera *et al.*, 1969; Kilpatrick, 1974) showed that, in the 3-6 months after diagnosis of thyrotoxicosis, LATS levels remain unchanged or fall in the majority of patients treated with antithyroid drugs (Fig. 5). In patients treated with radioiodine, the results are significantly different, many patients showing increased LATS levels or appearance of LATS for the first time (Fig. 6). Subtotal thyroidectomy has a significant tendency to increase LATS levels (Fig. 7), but the magnitude of the effect is less than that with radioiodine treatment, and after 4 months LATS levels fell in the majority of patients (Mukhtar *et al.*, 1975).

These effects are all intelligible on the basis of the concept that destruction of thyroid cells provides an antigenic stimulus to LATS production, the prolonged damaging effect of radioiodine providing a

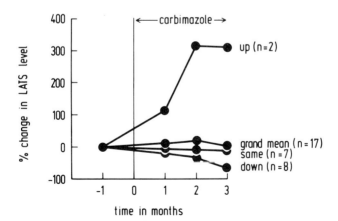

FIG. 5. The percentage change in LATS levels in 17 thyrotoxic patients treated with carbimazole. Reproduced, with permission, from Kilpatrick (1974).

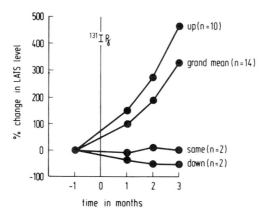

FIG. 6. The percentage change in LATS levels in 14 thyrotoxic patients treated with ^{131}I therapy. Reproduced, with permission, from Kilpatrick (1974).

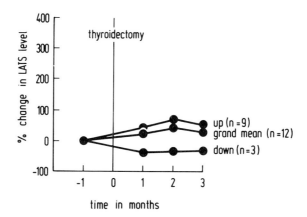

FIG. 7. The percentage change in LATS levels in 12 thyrotoxic patients treated by subtotal thyroidectomy. Reproduced, with permission, from Kilpatrick (1974).

greater stimulus than the acute damage of thyroid surgery. Additionally, the stress of surgical operation with greatly increased corticosteroid production could be expected to have an immunosuppressive effect on LATS production. With two opposing effects occurring, it is understandable that subtotal thyroidectomy sometimes produces dramatic remissions of exophthalmos (see Section IX) and sometimes dramatic exacerbations.

E. Chemical Properties of LATS

1. *Fractionation of Serum Proteins*

a. *LATS in the γ-Globulins.* The first successful study of the chemical properties of LATS was by H. D. Purves, who showed it to be in the γ-globulin fraction when serum proteins from untreated thyrotoxic patients were fractionated on a carboxymethyl cellulose column (Purves and Adams, 1961). Subsequently, T. H. Kennedy confirmed this finding, when he fractionated the serum proteins by precipitating the γ-globulins with 27% ethanol at $-7°C$. Five separate fractionations were made of three separate high-potency LATS sera; the mean recovery of LATS in the γ-globulins was 86% (73–99% for $p = 0.05$). The supernatant fractions contained the albumin and only 3 to 7% of the LATS activity (Adams and Kennedy, 1962). The advent of Sephadex G-200 fractionation columns enabled further demonstration of association of LATS with the γ-globulins (McKenzie, 1962b).

b. *TSH Is Separable from LATS.* Thyroid-stimulating hormone is a rugged, soluble, little protein that can be separated easily from the bulk of the serum proteins by application of procedures that take advantage of its resistance to denaturation. Thus, Bates *et al.* (1959) were able to concentrate serum TSH 30- to 40-fold with an alcohol percolation method in which freeze-dried serum was powdered, mixed with a diatomaceous earth (Hyflo), suspended in 95% ethanol, and packed into a column. After percolation with 76% ethanol to remove some inactive material, the TSH was extracted in high yield (e.g., 87%) by percolation with 38% ethanol containing 8% NaCl. Applying this method, Purves showed that LATS was not extracted, then, having mixed LATS and TSH, he selectively extracted the TSH (Purves and Adams, 1961).

Another TSH extraction method, based on Ciereszko's (1945) observation that pituitary TSH is soluble in 50% acetone but insoluble in 75% acetone, was developed by T. H. Kennedy and used extensively to establish serum TSH levels in various states (see Section III). This method, too, readily separates TSH from LATS (Adams and Kennedy, 1965).

2. *In Vitro Reactions of LATS*

a. *Not Neutralizable with Antiserum to TSH.* In the 1930s, when the various anterior pituitary hormones were being discovered by observation of the effects of injecting laboratory animals with extracts of pituitary tissue, it was noted that on repetition the injections tended to become less effective. J. B. Collip put forward the concept that each hormone had a corresponding antihormone, which maintained equilibrium by opposing the action of the hormone. However, the animal providing the pituitary extract and the animal receiving the injections often belonged to different species, and it became apparent that antihormones were antibodies with specificity for cross-species differences in the hormone molecules. With the advent of the adjuvants of Freund *et al.* (1948) and radioisotopes, some perceptive investigators saw the possibility of developing a method for measuring hormones by radioimmunoassay, ultimate success falling to Berson *et al.* (1956). Meanwhile, a fringe benefit was the demonstration that antisera to bovine TSH will neutralize TSH in human blood, but not LATS (Werner *et al.*, 1960; McKenzie and Fishman, 1960; Adams *et al.*, 1962a).

  b. Heat Resistance. Seeking evidence of the γ-globulin identity, and hence autoantibody nature, of LATS, McGiven *et al.* (1965) compared the heat stability of autoantibodies to thyroglobulin (thyroglobulin autoantibodies, TGaab) with that of LATS and TSH. By applying heat to TGaab for 10 minutes, at various temperatures, it was possible to construct a regular curve of residual activity versus temperature. At 60°C, 65% of the TGaab activity remained; at 65°C, 23%; at 70°C, 1.9%; and at 75°C, 0.026%. Heating for 10 minutes at 70°C reduced LATS potency to less than 10% ($p < 0.001$), comparable to the effect on TGaab, whereas TSH potency was reduced only to 45% (79; 26 for $p = 0.05$). Thus LATS was found to resemble TGaab and to differ from TSH in its susceptibility to heat.

  c. Neutralizable with Antiserum to γ-Globulins. Meek *et al.* (1964) and Kriss *et al.* (1964), in their studies of the chemical nature of LATS, showed that antiserum to human 7 S γ-globulin made in rabbits or sheep, will neutralize LATS, but not TSH. This was confirmed by Adams and Sharard (1965).

  d. Neutralizable with Thyroid Homogenate. The concept that LATS is a thyroid autoantibody presumes its reaction with a thyroid cell autoantigen. Finding that it was not possible to demonstrate neutralization of TSH by incubation with thyroid gland homogenate, the author was discouraged from making similar studies with LATS. However, Kriss *et al.* (1964) had no such inhibition. With dog tissue homogenates, they showed that thyroid tissue would reduce LATS potency significantly and that other tissues, including kidney, liver, adrenal, and spleen, were at least 10 times weaker in this activity. This fundamentally important observation, which was to provide the basis of much subsequent progress, was soon confirmed (Beall and Solomon,

1965, 1966; Sharard and Adams, 1965; Dorrington *et al.,* 1966). The nature of the LATS autoantigen is considered in Section VI.

3. *LATS in Isolated IgG*

In an elegant study using polyacrylamide gel electrophoresis to analyze protein components, Meek *et al.* (1964) isolated γ-globulin from potent LATS sera by precipitation with ammonium sulfate followed by fractionation on DEAE-cellulose columns, achieving an approximately 10-fold purification of the LATS in a preparation containing only γ-globulin. Similarly, Kriss *et al.* (1964) isolated γ-globulin from LATS sera by fractional precipitation with acid potassium phosphate, followed by filtration through DEAE-Sephadex columns, achieving an 8-fold purification. Additionally, Kriss *et al.* (1964) showed that the components of their LATS concentrate had the sedimentation velocity of 7 S molecules and that on fractional centrifugation through a sucrose gradient the LATS activity and protein concentration coincided well.

Changing to modern nomenclature, one can state that Kriss *et al.* (1964) demonstrated that LATS was present in isolated 7 S immunoglobulin (IgG). Their claim to have "isolated" LATS was the only blemish in an outstanding research contribution. At the time of writing, isolation of TSaab, which would have to involve affinity chromatography with the specific antigen, remains to be achieved.

4. *Fragmentation of LATS Immunoglobulin G*

At the time when it was becoming apparent that LATS might be an autoantibody, the classic work of R. R. Porter and G. M. Edelman on myeloma proteins was leading to establishment of the exact chemical structure of antibody molecules. The chemists were wary of using the name "antibody" for myeloma proteins, since they arise from plasma cell tumors and usually have no known complementary antigen. The term "γ-globulin," referring to relative electrophoretic immobility, was unsatisfactory since both myeloma proteins and antibodies may be β-globulins. Hence the new name "immunoglobulin" was introduced and has become established, although it can now be seen to be superfluous because it is synonymous with "antibody."

Meek *et al.* (1964) split LATS-containing immunoglobulin into its constituent heavy (A) and light (B) polypeptide chains by reduction and alkylation (Edelman and Poulik, 1961), finding the biological activity to survive reduction and to be present in isolated heavy chains but not light chains. They also applied proteolysis with papain (Fleischman *et al.,* 1972) and found activity in piece I (Fab) but not in piece

III (Fc). These findings were in accord with those from similar treatment of known antibodies and so provided strong evidence for an autoantibody nature for LATS.

Meanwhile, supported by G. M. Wilson, who played a role similar to that of Purves in Dunedin and Astwood in Boston, D. S. Munro had begun a sustained study of the chemistry of LATS, with the aid of K. J. Dorrington and B. R. Smith. These investigators confirmed the finding that thyroid-stimulating activity is present in the Fab fragment from papain hydrolysis and absent from the Fc fragment (Dorrington *et al.*, 1965). Moreover, they showed that the time course of response to the Fab fragment was shorter than that to the intact LATS molecule. They suggested faster renal clearance of the smaller molecule as an explanation. Making further digests with pepsin, Dorrington *et al.* obtained a 5 S fragment, containing the two antigen combining sites, which they were able to reduce to two 3.5 S fragments, containing one combining site each. The time course of the thyroid-stimulating activity in these fragments was again proportional to their molecular size. The culmination of research into the chemical nature of LATS was provided by the data of Smith *et al.* (1969) shown in Table I. A highly potent LATS serum (from Mrs. C) was subjected to reduction and alkylation fol-

TABLE I

RECONSTITUTION OF LATS BY RECOMBINATION OF ITS CONSTITUENT HEAVY (H) AND LIGHT (L) POLYPEPTIDE CHAINS[a]

Sample	Assay concentration (mg/ml)	LATS assay, mean blood ^{131}I (% initial value ± SE)	
		At 3 hours	At 10 hours
LATS-IgG	1.0	549 ± 40	1133 ± 148
LATS-IgG	0.1	225 ± 46	477 ± 56
H chain	9.0	916 ± 81	338 ± 53
H chain	4.0	518 ± 35	211 ± 18
L chain	3.0	78 ± 8	98 ± 10
H chain + L chain (3:1)			
mixed and assayed	5.0	422 ± 63	193 ± 26
at pH 7.4.	0.5	103 ± 9	114 ± 13
H chain + L chain (3:1)			
mixed at pH 2.4 and	5.0	673 ± 64	1352 ± 100
assayed at pH 7.4	0.5	136 ± 21	335 ± 23
Phosphate saline	—	88 ± 5	129 ± 6

[a]Reproduced, with permission, from B. R. Smith *et al.* (1969).

lowed by separation of the heavy and light chains by gel filtration. The heavy chains showed thyroid-stimulating activity of shortened time course, the light chains were inactive. The separated heavy and light chains failed to recombine when mixed at pH 7.4, but, when the pH was reduced to 2.4, substantial recombination occurred, with recovery of more than 20% of the original activity and restoration of the prolonged time course (Table I). No autoantibody has had its immunoglobulin nature more rigorously established.

III. Thyroid-Stimulating Hormone (TSH) Levels in Blood

A. Adaptation to Iodine Deficiency and Its Consequences

Our dependence on thyroid hormone has been mentioned (Section I,A). For reasons still hidden deep in the basics of chemistry, both the thyroid hormones, thyroxine (T_4) and triiodothyronine (T_3), need iodine atoms in their molecules. This makes us vulnerable to deficiency of iodine, which is a trace element. In seawater, from whence our ancestors emerged, the level of iodine is about 20 μg/kg. Some seaweeds concentrate iodine 10,000-fold to levels of 200 mg/kg. The thyroid gland concentrates iodine, similarly, to levels around 500 mg/kg. In freshwater, iodine levels are lower than in seawater, e.g., 1 μg/kg. In soil, levels up to 1 mg/kg occur, but in many parts of the world, especially mountainous and recently glaciated regions, soil levels are low, causing iodine deficiency in the inhabitants. In primitive animals, thyroid hormone formation occurs in the gut lumen. In higher animals there is a specialized thyroid gland, responsive to stimulation by TSH from the pituitary gland's thyrotroph cells (Purves, 1966), which in turn are responsive to neural modulation by TSH-releasing hormone (TRH) from the hypothalamus (Scanlon *et al.*, 1978). This control system provides not only a better regulated supply of thyroid hormone, but also a powerful defense against hypothyroidism. Additionally, when thyroidal iodine becomes low, iodination of tyrosine becomes less complete, producing more monoiodotyrosine in proportion to diiodotyrosine, which in turn leads to increased production of triiodothyronine (T_3) compared to thyroxine (tetraiodothyronine, T_4) (Kennedy and Purves, 1956). Since T_3 with its three iodine atoms is three times more potent than T_4 with its four iodine atoms (Gross and Pitt-Rivers, 1953; Pitt-Rivers and Cavalieri, 1964), this effect enables four times as much thyroid hormone to be made from the same amount of iodine.

In the absence of TSH, the thyroid continues to function at a low level (Purves, 1964), which is why hypothyroidism secondary to hypopituitarism is less severe than primary hypothyroidism. TSH secretion, which is under negative feedback control by blood thyroid hormone levels (combined effect of T_4 and T_3), is capable of dramatic increase (see Section III,C). Because the control system incorporates a feature that is called "gain" in electrical theory (Purves, 1964), clinically unimportant reductions in blood thyroid hormone levels can provoke disproportionately large increases in TSH secretion rates. Thus, widely ranging TSH levels are found in clinically euthyroid people; the greater the iodine deficiency or thyroid gland impairment, the higher the TSH level. High TSH levels cause increased thyroid cell growth, in both size and numbers, as well as increased iodine uptake and thyroid hormone production. The T_4 to T_3 switch and the TSH effect make hypothyroidism rare, but the continual, strong stimulation of the thyroid cells by TSH exacts a toll in the form of endemic goiter (Stanbury, 1969; Ibbertson, 1979). It is my belief that goiters that fail to regress when iodine sufficiency causes TSH levels to return to normal are benign tumors, biochemically defective because their genome has been altered by somatic mutations occurring in the stimulated thyroid cells (Adams, 1978b). Endemic goiter once affected millions of people, but it is now being abolished through application of the principle of iodine prophylaxis (Marine and Kimball, 1921; Hetzel, 1970).

B. INFORMATION FROM MEASUREMENT OF HIGH TSH LEVELS

1. Distinction of TSH from LATS

Once bioassays attained adequate specificity, it became apparent that levels of TSH in the blood of hypothyroid animals and people were measurable and were above the normal level, which was not measurable (see Section II,A). In untreated thyrotoxicosis, levels were also undetectable (Hertz and Oastler, 1936), suggesting that pituitary function is normal in this condition. After his discovery of antithyroid drugs, Astwood (1949) observed the occurrence of thyroid enlargement in thyrotoxic patients who had been rendered hypothyroid by overtreatment. He recognized this as evidence of a normal pituitary response to hypothyroidism, from which he concluded that abnormal TSH secretion by the pituitary was not the cause of thyrotoxicosis. However, when more sensitive bioassays in responsive laboratory animals detected strong activity in some patients with exophthalmos (De Robertis, 1948; Purves and Griesbach, 1949; D'Angelo et al., 1951) the situation was baffling until there was awareness of the existence of LATS. In both the original guinea pig assay and the McKenzie mouse adaptation it is easy to distinguish TSH from LATS, both by the time course of the response and by incorporating neutralization tests with antiserum to TSH (Section II,E,2,a). From the beginning it was consistently observed that the high TSH levels in hypothyroid people would fall with thyroid hormone treatment, but that LATS levels would not (Adams, 1958).

2. Normal Control of TSH Secretion in the Presence of LATS

The ease with which TSH in blood can be separated from co-present LATS has been mentioned (Section II,E,1,b). Encountering a patient with thyrotoxicosis who developed a high LATS level and became hypothyroid after ^{131}I therapy, T. H. Kennedy and I studied her TSH levels in various clinical states by making 6-fold and 12-fold TSH concentrates of her serum (Adams and Kennedy, 1965). In the untreated thyrotoxic state the serum TSH level was undetectable at <9 μU/ml. In the hypothyroid state the level was 85 μU/ml (147; 47 for $p = 0.05$), falling to an undetectable level (<18 μU/ml) with thyroxine treatment. LATS was undetectable before administration of the ^{131}I therapy, but was high (mean 10-hour assay response was 983%) in the untreated hypothyroid state and did not change with the thyroxine treatment. Thus, there was normal reaction of the pituitary's TSH secretion mechanism to changing blood thyroid hormone levels in the presence of a high and unchanging LATS level, a finding incompatible with the concept that LATS was TSH abnormally bound to a plasma protein (Major and Munro, 1962). The first appearance of LATS after ^{131}I treatment is not unusual and is discussed in Section IX.

C. THE EUTHYROID TSH LEVEL

1. Raised in Iodine Deficiency

On direct bioassay of serum, the only TSH levels detectable are those occurring in hypothyroidism, of the order of 100–1000 μU/ml (Table II). T. H. Kennedy and I set out to find the level in euthyroidism by collecting large volumes of pooled serum from groups of euthyroid people and making TSH extracts of sufficient purity to enable the making of concentrates potent enough to assay. At this time, it had been shown that iodine-deficient people in the Andes had hyperactive thyroid glands as measured by ^{131}I uptake and secretion (Stanbury et al., 1954). It was believed that this hyperactivity was mediated by increased blood TSH

TABLE II

SERUM TSH LEVELS IN RELATION TO THYROID STATUS AND IODINE INTAKE

Group	Serum TSH (μU/ml)	
	Mean	Range
Hypothyroidism[a]		
Babies (3)[b]	632	242–1167
Adults (22)	190	29–393
Euthyroidism		
Extreme iodine deficiency, urinary ^{127}I 5 μg/day,		
New Guinea people (22)[a,c]	57	<4–200
Severe iodine deficiency, urinary ^{127}I 20 μg/day,		
Nepalese people (9)[d]	22	<3–348
Iodine sufficiency,[e]		
urinary ^{127}I 200–400 μg/day, U.S. and New		
Zealand people (10)	1.01	0.35–2.6
Treated with T_4, 0.4 mg for 3–4 days (7)	0.31[f]	—
Treated with thyroid siccum 120 mg/day for		
4 months (1)	0.07[f]	—

[a] Adams *et al.* (1971).

[b] Number of people is given in parentheses.

[c] Adams *et al.* (1968).

[d] Samples were provided by Professor H. K. Ibbertson (see Ibbertson, 1979).

[e] Adams *et al.* (1972).

[f] Maximal value, immunoassay in nonspecific range; true value could be lower.

levels, but this had not been demonstrated. In New Guinea, A. Querido and his colleagues were investigating people suffering from very severe endemic goiter. These people proved to be the most iodine-deficient ever encountered on this planet, with urinary ^{127}I excretions averaging less than 5 μg/day (Choufoer *et al.*, 1963, 1965), compared to values of 200–400 for iodine-sufficient people in the United States and New Zealand (Table II).

As a preliminary to the more difficult measurement of serum TSH levels in euthyroid, iodine-sufficient people, Kennedy and I collaborated with Querido's group to make the first measurements of TSH levels in an iodine-deficient population, the New Guinea people, by using bioassay of concentrated extracts (see Section III,C,2,a) of single or pooled sera when direct assay of single serum samples was negative (Adams *et al.*, 1968). Some of the New Guinea people were clinically hypothyroid, and these were found to have high TSH levels, comparable to those of similar people in New Zealand. The clinically euthyroid people had low plasma T_4 values, depending on raised plasma T_3 for their euthyroidism (Ibbertson, 1979) (see Section III,A). In one clinically euthyroid subject the serum TSH level was in the range for hypothyroidism at 194 μU/ml, but in all the others it was undetectable on direct assay. However, assay of 6-fold (10-fold volume reduction with 60% recovery) concentrates showed the serum TSH levels to range from 123 μU/ml to less than 41, with a mean value for the whole group of 54 μU/ml (Adams et al., 1968). Subsequent studies of these sera by radioimmunoassay, in collaboration with R. D. Utiger, gave figures in agreement with those from bioassay, the combined estimate of the mean level being 57 μU/ml, with a range from <4 to 200 (Adams et al., 1971) (Table II).

An interesting comparison was afforded by serum samples from severely goitrous people in Nepal, studied by a team led by H. K. Ibbertson (1979). These people had more iodine than those in New Guinea, but were still grossly deficient, with urinary ^{127}I excretions averaging 20 μg/day. Two clinically hypothyroid subjects had TSH levels in the hypothyroid range at 561 and 424 μU/ml. Of nine clinically euthyroid subjects, one showed a high level at 348 μU/ml. In the remaining eight, immunoassay of TSH concentrates showed values ranging from <3 to 20, with a mean of 5, rising to 22 μU/ml with inclusion of the subject with the high level (Table II).

2. The Level in Iodine-Sufficient People

a. *TSH Extraction Method.* The first measurements of the serum TSH level in euthyroid, non-iodine-deficient people were made by bioassay of concentrated extracts made from pooled serum obtained from groups of people (Adams and Kennedy, 1968; Adams et al., 1969). Kennedy used a two-stage procedure for extracting the TSH. The first stage, in outline, involved precipitation of the bulk of the serum proteins with 50% acetone, the TSH remaining in the supernatant, from which it was precipitated by raising the acetone concentration to 75%. From this second precipitate the TSH was extracted with water and ammonium acetate solution. The extract contained about one-fiftieth of the original serum protein with about 60% of the TSH, giving a 30-fold purification. This was insufficient, so Kennedy developed a second-stage procedure, which was similar to the first but performed at acid pH. The recovery of TSH through the second-stage procedure was also about 60%, with one-tenth of the protein, giving a further 6-fold purification. Thus, through the two stages there was a 500-fold reduction in protein content with recovery of about 35% of the serum TSH, giving a purification factor of about 180.

b. Bioassay of Extracts of Pooled Euthyroid Sera. A group of 22 euthyroid volunteers, 11 men and 11 women, were bled to provide a pool of 1500 ml of serum. Subsequently, each person took 0.4 mg of thyroxine daily for a week, at the end of which time each subject was bled again to provide another serum pool of 2000 ml. The TSH was extracted from the serum pools by the two-stage procedure, to give concentrates in volumes of 3.0 ml, which were assayed. To establish the specificity of any activity found, a portion of each concentrate was incubated with neutralizing antiserum to TSH before assay, and assay responses were measured at both 2 hours and 10 hours after injection of test materials. To enable measurement of the amount of any activity found, standard human TSH was assayed concurrently in a range of doses differing from each other by a factor of 4.

The concentrate from the untreated euthyroid people elicited a significant response at 2 hours, reduced at 10 hours ($p<0.02$) and abolished by the incubation with antiserum to TSH ($p<0.05$). This established the activity as due to TSH. A three-point assay calculation against the bracketing doses of standard TSH, with corrections for volume reduction and recovery (35%) indicated a TSH level in the original pooled serum of 0.35 μU/ml. There was no activity in the concentrate from the thyroxine-treated people, and, allowing for the somewhat greater volume reduction employed, the TSH content of the pooled serum was calculated as being significantly less than 0.26 μU/ml ($p<0.05$).

c. Immunoassay of Extracts of Individual Euthyroid Sera. The invention of radioimmunoassay by Berson *et al.* (1956) has been mentioned (Section II,E,2,a). Its application to the measurement of TSH was pioneered by Odell *et al.* (1965) and Utiger (1965). Unfortunately, the sensitivity is insufficient for direct measurement of the euthyroid level (Adams *et al.*, 1972). However, the small volumes of sera required for immunoassay and the greater sensitivity over the bioassay make possible measurement of euthyroid levels in extracts of sera from individual people. Such measurements were made by Adams *et al.* (1972) using Kennedy's one-stage TSH extraction procedure. It was necessary to take 150 ml of blood from each person to provide 40 ml of serum for reduction to 1 ml of concentrated extract. With recovery of 60%, the concentration of TSH was 24-fold. The mean serum TSH level found in 10 euthyroid subjects was 1.01 μU/ml, the individual values ranging from 0.35 to 2.6 (Table II). Treatment of the subjects with thyroid hormone reduced the TSH level significantly ($p<0.005$), whereas such treatment had no effect on values determined by direct immunoassay of unfractionated serum. The study demonstrated that immunoassay values below about 5 μU/ml. are caused by nonspecific reaction and do not indicate TSH content.

D. The TSH Level in Untreated Thyrotoxicosis

1. *Bioassay of an Extract of Pooled Thyrotoxic Sera*

With the development of Kennedy's TSH extraction method, it at last became feasible to attempt a comparison of TSH levels in the blood of euthyroid and untreated thyrotoxic people (Adams *et al.*, 1969). Large blood samples were taken from 39 patients with unequivocal thyrotoxicosis, before the institution of any therapy. This provided a pool of 2680 ml of serum, which was reduced to 3.0 ml of concentrated extract by Kennedy's two-stage procedure (Table III). For comparison,

TABLE III

DEMONSTRATION OF BELOW NORMAL TSH LEVEL IN THE BLOOD OF UNTREATED THYROTOXIC PEOPLE[a]

Starting material	Volume of TSH concentrate (ml)	Material assayed (dose/mouse)	No. of mice	Mean 2-hr response
2545 ml of pooled serum from 19 euthyroid people	3.0	Concentrate, 0.27 ml		
		+0.03 ml saline	5	49± 12
		+0.03 ml antiserum[b]	4	−5± 4
2680 ml of pooled serum from 39 untreated thyrotoxic people	3.0	Concentrate, 0.27 ml		
		+ 0.03 ml saline	5	−9± 3
		+ 0.3 ml antiserum	4	−10± 3

3-Point assay calculation:

$$b = \frac{125 - 39}{\log 4} = 143$$

$$X = \frac{Y-a}{b} = \frac{49-39}{143} = 0.06993$$

antilog = 1.175

TSH standard[d] in saline

12 μU in 0.3 ml	9	−4± 8
48 μU in 0.3 ml	3	39± 17
192 μU in 0.3 ml	8	125± 15

Recovery of TSH through concentration procedure = 38%

Potency of euthyroid serum $= 48 \times 1.175 \times \frac{3.0}{0.27} \times \frac{100}{38} \times \frac{1}{2545} = 0.65$ μU/ml (1.8, 0.24, $p = 0.05$).

Significance of difference between euthyroid and thyrotoxic concentrates is $p < 0.01$.

[a] From Adams *et al.* (1969), with permission.
[b] Rabbit antiserum to human pituitary TSH.
[c] Standard error of mean.
[d] Human Thyrotrophic Hormone Research Standard A, 1966, National Institute for Medical Research, London.

a pool of 2545 ml of serum from 19 euthyroid people was extracted similarly to make the euthyroid concentrate, also of 3.0 ml. The assay is shown in Table III. The euthyroid concentrate showed activity that was significantly reduced by incubation with antiserum to TSH ($p<0.01$). The thyrotoxic concentrate failed to elicit a response, its effect differing significantly from that of the euthyroid concentrate ($p<0.01$). The potency of the euthyroid concentrate was determined by applying the formula for a three-point assay. With adjustment for the volume reduction and the recovery (38%), the TSH content of the euthyroid serum pool was calculated to be 0.65 μU/ml, with confidence limits of 1.8 and 0.24 for $p=0.05$ (Table III). This value is in agreement with the mean (1.01 μU/ml) found subsequently on immunoassay of TSH concentrates from individual euthyroid people (Table II).

The sensitivity of the TSH assay shown in Table III was less than usual. This was because the author, anxious to improve sensitivity, had increased the daily thyroxine dosage to the assay mice from 5 μg to 10 μg. The effect was the reverse of that intended, as iodide from excessive thyroxine has an inhibitory effect on the sensitivity of the mouse thyroid to TSH and LATS (Sharard et al., 1970; Florsheim et al., 1970; Shishiba et al., 1974). Fortunately, the degree of concentration applied to the euthyroid serum pool was sufficient to make the lack of sensitivity unimportant, but the incident is illustrative of the hazards that beset original work.

2. Immunoassay of Extracts of Individual Thyrotoxic Sera

In the course of an investigation of iodine-induced thyrotoxicosis in Tasmania (see Section V,E), the TSH content of individual sera from 20 cases of untreated thyrotoxicosis was studied by immunoassay of Kennedy's one-stage TSH extracts (Adams et al., 1975). The patients included cases of toxic adenoma as well as cases of Graves' disease. Each was bled 150 ml to provide 45 ml of serum, which was reduced to 1 ml of extract, a 27-fold concentration, allowing for the 60% recovery. No extract showed a TSH content above the nonspecific limit of 5 μU/ml. The calculated serum values ranged from a spurious 0.15 to <0.06 μU/ml. Similar extracts from three euthyroid controls showed 15.9, 21.9, and 18.9 μU/ml, giving serum values of 0.59, 0.81, and 0.70 μU/ml.

3. Implications of Findings with TSH

Thus, there is comprehensive evidence that serum TSH levels are below normal in the hyperthyroidism of Graves' disease as well as in toxic adenoma. This is in accord with cytological evidence that the pituitary thyrotrophs are inhibited in Graves' disease (Murray and Ezrin, 1966) and with the everyday experience that in this disorder there is no response to TSH-releasing hormone (TRH) (Scanlon *et al.*, 1978). This evidence is an important complement to that concerning the pathogenic role of thyroid-stimulating autoantibodies, presented in Section V.

E. Diagnostic Measurements of TSH

It is unfortunate that the immunoassay for TSH, which is inexpensive and suited to the performance of large numbers of tests, lacks the sensitivity to distinguish normal from subnormal levels, as this would be a more convenient test for mild hyperthyroidism than the currently used TRH test. From the data referred to above, and with recent advances in technology, it seems possible that a TSH-extraction-microimmunoassay system could be devised that would enable distinction between normal and lower blood TSH levels in more conveniently sized (20–30ml) samples of blood. Patel *et al.* (1971) have shown that the sensitivity of the TSH immunoassay can be increased by using smaller amounts of labeled TSH and antiserum.

IV. LATS Protector

A. A Puzzling New Autoantibody

Under the impression that the inability to demonstrate LATS in many severe cases of Graves' disease was due to a lack of sensitivity of the bioassay, together with variable degrees of thyroid gland impairment by coexistent autoimmune thyroiditis, I was anxious to find a means of distinguishing small responses to LATS from nonspecific effects in the assay (see Section II,C,3). When TSH present in strong protein solutions, such as serum, is assayed, demonstration of neutralization by specific antiserum is a satisfactory way of establishing the specificity of small responses. The discovery by Kriss *et al.* (1964) that LATS can be neutralized by incubation with thyroid gland homogenates suggested an analogous procedure for demonstrating the specificity of small responses to LATS. However, an attempt to utilize this device was foiled because LATS sera were found to show a variable resistance to neutralization with thyroid extracts, unrelated to LATS potency (Adams and Kennedy, 1967) (Table IV). Inclined to think of LATS as an entity of constant properties, albeit varying widely in titer

TABLE IV

VARIABLE NEUTRALIZATION OF LATS IN DIFFERENT SERA, ON INCUBATION WITH
THYROID EXTRACT[a]

Material assayed, dose/mouse made up to 0.5 ml with saline	No. of mice	Mean 17-hr response[b]	p for difference	Neutralization
Mrs. M. F.'s serum, 60 µl				
Alone	3	645 ± 50		
+30 µl of thyroid extract	5	22 ± 16	<0.001	Complete
Mr. L. M.'s serum, 450 µl				
Alone	6	422 ± 59		
+50 µl of thyroid extract	6	228 ± 22	<0.02	Partial
Mr. W. P.'s serum, 180 µl				
Alone	6	204 ± 20		
+50 µl of thyroid extract	7	246 ± 52	NS[c]	None
+200 µl of thyroid extract	7	34 ± 19	<0.001	Complete
Mrs. M. G.'s serum, 450 µl				
Alone	5	6 ± 10		
+50 µl of thyroid extract	5	5 ± 11		
Mrs. M. G.'s globulin, 450 µl of 9-fold concentrate				
Alone	5	442 ± 78		
+50 µl of thyroid extract	5	589 ± 48	NS	None
Saline, 500 µl	4	14 ± 4		

[a]Reproduced, with permission, from Adams and Kennedy (1967).
[b]Errors shown are standard errors of the means.
[c]NS, not significant.

among patients (a mistaken view, appropriate to hormones but not to antibodies) I suspected the existence of an interfering substance. In Table IV, it can be seen that serum from Mrs. M.G. was inactive on direct assay but showed LATS, resistant to neutralization, in a 9-fold globulin concentrate. This serum was mixed with a potent LATS serum (Mrs. M.F.) in the proportion of 8 volumes to 1, before addition of a minimal amount of thyroid extract and incubation at 36°C for 20 minutes. Neutralization of the LATS was blocked (Table V). Fractionation of Mrs. M.G.'s serum by ammonium sulfate precipitation and chromatography on DEAE-cellulose showed the blocking activity to be in the immunoglobulins (Table VI). Serum and immunoglobulin preparations from normal people were inactive, but in thyrotoxic people the blocking activity was found to be more prevalent than LATS itself (Adams and Kennedy, 1967).

What was this blocking agent? Since it was an immunoglobulin, reactive with a thyroid tissue component and present only in people with thyrotoxicosis, it appeared to be another thyroid autoantibody.

TABLE V

EFFECT OF SERUM FROM A THYROTOXIC PATIENT IN BLOCKING THE NEUTRALIZATION OF LATS
BY THYROID EXTRACT[a]

Material assayed, dose/mouse made up to 0.5 ml with saline	No. of mice	Mean 17-hr response[b]	p for difference
LATS serum, 50 µl (Mrs. M. F.)			
Alone	6	339 ± 63	<0.05
+50 µl thyroid extract	4	−32 ± 13	NS
+400 µl Mrs. M. G.'s serum	6	534 ± 93	NS
+400 µl Mrs. M. G.'s serum +50 µl thyroid extract	5	357 ± 34	
Mrs. M. G.'s serum, 400 µl	5	56 ± 21	
Saline	4	−12 ± 12	

[a] Reproduced, with permission, from Adams and Kennedy (1967).
[b] Errors shown are standard errors of the mean.

Because its presence did not in the least impair the stimulatory activity of LATS in the assay mouse, it clearly did not block the reaction between LATS and the thyroid *in vivo.* Yet it did so *in vitro,* protecting LATS from neutralization. Therefore, the name "LATS protector" was chosen. It was postulated that LATS possessed two sites reactive with the thyroid cell, one stimulatory, absent from LATS protector, the other binding, shared by LATS protector (Adams and Kennedy, 1967).

TABLE VI

ACTIVITY OF PURIFIED γ-GLOBULIN FROM A THYROTOXIC PATIENT IN BLOCKING THE
NEUTRALIZATION OF LATS[a]

Material assayed, dose/mouse made up to 0.5 ml with saline	No. of mice	Mean 17-hr response[b]	p for difference
LATS serum, 60 µl (Mrs. M. F.)			
Alone	5	810 ± 93	<0.001
+ 60 µl of thyroid extract	6	1 ± 5	
+180 µl of γ-globulin (Mrs. C. C.) +60 µl of thyroid extract	6	207 ± 31	<0.001 <0.001
γ-globulin 180 µl (Mrs. C. C.)	5	−14 ± 6	
Saline	5	−23 ± 8	

[a] Reproduced, with permission, from Adams and Kennedy (1967).
[b] Errors shown are standard errors of the means.

B. A LETTER FROM DEBORAH DONIACH

The LATS protector phenomenon might have lain fallow for years but for the intervention of Dr. Deborah Doniach, who wrote to the author as follows: "London, May 5th, 1967. I wonder why you assume that the new LATS blocking antibody is not active *in vivo?* It could be more species specific and therefore not show up in the mouse test, yet still have stimulating properties on the human thyroid."

C. DEMONSTRATION OF THE SPECIES SPECIFICITY OF LATS PROTECTOR

Dr. Doniach's brilliant insight could be seen immediately to be logically flawless. An obvious way to test it was to perform the LATS protector reaction with mouse thyroid tissue in place of human thyroid tissue. This posed a supply problem. A typical mouse thyroid gland weighs 1.5 mg compared to 50 g for a human thyrotoxic thyroid, which was our usual source of neutralizing extracts. In our first test we used an extract made from 1000 mouse thyroid glands—it failed to neutralize the LATS. We then decided to harvest thyroids of goitrous mice, after 3 months' treatment with 0.01% methylthiouracil, administered in the drinking water. This treatment succeeded in increasing the average mouse thyroid weight to 7 mg. Two mouse thyroid extracts were made; one from 203 goitrous mice, the other from 507 (Adams and Kennedy, 1971).

Table VII shows the findings when the mouse thyroid extracts were tested for reaction with two LATS protector sera. The mouse extracts significantly neutralized the test LATS, but did not show protector activity, fulfilling Dr. Doniach's prediction.

This finding was of critical conceptual significance. If LATS protector did not react with the mouse thyroid, its lack of stimulatory activity in the mouse bioassay had an explanation that left open the possibility of a stimulating reaction with the human thyroid. From being merely the cause of an obscure, peripheral phenomenon, LATS protector became a strong candidate for the causative role in autoimmune thyrotoxicosis. Section V tells how this possibility was explored.

V. THYROID-STIMULATING AUTOANTIBODIES (TSaab) AS THE CAUSE OF THE HYPERTHYROIDISM OF GRAVES' DISEASE

Armed with the awareness that thyroid-stimulating autoantibodies could show a deceptive variation in species specificity (Section IV), the author and his colleagues set out to study the incidence and role of LATS protector, which could now be seen as a possible human

TABLE VII
ABSENCE OF LATS PROTECTOR EFFECT WHEN MOUSE THYROID EXTRACT WAS USED INSTEAD
OF HUMAN THYROID EXTRACT[a]

Assay	Materials assayed, dose/mouse, made up to 500 μl with saline	No. of mice	Mean response[b]	
1	LATS serum Wo, 17 μl	6	404	$p<0.01$
	LATS + human thyroid extract P, 50 μl	6	1	
	LATS + human thyroid extract P, 50 μl,			$p<0.001$
	+ serum C, 363 μl	6	265	
	Serum C alone	6	-14	
2	LATS serum Wo, 25 μl	15	1089	$p<0.001$
	LATS + mouse thyroid extract, 135 μl	9	588	
	LATS + mouse thyroid extract, 135 μl,			NS
	+ serum C, 340 μl	8	629	
	Serum C alone	3	24	
3	LATS serum Wo, 30 μl	5	1509	$p<0.001$
	LATS + human thyroid extract P, 65 μl	5	550	
	LATS + human thyroid extract P, 65 μl,			$p<0.01$
	+ serum C, 410 μl	5	1100	
	LATS + serum C, 410 μl	5	1165	
4	LATS serum Wo, 12.5 μl	10	600	$p<0.001$
	LATS + human thyroid extract H, 8 μl,	10	240	
	LATS + human thyroid extract H, 8 μl,			$p<0.01$
	+ serum Wb, 350 μl	10	376	
	Serum Wb alone	5	7	
5	LATS serum Wo, 12.5 μl	20	625	$p<0.002$
	LATS + mouse thyroid extract, 125 μl	16	360	
	LATS + mouse thyroid extract, 125 μl,			NS
	+ serum Wb, 260 μl	16	311	
	Serum Wb alone	12	-6	

[a] Reproduced, with permission, from Adams and Kennedy (1971).
[b] Percentage increase in mouse blood ^{125}I 17 hours after injection of the test materials.

thyroid-stimulating autoantibody, not cross-reactive with the mouse thyroid and therefore invisible in the LATS bioassay.

A. INCIDENCE OF TSaab

From the time of its discovery, LATS protector was noted to be absent from normal people and present in thyrotoxic people more frequently than LATS (Adams and Kennedy, 1967). After recognition of its possible causative role, LATS protector was tested for (see Section VII) in 20 diagnostically unequivocal, LATS-negative cases of thyrotoxicosis (Adams and Kennedy, 1971). In 14 of the cases, LATS protector was found on test of the serum. In the remaining 6 cases the serum was negative, but significant activity was present on test of a 10-fold immunoglobulin concentrate. No case was negative.

In collaboration with R. D. H. Stewart, Kennedy and I made a more comprehensive study, involving 50 consecutive cases of diffuse toxic goiter (Adams et al., 1974a). LATS and LATS protector were tested for in serum samples and, if these were negative, in 10-fold (volume reduction) immunoglobulin concentrates (Table VIII). Clinical diagnosis was supplemented by measurements of serum thyroxine, corrected for variation in the capacity of the binding proteins (free thyroxine index, Clark and Horn, 1965), and measurements of thyroid ^{131}I uptake at 1 hour, expressed as the rate factor (k_1) of Oddie et al. (1955). As usual, because the severity of thyrotoxicosis shades imperceptibly into the normal state, the diagnosis was in doubt in some cases, seven of which are included in Table VIII. One doubtful case showed LATS, another showed LATS protector, the remainder were negative for TSaab, forming group III in Table VIII. Details of the individual cases are reported in the paper by Adams et al. (1974b).

From Table VIII, it can be seen that LATS was present in 15 patients (30%), all of whom also had LATS protector (see Section VII for description of measurements of TSaab). LATS protector alone was present in 30 patients (60%), making a total incidence of 45 out of 50 (90%). The group of patients with LATS did not differ significantly in any feature from the group with LATS protector only, but the LATS group showed more exophthalmos (67% versus 40%) together with higher mean values for free T_4 index and thyroid ^{131}I uptake. The last two differences resulted from fewer mild cases in the LATS group. All three differences could be significant in a larger series.

The group of five patients without TSaab differed from the other two groups in having significantly lower mean values for free T_4 index ($p < 0.005$) and thyroid ^{131}I uptake ($p < 0.01$), together with significantly larger thyroid size ($p < 0.005$). When this difference in the two-dimensional scan area is adjusted to three dimensions, the magnitude becomes a factor of approximately 2. The author feels that at least some of these five cases had diffuse, autonomously functioning adenomas (toxic adenomas). Deborah Doniach would suspect the presence of TSaab that stimulate thyroid growth rather than thyroid secretion (Doniach and Marshall, 1977). This is discussed further in Sections V,E and VIII.

TABLE VIII

INCIDENCE OF TSaab AND RELATIONSHIP TO INDICES OF THYROID ACTIVITY IN 50 CONSECUTIVE CASES OF DIFFUSE TOXIC GOITER[a]

Group	TSaab present	No. of patients	Mean age	Sex F:M	No. with exophthalmos	Thyroid size[b]	Free T$_4$ index[c]	Thyroid ^{131}I uptake[d]
I	LATS and LATS protector	15 (30%)	45	12:3	10 (67%)	22.9±1.9[e]	29.5±2.3	14.6±1.4
II	LATS protector only	30 (60%)	45	25:5	12 (40%)	21.6±1.6	27.3±1.7	11.1±1.6
III	Neither	5 (10%)	51	4:1	1 (20%)	33.6±2.0	15.0±1.3	2.3±0.5
		50 (100%)		41:9	23 (46%)			

[a] Adams et al. (1974a), with permission.

[b] Area in square centimeters measured by planimetry of ^{m}Tc pertechnetate scan.

[c] Serum T$_4$ by protein-binding assay × T$_3$ resin uptake ÷ 100 (Clark and Horn, 1965). Normal range up to 13.5.

[d] Rate factor (k_1) from 1 hour uptake (Oddie et al., 1955). Normal range 0.8 to 2.0 (× 10^{-3}/minute).

[e] Standard error of mean.

Looking at Table VIII, one can see how the advent of LATS protector has transformed the evidence for a causal role of TSaab in Graves' disease. With measurement of LATS only, the incidence is 30%, with exclusion of many severe cases, but with measurement of LATS protector the incidence of TSaab rises to 90%, including all but marginal cases. The data suggest that, as performed in this series, the sensitivity of LATS protector measurement must approximate, or even reach, that needed for detection of minimal pathogenic levels.

B. CORRELATION BETWEEN TSaab LEVELS AND THYROID GLAND
   ACTIVITY

A scattergram of the relationship between LATS protector levels in individual patients and their thyroid ^{131}I uptake (k_1, see Section V,A) is shown in Fig. 8. The 30 patients are those with LATS protector, but no LATS, forming group II in Table VIII. There is a significant correlation between the LATS protector and k_1 values, with $r = 0.68$ and $p < 0.001$.

The relationship between LATS and thyroid uptake was studied in 20 thyrotoxic patients, including the 15 cases forming group I in Table VIII. The scattergram is shown in Fig. 9 (Adams *et al.*, 1976). There is

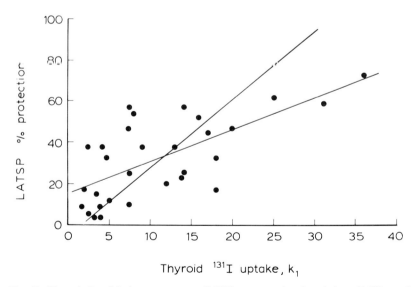

Thyroid ^{131}I uptake, k_1

FIG. 8. The relationship between serum LATS protector level and thyroid ^{131}I uptake rate factor (k_1) in 30 LATS-negative patients with diffuse toxic goiter. The correlation coefficient (r) = 0.68, with $p < 0.001$. Reproduced, with permission, from Adams *et al.* (1974a).

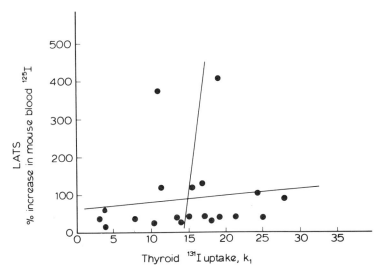

FIG. 9. Lack of correlation between LATS level and thyroid ^{131}I uptake rate factor (k_1) in 20 thyrotoxic patients. The correlation coefficient $(r) = 0.11$, not significant. Reproduced, with permission, from Adams *et al.* (1976).

not a significant correlation between the LATS and k_1 values, with $r = 0.11$. However, measurements of LATS protector (see Section VII) in these same patients did show a correlation with thyroid uptake, with $r = 0.66$ and $p<0.005$ (Fig. 10) (Adams *et al.*, 1976).

The data shown in Figs. 8–10 provide strong evidence that LATS protector is the direct cause of the hyperthyroidism in Graves' disease. What of LATS? In a series of 55 patients, Carneiro *et al.* (1966) found a significant correlation between LATS level and thyroid size $(r = 0.4, p<0.01)$ and a stronger correlation between LATS level and 48-hour plasma protein-bound ^{131}I $(r = 0.55, p<0.001)$. Other studies with smaller numbers of patients have failed to show correlation between LATS and thyroid activity. It is to be expected that LATS, which is a measurement of cross-reactivity with the mouse, should show a weaker correlation with thyroid activity than LATS protector. The finding (Fig. 10) that the presence of varying amounts of LATS did not impair the correlation between thyroid activity and LATS protector led us to postulate that LATS does not stimulate the human thyroid (Adams *et al.*, 1976). However, this interpretation shows the endocrinologist's bias toward thinking of TSaab in terms of the relative constancy of hormone molecules instead of the wide diversity of antibody molecules. We now think of LATS (cross-reactivity with the mouse) more as a vari-

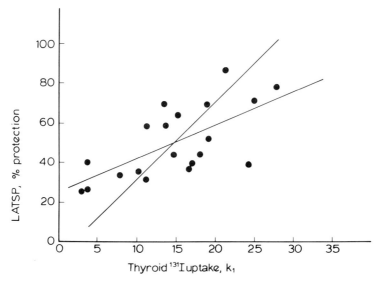

FIG. 10. Correlation between LATS protector level and thyroid ^{131}I uptake rate factor (k_1) in 20 thyrotoxic patients with detectable LATS levels. The correlation coefficient (r) = 0.66, with $p < 0.005$. Reproduced, with permission, from Adams *et al.* (1976).

able characteristic of human-reactive TSaab clones, rather than as the occurrence of separate clones. This is discussed further in Section VIII.

C. THE STIMULATING ACTIVITY OF LATS PROTECTOR

1. *In Vitro Effects of LATS Protector*

Shishiba *et al.* (1973) were the first to confirm the existence of LATS protector. Additionally, by demonstrating that LATS protector, applied to slices of human thyroid tissue, caused an increase in the number of intracellular colloid droplets, these investigators were the first to obtain evidence that LATS protector is a stimulator of the human thyroid. Onaya *et al.* (1973), also using human thyroid slices, found colloid droplet-forming activity in 42 of 51 LATS-negative sera from thyrotoxic people. Furthermore, these investigators showed that LATS-negative sera from thyrotoxic patients differed significantly from normal sera in causing accumulation of cyclic AMP when applied to human thyroid slices.

2. *Infusions of LATS Protector into Monkeys*

Concurrently with the *in vitro* studies described in Section V,C,1, evidence of a thyroid-stimulating effect *in vivo* was being sought in studies involving infusions of LATS and LATS protector into rhesus monkeys (Knight and Adams, 1973a). The animals were prepared similarly to the LATS assay mice, by being given tracer doses of ^{125}I iodide followed by triiodothyronine (T_3) in their drinking water to suppress their endogenous TSH secretion. Surprisingly, although an infusion of LATS had a powerful effect in raising the blood ^{125}I level in one of the monkeys, three infusions of potent LATS protector sera were inactive. This indicates the existence of a considerable evolutionary gulf between the rhesus monkey and *Homo sapiens*.

3. *Infusions of LATS Protector into Men*

At a time when it was established that there is a close correlation between the presence of LATS and the occurrence of Graves' disease, but the incomplete incidence made a causative relationship uncertain, Arnaud *et al.* (1965) studied the effect of infusions of plasma from patients with Graves' disease on organic iodine metabolism in human recipients and concluded that the infused plasma contained a thyroid-stimulating principle distinct from TSH.

To test whether this thyroid-stimulating principle was LATS protector, Adams *et al.* (1974c) performed similar studies, using four LATS protector sera of varying potency and devoid of LATS activity. The recipients, senior members of the staff of the University of Otago Medical School, were prepared analogously to the assay mice, being given 100–300 μCi of [^{125}I]iodide followed by continuous treatment with 80–100 μg of T_3 per day in divided dosage. Figure 11 shows the study using the most potent LATS protector serum (72% protection) obtained from Mrs. M.P., with very severe thyrotoxicosis. A control infusion of 280 ml of plasma from a normal person can be seen to have no effect on the blood ^{125}I level, but the LATS protector infusion produced a highly significant and prolonged increase in the recipient's blood ^{125}I level $(p<0.001)$. It is noteworthy that the concentration of LATS protector achieved in the recipient (280 ml into a distribution space of 5 liters) was equivalent to only 1/18th of the concentration circulating in the thyrotoxic donor. Infusions of two moderately strong LATS protector sera (57% and 52% protection) into two other volunteers elicited highly significant $(p<0.001)$, smaller effects, whereas a weak LATS protector serum (17% protection) had a corresponding weak, albeit significant $(p<0.02)$, effect.

The results of this infusion study conformed closely to expectation, providing strong direct evidence that LATS protector has a stimulatory effect on the human thyroid, in confirmation of the *in vitro* evidence and the strong indirect evidence. Figure 12 shows the current concept of the pathogenesis of Graves' disease, with TSaab from forbidden clones of immunocytes acting on the thyroid gland to cause stimu-

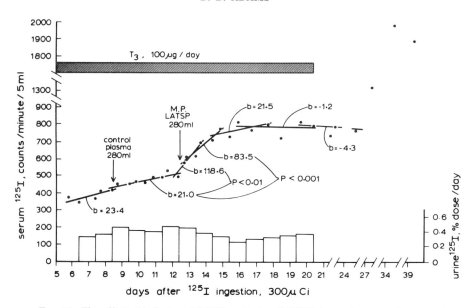

FIG. 11. The effect of infusion of LATS protector (LATSP) into a human volunteer. A control infusion of normal plasma has had no effect on the slowly rising blood ^{125}I level, but the LATSP infusion has caused a prominent and significant rise, indicating the occurrence of thyroid stimulation. Reproduced, with permission, from Adams *et al.* (1974c).

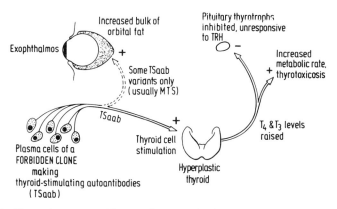

FIG. 12. The pathogenesis of Graves' disease. TSaab from forbidden clones of immuno-cytes stimulate the thyroid cells, causing overproduction of thyroid hormones (T_4 and T_3) and the manifestations of thyrotoxicosis. The thyrotroph cells of the anterior pituitary are inhibited by the high blood thyroid hormone level, so TSH secretion ceases and response to TRH is absent. Indirect evidence suggests that some variants of TSaab react with receptors on fat cells in the orbit to cause exophthalmos. MTS = mouse thyroid stimulator. Reproduced, with permission, from Adams (1978b).

lation, with overproduction of thyroid hormone, which in turn causes autoimmune thyrotoxicosis. TSH secretion from the pituitary gland's thyrotroph cells is inhibited by negative feedback action of the raised thyroid hormone levels, so blood TSH levels are below normal and there is no response to injections of TRH. Some variants of TSaab (usually cross-reactive with the mouse, i.e., LATS) appear to be responsible for exophthalmos through an action on fat cells in the orbit (see Section VIII,C,4).

D. NEONATAL THYROTOXICOSIS

Some mothers, with past or present thyrotoxicosis, give birth to babies that suffer from a transient form of the disorder, which disappears by 3 months of age (Sclare, 1960). Sometimes the condition is so severe that the baby dies before or soon after birth. If the mother is receiving antithyroid drug treatment, the baby may be euthyroid at birth and not show thyrotoxicosis until several days later. When the mother is not on antithyroid drugs, the baby is thyrotoxic from birth. The baby may show exophthalmos, if this disorder is present in the mother.

All these features are explicable by the concept that neonatal thyrotoxicosis is caused by transplacental passage of TSaab (Major and Munro, 1960; Adams *et al.*, 1964). Antithyroid drugs also cross the placenta, so when administered to the mother they provide treatment for the fetus, explaining the delayed onset of the thyrotoxicosis in babies of antithyroid drug-treated mothers. LATS was first demonstrated in the blood of babies with neonatal thyrotoxicosis by McKenzie (1964). Sunshine *et al.* (1965) measured its half-life, finding it to be 6 days.

As with adult thyrotoxicosis, LATS is not demonstrable in many cases of the neonatal condition, but Dirmikis and Munro (1975) have shown that high maternal levels of LATS protector accurately predict the occurrence of neonatal thyrotoxicosis in the baby. In a series of 18 thyrotoxic or exthyrotoxic mothers, all those with LATS protector levels of 20 units/ml or more had thyrotoxic babies, whereas the disorder did not occur in babies of mothers with levels of 5 units/ml or less. This is strong additional evidence of the pathogenic role of LATS protector in Graves' disease.

In pregnant women with present or past thyrotoxicosis, fetal pulse rate should be monitored frequently toward the end of pregnancy, so that if neonatal thyrotoxicosis occurs treatment with an antithyroid drug or propranolol can be instituted prenatally via the mother and continued after birth.

E. Iodine-Induced Thyrotoxicosis (Jod-Basedow Disease)

Thyrotoxicosis induced by administration of iodine was first re-
corded by Coindet (1821) in six goitrous patients. The condition came
to be called Jod-Basedow disease in Europe, where thyrotoxicosis was
named after its local discoverer, von Basedow. In the United States,
Kimball (1925) observed the phenomenon after introduction of iodized
salt for goiter prophylaxis, and, not for the last time, the safety of this
overwhelmingly beneficial procedure was questioned (Hartsock, 1926).
Most people do not develop thyrotoxicosis, no matter how much
iodide they ingest. Apart from the TSH-mediated negative feedback
control of blood thyroid hormone levels (which might be too slow to
protect against an "overshoot" of thyroid hormone production after
ingestion of a large amount of iodide) there are two iodide-mediated
effects that occur in the thyroid gland and are presumably protective.
First, in dosages greater than 1 mg per day, iodide has an inhibitory
effect on the incorporation of iodine into tyrosine molecules, partially
blocking the so-called organification of iodine (Wolff et al., 1949; Wolff,
1969). Second, in high dosage, iodide also has an inhibitory effect on
thyroid hormone secretion in Graves' disease (Adams and Purves,
1951; Solomon, 1954; Greer and DeGroot, 1956; Goldsmith et al., 1958)
and in normal people (Mercer et al., 1960).
A recent occurrence of the Jod-Basedow phenomenon was in Tasmania after addition of iodate to the bread to correct endemic goiter
caused by a relatively mild iodine deficiency (Connolly et al., 1970). By
this time, techniques were available for detecting areas of localized
autonomy in goiters by scanning after administration of ^{131}I, and also
for measurement of serum TSH and TSaab, enabling a detailed study
of the pathogenic mechanisms (Adams et al., 1975). Thirty cases of
thyrotoxicosis, occurring when the incidence was double that preceding the iodate prophylaxis, were investigated. All had raised serum
protein-bound iodine, and all were found to have below-normal serum
TSH levels on immunoassay of concentrated extracts. The patients
were grouped according to thyroid scan findings. In eight patients, the
presence of autonomous nodules was demonstrated by thyroid scan
appearances, before and after injections of TSH. These cases were of
relatively mild severity, and none showed TSaab. They conform to
Plummer's (1913) description of toxic adenoma. The remaining 22 patients had uniform or diffusely irregular scans without evidence of
local autonomy. This group included the more severe cases, several
with exophthalmos, and showed TSaab in 16 cases (73%), many of
whom had nodular goiters.

The high proportion of cases of toxic adenoma, 27% (possibly up to 47% if all TSaab-negative cases were included) is typical of a population with endemic goiter and is reminiscent of the situation in New Zealand before iodide supplementation (Purves, 1974). It seems likely that the increased incidence of thyrotoxicosis in Tasmania involved both types of the disorder. In mild Graves' disease, a subclinical level of TSaab could clearly become pathogenic when correction of iodine deficiency increased thyroid gland efficiency in making thyroid hormone. Similarly, an autonomously functioning tumor would increase its thyroid hormone output on correction of a previous iodine deficiency and could thus become pathogenic.

It can be stated that people who develop thyrotoxicosis on administration of iodine have one of two possible defects, either (a) TSaab, at a previously subpathogenic level; or (b) defective thyroid tissue resulting from a genetic mutation, or a somatic mutation to a benign tumor, with defective biochemical function that causes insensitivity to TSH deprivation. It seems clear that endemic goiters are benign tumors that have arisen through the occurrence of somatic mutations in thyroid cells under long-continued stimulation by TSH. Fear of Jod-Basedow disease should never inhibit goiter prophylaxis by iodide supplementation, as cases of toxic adenoma become a rarity with disappearance of goiter in general and the probable slight increase in incidence of manifest autoimmune thyrotoxicosis is unimportant compared to the morbidity caused by endemic goiter.

F. The Mechanism of Restoration of Euthyroidism in Treated Thyrotoxicosis

Thoughtful surgeons used to marvel at the regularity with which a seven-eighths subtotal thyroidectomy would restore, not near, but exact euthyroidism to a thyrotoxic patient. One would expect the result to be at best slight hyper- or hypothyroidism, but this is the exception rather than the rule. The reason is now clear, as shown in Fig. 13. The thyroid gland does not have the capacity to increase its rate of secretion of thyroid hormone by an astronomically large factor, and it is only in cases of quite exceptional severity (e.g., Mrs. C, see Section II,D,1) that stimulation by TSaab causes *maximal* thyroid secretion. Reduction of the thyroid gland by seven-eighths will lower thyroid hormone output correspondingly, and this is usually sufficient to produce a subnormal rate of thyroid secretion. Therefore T_4 and T_3 levels in the blood become subnormal, causing resumption of TSH secretion by the thyrotrophs, and, as this secretory activity is regulated, exact

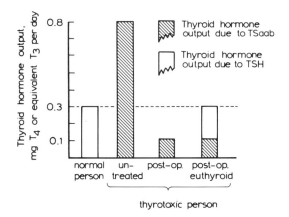

Fig. 13. The mechanism by which reduction in thyroid efficiency can restore exact euthyroidism in thyrotoxic patients, despite continuing presence of TSaab. Subtotal thyroidectomy, tissue destruction with ^{131}I, or antithyroid drug block have equivalent effect in reducing thyroid efficiency until thyroid secretion is below normal, whereupon the action of the TSaab is supplemented by a regulated secretion of TSH, with restoration of euthyroidism. Reproduced, with permission, from Adams (1965).

euthyroidism is restored. Destructive therapy with radioactive iodine and biochemical block with antithyroid drugs act analogously by also causing the reduction in thyroid efficiency (Purves, 1964) necessary to restore control by TSH. Effects of the various modes of therapy on TSaab production are discussed in Section IX.

VI. The Site and Mode of Action of TSaab

A. LATS Is a Superior Thyroid Stimulator to TSH

In many bioassays the effect measured is relatively insensitive to change in dosage, which is one reason why it is customary to make logarithmic increments in dosage while measuring the response in natural numbers. In the McKenzie bioassay for TSH, and its guinea pig predecessor, the response is unusually sensitive to change in dosage, so that natural increments in dosage are preferable to logarithmic, when working with low dosage (Adams and Purves, 1957). As mentioned (Section II,B), this suggests that the parameter measured (secretion of ^{125}I from the thyroid into the blood) is a primary effect of TSH and that the mechanism stimulated contains an amplification device to make it particularly sensitive to change in the stimulus. When LATS was discovered, it seemed remarkable in that far from being a somewhat inferior mimic of the hormone that nature had provided to stimulate the thyroid, LATS proved to be a vastly superior stimulator (see Section II,D,4 and Figs. 3 and 4). This suggested strongly that LATS acts on the mechanism designed to respond to TSH. An early explanation for both the longer and stronger action of LATS over TSH was the finding of its much longer stay in the circulation (Fig. 2).

B. LATS ACTION IS NOT MEDIATED BY COMPLEMENT

Evidence that the action of LATS is stimulatory, not cytotoxic is mentioned in Section II,D,1. In accord with this, Beall and Solomon (1966) found that *in vitro* reaction between LATS and its thyroid antigen did not fix complement. Additionally, Kohler *et al.* (1967) showed that LATS sera that had been heated to inactivate their contained complement were fully active in mice congenitally lacking a complement component (C5), which is essential for complement activity.

C. TSaab ACTIVATE ADENYLATE CYCLASE

A fascinating field of biochemical research has been the elucidation of the various mechanisms by which circulating hormones specifically stimulate certain cells, epitomized by E. W. Sutherland's identification of cyclic adenosine monophosphate (cyclic AMP, cAMP) as a secondary, intracellular messenger, mediating a hormonal stimulus. The current concept of the manner in which TSH stimulates the thyroid cell, built on clear and detailed evidence (Sutherland and Robinson, 1966; Klainer *et al.*, 1962; Dumont, 1971) shows that the hormone binds to a specific receptor on an allosteric molecule in the cell membrane. The term "allosteric," literally "another space," was coined by J. Monod, J.-P. Changeux, and F. Jacob of the Pasteur Institute to describe an enzyme that possesses, in addition to its catalytic site, another site to which a modulatory molecule binds. The phenomenon can be seen as fundamental to many regulatory processes in biology, including the activation of a binding site for complement by the reaction of the specific epitope with the paratope of an immunoglobulin molecule.

The catalytic site associated with the receptor for TSH, known as adenylate cyclase, catalyzes the conversion of adenosine triphosphate (ATP) to cAMP, which activates a protein kinase and so initiates an amplification cascade of enzyme activity within the thyroid cell.

It was of great interest to know whether LATS activates adenylate cyclase. First evidence came from Bastomsky and McKenzie (1968), who found that mice treated with theophylline showed increased responsiveness to LATS. Since theophylline is an inhibitor of phosphodiesterase, the enzyme that degrades cAMP, the effect was presumptive evidence that LATS acts through the adenylate cyclase mechanism. Definitive evidence came from two sources. Kaneko *et al.* (1970) showed that LATS increases cAMP levels and conversion of ^{3}H-labeled adenine into ^{3}H-labeled cAMP in canine thyroid slices. Using bovine and canine thyroid homogenates, Levey and Pastan (1970) also showed that LATS stimulates adenylate cyclase activity. These findings have been confirmed and amplified and used as a basis for measuring TSaab (see Section VII).

Evidence that the stimulatory activity of LATS protector on the human thyroid is also mediated by adenylate cyclase was first provided by Onaya *et al.* (1973), who found increased cAMP in human thyroid slices after incubation with LATS-negative sera from thyrotoxic subjects. This finding was highly predictable, once it was realized that the essential difference between LATS and LATS protector was one of species specificity. Measurement of cAMP accumulation in human thyroid slices is used for routine measurement of TSaab by McKenzie *et al.* (1978), who found positive results in 93% of a series of 43 cases of untreated thyrotoxicosis (see Section VII).

D. LACK OF ALLOTYPIC VARIATION IN THE THYROID AUTOANTIGEN FOR TSaab

A foundation of the modern concept of autoimmune disease is the consistent finding that autoantibodies react with normal, unaltered antigens in other members of the species, the autoreaction being due to an abnormality of immune specificity (i.e., the presence of a forbidden clone of B cells or T cells) and not due to an abnormality of antigen specificity (Adams, 1978a; Volpé, 1978) (see Section IX). However, from time to time there have been suggestions that minor alterations of autoantigen specificity are implicated in autoimmune diseases. The precision with which the TSaab can be measured makes these autoantibodies especially favorable for testing for minor variations in autoantigen specificity. In an extensive search for allotypic variation, Knight (1977) tested LATS sera from 13 patients against thyroid extracts from 10 patients. The thyroid extracts varied in neutralizing potency (TSH receptor content), and the sera varied in the amount of thyroid extract needed to neutralize a unit of LATS activity (variable LATS protector content, see Table IV) but there was no variation ascribable to especially strong or weak reactions between individual thyroid extracts and individual LATS sera. This evidence indicates that the autoreaction of TSaab with the thyroid gland does not depend on allotypic variation in the thyroid antigen. It follows that the autoantigen for TSaab is a structure universally present in man.

A study has been made of the properties of the insulin receptor on cells from patients suffering from insulin resistance due to autoantibodies to the receptor (Muggeo *et al.*, 1979). The receptors showed no abnormality, once again illustrating the principle that in autoimmune disease the abnormality lies in the specificity of host immunocytes, not host antigens.

E. TSaab BIND TO THE TSH RECEPTOR

1. *Demonstration of Binding of Isotopically Labeled TSH to a Thyroid Cell Component*

After the important concept of "hormone receptors" as identifiable molecular entities had been experimentally validated with catecholamines and certain peptidic hormones, it proved difficult to demonstrate *in vitro* binding of labeled TSH to thyroid tissue. The first success was when Schell-Frederick and Dumont (1970) demonstrated absorption of ^{125}I-labeled TSH to isolated bovine thyroid cells and reversal with excess unlabeled TSH. One problem with thyroid tissue is its paucity of cells, a nonhyperplastic gland having only thin layers of cells in the form of acini containing large masses of colloid.

In a superb series of experiments, S. W. Manley and J. R. Bourke, working in the department of R. W. Hawker, steadily surmounted manifold difficulties to succeed in exploring the reaction between first TSH, and later LATS, and the thyroid cell. These studies began with the utilization of K. E. Kirkham's (1962) *in vitro* bioassay for TSH. Slices of hyperplastic thyroid tissue from propylthiouracil-treated guinea pigs were used for this assay, so the investigators had available an excellently viable cell-rich preparation of thyroid tissue to use for tests of binding of ^{125}I-labeled TSH. Reversible, saturable, high-affinity (3.8×10^8 liters/mol), tissue-specific (not with kidney, adrenal, liver, testis, or salivary gland slices) binding was demonstrated (Manley *et al.*, 1972).

The next experiments involved the use of subcellular thyroid preparations (Manley *et al.*, 1974a). Hyperplastic guinea pig thyroid tissue was gently homogenized, filtered through a single layer of thin cotton cloth, and centrifuged at 800 g for 10 minutes. The supernatant was centrifuged at 10,000 g for 20 minutes to provide a pellet (10 K fraction) that was resuspended in 10 mM Tris-HCl (pH 7.4) with 1 mg of bovine serum albumin per milliliter as carrier protein. Bovine TSH (25 IU/mg) was labeled with ^{125}I by the chloramine-T method (Greenwood *et al.*, 1963). After preliminary purifications on cellulose and Sephadex columns, the labeled hormone was submitted to a critically important further purification by adsorption to the 10 K thyroid preparation and elution with 2 M NaSCN. The receptor-purified, labeled TSH and 10 K thyroid preparation were incubated together at 37°C for 30 minutes, then the bound hormone was separated from the free hormone by centrifugation after addition of a cold (4°C) solution of bovine γ-globulin and polyethyleneglycol.

Figure 14 shows saturation curves for binding of ^{125}I-labeled TSH (bound:free ratio) against dose of unlabeled TSH in the mixture. The various symbols indicate the values obtained with unlabeled TSH of

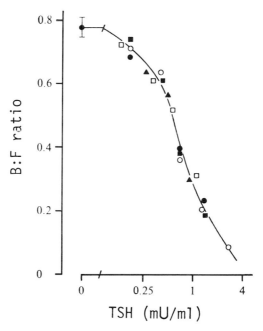

Fig. 14. Saturation curves for binding of ^{125}I-labeled TSH (bound:free ratio) to the TSH receptor in a particulate preparation of thyroid tissue. The various symbols indicate findings with TSH preparations of widely varying purity. The concordance of the various curves indicates that the effect is dependent on TSH content, not protein concentration. Reproduced with permission from Manley *et al.* (1974a).

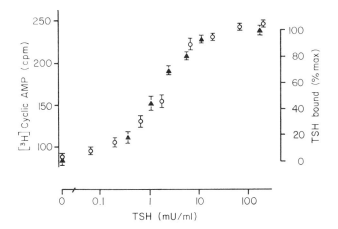

FIG. 15. The effect of dosage of TSH on formation of cyclic AMP (○) and saturation binding of labeled TSH (▲) by a particulate preparation of thyroid tissue. The concordance of the curves indicates that TSH binding is related to adenylate cyclase stimulation. Reproduced, with permission, from Manley *et al.* (1974a).

varying degrees of purity, ranging from 25 IU/mg to 3 IU/mg. It can be seen that the bound:free ratio was progressively depressed by increasing dosage of unlabeled hormone, and that the efficiency of the various TSH preparations in saturating binding was related to their bioassay potencies, not their protein content. Figure 15 shows the effect of increasing TSH dosage on the binding of labeled TSH, together with the effect on adenylate cyclase activity in the 10 K thyroid preparation. The remarkable correspondence of the two effects is strong evidence of a causal relationship between binding of TSH and stimulation of adenylate cyclase.

Meanwhile, using a very different thyroid preparation, from human thyroid tissue, Mehdi and Nussey (1975) also demonstrated saturable binding of ^{125}I-labeled TSH. The thyroid preparation was made by discontinuous sucrose-density-gradient centrifugation, the most active TSH-binding fraction being at the interface of 1.23 *M* and 0.8 *M* sucrose layers.

2. *Competitive Binding by LATS*

Using the 10 K particulate fraction of hyperplastic guinea pig thyroid tissue (Section VI,E,1), Manley *et al.* (1974b) proceeded to demonstrate inhibition of binding of labeled TSH by LATS in the form of purified immunoglobulin. The LATS IgG also stimulated adenylate cyclase activity. Figure 16 shows saturation curves for the inhibition of

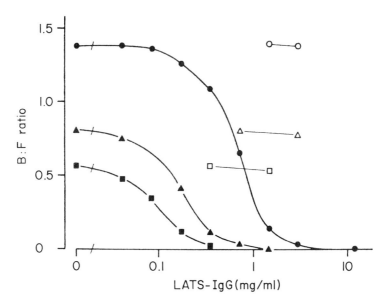

FIG. 16. The inhibitory effect of immunoglobulin-containing LATS on receptor-binding of ^{125}I-labeled TSH by a particulate preparation of thyroid tissue. Filled symbols indicate the findings with constant LATS and labeled TSH dosage and three different concentrations of the receptor preparation. Open symbols indicate the findings with control immunoglobulin. Reproduced, with permission, from Manley *et al.* (1974b).

[^{125}I]TSH binding by LATS (filled symbols) in contrast to the lack of effect of control immunoglobulin (open symbols). Curves for three different concentrations of receptor are shown, and it is noteworthy that the amount of LATS needed to inhibit TSH binding was proportional to the amount of receptor present, implying that the inhibition involved not a simple concentration-dependent effect, but a binding interaction between LATS and the receptor preparation. Scatchard plots of saturation data for TSH binding in the presence and in the absence of LATS indicated that the inhibiting effect of LATS was due not to a diminished binding affinity, but to a reduction in the number of binding sites available for combination with TSH. Finally, Manley *et al.* (1974b) used nonionic detergent (Triton X-100) to solubilize complexes of receptor and labeled TSH to enable determinations of molecular weight by gel filtration. Two sizes of complex were found, one of molecular weight 150,000, the other of 500,000. The presence of LATS did not alter these molecular weights, providing evidence against simultaneous combination of LATS and labeled TSH with the same receptor molecule.

Mehdi and Nussey (1975), using their human thyroid membrane preparation, were also able to show that LATS-IgG exerts a saturable inhibition of binding of ^{125}I-labeled TSH. These workers went on to show a correlation between the presence of TSH-binding inhibitory activity and LATS bioassay activity in sera from 10 thyrotoxic patients. Of 10 LATS-negative patients with Graves' disease, 3 showed strong inhibitory activity and 7 were negative, suggesting lower sensitivity than that of the LATS protector bioassay method.

3. A Receptor Assay for TSaab

The work of Manley et al. (1974b) and Mehdi and Nussey (1975) provided the basis of a receptor assay for both TSH and TSaab. The former was found to be of lower sensitivity and lesser convenience than the immunoassay, so has not been used. Development of the TSaab receptor assay required an active clinical environment and this was provided by Reginald Hall, who supported B. R. Smith in applying the fundamental discoveries. Smith used human thyrotoxic thyroid tissue obtained at subtotal thyroidectomy operations. The methods of Manley et al. were used to prepare a particulate receptor preparation and to purify ^{125}I-labeled TSH by absorption to and elution from the thyroid receptor preparation. Figure 17 shows the findings when immunoglobulins from various groups of patients were assayed (Smith and Hall, 1974a). The majority of the Graves' disease patients are clearly distinguishable from the control groups. A subsequent technical improvement was the replacement of the chloramine-T method of labeling the TSH by a method using lactoperoxidase (Mukhtar et al., 1975). The receptor assay of Smith and Hall for TSaab has come into widespread use for diagnosis. It is discussed further in Section VII.

F. KINETICS OF THE REACTION BETWEEN TSaab AND THE TSH RECEPTOR

Figure 1 shows the gross difference in time course of action of LATS and TSH, after a single injection into an assay mouse. Figure 2 shows that LATS has a grossly prolonged life in the circulation compared to TSH, which offers an explanation for the prolonged action of LATS. If this were the entire explanation, the two stimulators should have identical time courses in in vitro reactions. There has been controversy as to whether this is so (Doniach and Marshall, 1977).

Delayed responses to TSaab compared to TSH in in vitro systems have been reported by workers using human thyroid slices (Fig. 18) (McKenzie and Zakarija, 1977), dog thyroid slices (Kaneko et al., 1970), intact mouse thyroid lobes (Kendall-Taylor, 1972), and crude

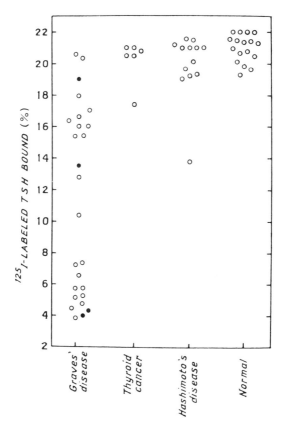

FIG. 17. The effect of immunoglobulins from patients with Graves' disease, Hashimoto's disease, and thyroid cancer on binding of ^{125}I-labeled TSH human thyroid membranes. Reproduced, with permission, from Smith and Hall (1974a).

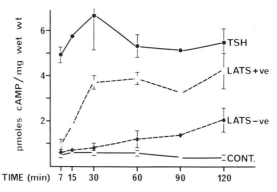

FIG. 18. Time course of effect of TSH and TSaab (LATS+ve and LATS−ve) in an *in vitro* assay based on measurement of cyclic AMP production in human thyroid slices. Dosage of TSH was very high at 50 mU/ml. This probably accounts for the faster action of TSH than of LATS (see text). Reproduced, with permission, from McKenzie and Zakarija (1977).

human plasma membrane preparations (Orgiazzi et al., 1976). However, in all these studies it seems likely that the molar concentrations of TSH applied were much greater than those of the TSaab, and this has been shown to cause a more rapid onset of effect (Shishiba et al., 1970). In the study by McKenzie and Zakarija (Fig. 18), for example, the dose of TSH used was 50 mU/ml, which is 50 times greater than the maximal blood levels of TSH occurring in hypothyroidism and 50,000 times greater than the euthyroid level. In mild thyrotoxicosis, the effect of the TSaab barely exceeds that of the euthyroid TSH level, and, because the long stay of TSaab in the circulation provides a large quantitative advantage over TSH, it is likely that the molar concentrations of TSaab in thyrotoxicosis are usually much less than the molar concentrations of TSH in myxedema. In Fig. 18, the immunoglobulin from the LATS–ve thyrotoxic patient could well have a lower content of human-reactive TSaab than the immunoglobulin from the LATS+ve patient (see Section V,A), which in turn would be expected to have a much lower molar concentration of stimulating molecules than the TSH preparation, accounting for the progressive increase in speed of onset of the effect from the LATS negative, to the LATS positive, to the TSH preparations.

Manley et al. (1974b) suggested that LATS might react with the receptor more slowly than TSH, on the basis of observed differences in the time course of dissociation of ^{125}I[TSH] from receptor combination after addition of unlabeled TSH or LATS. However, again the effect seems to be one of concentration, as the amount of TSH used was 16 mU/ml, and a 3 mg/ml concentration of LATS-IgG was appreciably faster in action than a 1.5 mg/ml concentration.

Over the years, D. H. Solomon has played a major role in fostering research on the TSaab, and from his laboratory has come a convincing and elegant comparison of the kinetics of TSH and TSaab action (Shishiba et al., 1970). Using an ionization chamber devised by W. D. Davidson, the investigators were able to monitor $^{14}CO_2$ production from canine thyroid slices, minute by minute. They observed that 1 Kriss Unit of LATS (a large dose in the McKenzie bioassay, see Section VII) was equivalent to 0.2 mU of TSH, and that at these equivalent dosages the latency of LATS action was 9 or 10 minutes, whereas that of TSH was 13 or 15 minutes. Shishiba et al. (1970) concluded that LATS is not slower in onset of action than TSH and may even be slightly faster. These perceptive authors have pointed out that the only major differences in speed of onset of LATS and TSH actions relate to speed of transcapillary movement (TSH being faster than LATS) and intravascular half-life (that of TSH being much shorter than that of

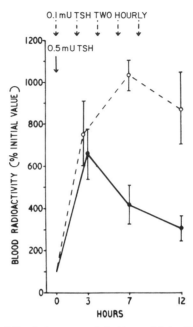

F<small>IG</small>. 19. The effect of five intravenous injections of 0.1 mU of TSH (O---O) given at 2-hourly intervals compared to the effect of a single injection of 0.5 mU of TSH, in the McKenzie bioassay. Reproduced, with permission, from Major and Munro (1962).

LATS). Studies of actions on the thyroid gland itself have unfolded a succession of similarities or identities (Scott *et al.*, 1962; Brown and Munro, 1967; Burke, 1968; Onaya and Solomon, 1969).

Knight and Adams (1973b) have studied interactions between fixed amounts of LATS, LATS protector, and thyroid receptor, incubated together in various combinations and order before assay for LATS and LATS protector activity. The findings, with both antibodies, indicated that the amount bound to the receptor after 10 minutes of incubation was as great as that after 60 minutes. After 5 minutes of incubation, the neutralization of LATS by receptor was 78% complete compared with a 93% maximum. With LATS protector, 5 minutes of incubation with the receptor gave as much protection of subsequently added LATS as did incubation for 1 hour or 6 hours. After either antibody had reacted with the receptor for 1 hour, addition of the other, even for 24 hours, caused no displacement, the neutralization or protection remaining the same as after 1 hour. The observations indicate that both LATS and LATS protector react with the receptor quickly and, unlike TSH, irreversibly.

Using the McKenzie bioassay, Major and Munro (1962) demonstrated very clearly how a prolonged action increases the potency of a thyroid stimulator, by comparing the effect of a dose of 0.5 mU of TSH given as a single injection to its effect given as five 2-hourly injections of 0.1 mU (Fig. 19). It can be seen that the maximum rise in mouse blood ^{131}I level was higher and, by integration, that the total output of ^{131}I was much greater. The hazard posed by autoantibodies reactive with a physiological receptor is apparent, since their prolonged stay in the circulation powerfully enhances their potency so that minute amounts may have deleterious effects.

G. Conclusions

Detailed evidence indicates that TSaab stimulate the thyroid cell by reacting with its surface receptor for TSH, causing activation of adenylate cyclase inside the cell membrane. The autoantibodies appear to react with the receptor at least as fast as TSH, but appear to differ from the hormone in binding more irreversibly. These effects provide a full explanation for the pathogenic action of the TSaab in causing thyrotoxicosis.

In the course of ingenious studies of the structure and function of cell membrane components, Kohn (1978) and his colleagues have found evidence that the TSH receptor is a ganglioside and that carbohydrate molecules are involved in the determination of its specificity. Future work in this field is likely to provide interesting detail on the molecular mechanisms involved in the activation of adenylate cyclase by TSH and TSaab.

VII. Measurement of TSaab

A. Introduction

At present there is no entirely satisfactory method of measuring TSaab for clinical purposes. The bioassay for LATS protector (Table IX), performed on 10-fold concentrates of serum immunoglobulins and using materials of adequate quality, seems still to be the most sensitive and dependable method (Table VIII, see Section V) (Knight et al., 1980b; Ozawa et al., 1979), but it is relatively laborious and expensive and requires 40 ml of test serum. The in vitro assays lack these disadvantages but cannot yet provide dependable diagnostic information on doubtful cases of thyrotoxicosis. The best hope for improvement would

TABLE IX
Measurement of LATS Protector by Bioassay in the Mouse[a]

Material assayed, dose/mouse made up to 500 μl with euthyroid serum	No. of mice	LATS response[b] ± SEM
Assay I		
LATS serum Archer, 20 μl, + (euthyroid serum)	6	788 ± 125
LATS + (17 μl Vaaulu thyroid + euthyroid serum)	8	90 ± 27 $p<0.001$
LATS + (thyroid + test serum Matthews)	8	637 ± 275 $p<0.01$
Test serum Matthews alone	3	43 ± 34
Percent protection for Matthews serum $= \dfrac{637-90}{788-90} \times 100 = 78\%$		
Assay II		
LATS serum Woofe, 25 μl, + (euthyroid serum)	6	913 ± 167
LATS + (50 μl of Heenan thyroid + euthyroid serum)	6	31 ± 19 $p<0.001$
LATS + (thyroid + test serum Summers)	6	973 ± 83 $p<0.001$
Test serum Summers alone	6	302 ± 69
Percent protection for Summers serum $= \dfrac{973-302-31}{913-31} \times 100 = 72\%$		

[a] Reproduced, with permission, from Knight (1977).

[b] Response is mean percentage increase in mouse blood ^{125}I level at 17 hours after injection of test materials.

TABLE X

Assays and Names for Thyroid-Stimulating Autoantibodies (TSaab)[a]

Method	Names used for TSaab activity[b]	Acronym[b]
Mouse bioassay	*Long-acting thyroid stimulator	*LATS
	Mouse thyroid stimulator	MTS
Binding to human thyroid, indirectly detected using mouse bioassay	*Long-acting thyroid stimulator protector Human thyroid stimulator	*LATSP HTS
Competition with [^{125}I]TSH for binding to TSH receptor on human thyroid	*TSH-displacing activity TSH-binding inhibitor immunoglobulin Thyroid-stimulating immunoglobulin	*TDA TBII TSI
cAMP accumulation in human thyroid slices	*Thyroid cAMP accumulator	*TCA
Adenylate cyclase activity in human thyroid membranes	*Thyroid adenylate cyclase stimulator	*TACS
Colloid droplet formation in human thyroid or in mouse thyroid using LATSP principle	*Thyroid colloid droplet stimulator	*TCDS

[a] Reproduced, with permission, from Knight et al. (1980b).
[b] Preferred names are marked with asterisks.

seem to lie in the making of improvements to the receptor assay (Section VII,D,1).

Table X lists the various assays for TSaab, together with the corresponding names and acronyms. For a fuller description of the methods of measuring TSaab, including calculation of errors, see Knight *et al.* (1980b). Here, the methods are described in outline only.

B. BIOASSAY OF LATS

1. *Principle*

Iodine-deficient mice are injected with ^{125}I, as iodide, to label the thyroid hormone in their thyroid glands, and started on continuing treatment with T_3 (triiodothyronine) to suppress their thyroid secretion through inhibition of their endogenous TSH secretion by negative feedback. After the lapse of 3 days, the injected ^{125}I-labeled iodide has been largely cleared from the blood and the thyroid gland is full of labeled thyroid hormone, ready for release. Injection of LATS triggers this, with rise in the blood ^{125}I level, which is measured as the index of activity in the bioassay.

2. *Preparation of the Mice*

Young, female, random-bred mice are housed in groups of 24, each assay using 1 to 4 groups. The animals are kept on an iodine-low diet for 2 weeks, then injected subcutaneously with 4 μCi of carrier-free $[^{125}I]$sodium iodide and 1 μg of thyroxine, which is followed 5 hours later by continuous treatment with T_3 (0.4 μg/ml) in distilled drinking water. Three days later the mice are ready for use.

3. *Performance of the LATS Bioassay*

Simple apparatus (Knight *et al.*, 1980b) is used to facilitate warming the mice to induce peripheral vasodilation so that they can be bled readily by tail vein nick with a sharp razor blade. Using acetone-rinsed pipettes, samples of 50 μl of blood are obtained and placed in glass vials containing 1.6 ml of a dilute solution of KI and KOH. The vials are capped and counted in a Packard autogamma scintillation spectrometer. Immediately after the initial bleeding of the mice, the test materials are injected, intravenously or intraperitoneally (no significant loss of sensitivity), in a total volume of 500 μl. The injection of test materials is conveniently done between 3 and 4 PM. Next morning, between 9 and 10 AM, the test bleedings are made for determination of the change in blood ^{125}I level.

4. *Analysis of the LATS Bioassay*

Table IX illustrates the use of the assay. The response to LATS is the percentage increase in the blood ^{125}I level after the test injection. Sometimes, to avoid negative values, it is more convenient to express responses as percentages of the initial blood ^{125}I level. The essence of successful use of bioassays is the strict use of statistical analysis of error, as described by Knight *et al.* (1980b).

C. BIOASSAY OF LATS PROTECTOR

1. *Principle*

LATS protector does not react with the mouse thyroid. However, since it reacts with the TSH receptor of the human thyroid, in competition with LATS, it can be measured by its effect in protecting LATS from neutralization on incubation *in vitro* with a limited amount of a human thyroid receptor preparation, prior to determination of the residual LATS activity in the bioassay.

2. *Performance of the LATS Protector Bioassay*

Table IX illustrates the procedure, the sensitivity of which depends on the quality of the LATS serum used. As well as being of high potency (e.g., eliciting a response of about 1000% in a dosage of about 25 μl), the LATS serum used needs to be readily neutralizable, so that 50 μl or less of a potent human thyroid extract will cause about 90% neutralization of the dose used. Each thyroid preparation used has to be titrated against the LATS serum used to determine the proportions in which they must be mixed because the use of an excess of thyroid extract causes neutralization of all the TSaab, both LATS and LATS protector. Dirmikis (1974) has provided clear and detailed data on factors affecting measurement of LATS protector. It is helpful to construct a table of the ingredients for the two successive incubations, both for 1 hour, at 37°C (Knight *et al.*, 1980b). The first incubation is of the test serum or IgG preparation and the requisite amount of human thyroid extract, shown in parentheses in Table IX. The control incubation is of euthyroid serum or IgG with the same amount of the thyroid extract. For the second incubation, the LATS is added, then the mixtures are injected into the assay mice (Table IX).

3. *Analysis of the LATS Protector Bioassay*

LATS protector activity is calculated as a simple percentage, as shown in assay I of Table IX. When small amounts of LATS are present, incorporation of a simple subtraction enables determination of the amount of LATS protector present, as shown in assay II of Table IX. The accuracy of this correction is testified by the close correlation between the LATS protector values obtained and the values for thyroid ^{131}I uptake in the patients being tested (Fig. 10).

D. *In Vitro* ASSAYS FOR TSaab

1. *The Receptor Assay for TSaab (Smith and Hall, 1974a,b; Mukhtar et al., 1975)*

Hyperplastic, human thyroid tissue is obtained at subtotal thyroidectomy operations for thyrotoxicosis. A crude particulate preparation of the TSH receptor is made by homogenization, centrifugation at 800 g for 5 minutes at 4°C to discard a deposit, then centrifugation at 15,000 g for 10 minutes at 4°C to sediment the preparation to be used.

Highly purified bovine TSH (30 IU/mg) is labeled with Na[125]I by the lactoperoxidase method. The labeled TSH is purified by absorption to the TSH receptor preparation followed by elution with 2 M NaCl.

The assay is performed by incubating the TSH receptor preparation with test or control immunoglobulins for 10 minutes at 37°C, after which the labeled TSH is added, and incubation is continued for a further 60 minutes. After cooling and dilution with cold buffer, the receptors are sedimented by centrifugation at 25,000 g for 15 minutes. The amount of labeled TSH bound is determined by removing the supernatant and counting the pellet. Potency is expressed as the thyroid-stimulating immunoglobulin (TSI) index, defined as the amount of labeled TSH bound in the presence of the TSI, divided by the amount of labeled TSH bound in the presence of control immunoglobulins.

2. *The cAMP Accumulation Assay (McKenzie et al., 1978)*

This assay requires inactive human thyroid tissue, which can be obtained at operations for nontoxic goiter or for parathyroid tumor. The tissue is cut into 2-mm slices, which are incubated for 2 hours at 37°C in Krebs–Ringer bicarbonate buffer (with reduced calcium ion content) with glucose, theophylline, serum albumin, and the test immunoglobulins, in a gas phase of 95% oxygen and 5% CO_2, in stoppered glass vials. After this, the slices are homogenized in cold 6% trichloroacetic acid for extraction of cAMP, which is measured by radioimmunoassay, using kits from Schwarz-Mann, Orangeburg, New York.

3. The Colloid Droplet Assay (Shishiba et al., 1973, 1978; Onaya et al., 1973)

Slices of nonhyperplastic human thyroid tissue are incubated with the test serum or immunoglobulin preparation before fixation and counting of the intracellular colloid droplets visible in sections examined under light microscopy. The method is sensitive, specific, and reasonably accurate.

E. UNITS OF TSaab AND TSH RECEPTOR

Dorrington and Munro (1964) provided the first standard preparation of LATS, made from the serum of Mrs. C (see Section II,D,1). Today, an international standard preparation, LATS B, is obtainable from Dr. D. R. Bangham, National Institute for Biological Standards and Control, Holly Hill, Hampstead, London NW3 6RB, England.

Kriss devised a very convenient and satisfactory unit of LATS, which is that amount giving a response of 15, response being the mean net blood radioactivity of the test mice, divided by the mean net blood radioactivity of control mice, at the posttreatment bleeding (Kriss et al., 1964). Thus, 1 Kriss Unit is that amount eliciting a response of 1400%, when response is expressed as percentage increase in initial mouse blood radioactivity, as in this review.

A unit of LATS protector has been defined by Dirmikis and Munro (1975) as the amount blocking the binding of a unit of LATS.

In studies of the purification of the TSH receptor, as measured by reaction with LATS, we find it convenient to use a unit of receptor defined as the amount that will neutralize 25 μl of a standard LATS serum down to a potency equivalent to 12.5 μl. As the dose-response relationships for LATS and the receptor are different, to compare receptor preparations it is necessary to use four-point assays, with two concentrations of each receptor preparation, differing by a factor of at least 4, being incubated with a single concentration of the standard LATS.

VIII. FINE VARIATION IN THE PARATOPES OF THE TSaab AND ITS IMPLICATIONS

A. DEFINITION OF FUNCTIONAL COMPONENTS OF IMMUNOGLOBULIN MOLECULES

The establishment of the exact molecular structure of immunoglobulins, led by R. R. Porter and G. M. Edelman, has immensely clarified immunology, since the structure demonstrated all the features needed to make concrete an understanding of the function of these molecules that had previously been only inferential. Before describing certain important characteristics of the TSaab, it is necessary to define the molecular structures on which they depend.

Paratope: Jerne's (1974) term for the combining site of an antibody. Its specificity depends on amino acid sequences coded for by a heavy-chain V gene and a light-chain V gene.

Epitope: Jerne's (1974) term for the portion of the antigen molecule that combines with the paratope.

Idiotope: An antigen on the variable portion of an immunoglobulin, coded for by the same two V genes that code for the paratope.

Allotope: An antigen on the constant portion of an immunoglobulin molecule coded for by an immunoglobulin C (constant region) gene. Allotopes are not of functional significance but show a genetic polymorphism and so provide useful chromosomal markers for V genes, as these are closely linked to C genes.

B. Evidence of Clonal Variation in TSaab Specificity

1. *Evidence for Multiple TSaab Clones in Individual People*

Some thyrotoxic patients show LATS protector only, others show LATS together with varying amounts of LATS protector, as judged by varying resistance to neutralization of their LATS by thyroid extracts. It is clear, therefore, that TSaab clones differ in specificity from person to person, but within a single person LATS and LATS protector activities could be properties of a single paratope. However, from general knowledge of the polyclonal nature of antibodies it is to be expected that multiple clones exist in individual thyrotoxic patients. Some evidence of this has been provided by Knight (1977) in the form of neutralization curves obtained by incubating various LATS sera with a range of concentrations of human thyroid extracts, then determining the residual LATS potency. Our two LATS sera that provide the most sensitive tests for LATS protector showed steep, monocomponent neutralization curves down to zero response. In contrast, another LATS serum showed a very gradual slope until the response was reduced to 400%, after which no further reduction occurred. This serum appeared to contain at least two clones, one of which was reactive with the mouse thyroid but not with the human thyroid. Other LATS sera also appeared to have two or three components in the neutralization curves, suggesting the presence of multiple clones with differing affinities for the human receptor.

2. *Variation in Cross-Species Reactivities of TSaab Clones*

The first indication of variation in the specificity of TSaab came with the discovery of LATS protector, which indicated that 60–70% of thyrotoxic patients lack clones cross-reactive with the mouse (Table VIII). Further variation was discovered in the author's laboratory after Allison Knight had devised an autolytic method for making potent receptor preparations from hypoplastic bovine and ovine thyroid tissue (Knight and Adams, 1976). When LATS protector tests (see Section VII) were performed with sheep or beef thyroid receptor preparations in place of human, the results showed every possible variation. Some LATS protector sera were reactive with both the sheep and the beef receptors, some with the sheep only, some with the beef only, and some with neither. This revealed what we describe as a fine variation in the specificity of LATS protector paratopes (Knight and Adams, 1980). With an *in vitro* cAMP assay, Zakarija and McKenzie (1978) have observed a similar variation in the reactions of TSaab sera with thyroid tissue from the dog, guinea pig, calf, and mouse.

C. EXOPHTHALMOS AND PRETIBIAL MYXEDEMA

1. *Clinical Description*

These two extrathyroid components of Graves' disease have long intrigued clinicians. Pretibial myxedema may cause ulceration of the skin and it may belie the topological component of its name by affecting the lower leg and foot diffusely, when it becomes a not inconsiderable disability. However, since J. P. Kriss discovered the efficacy of applications of topical steroids (Kriss *et al.*, 1964) the condition has had a satisfactory treatment.

In thyrotoxic patients, the sympathetic nervous system is overactive. The most important effect of this is on the heart, but there is also retraction of the eyelids, causing stare and lid lag, which disappear when the patient is rendered euthyroid by any means and which can be abolished quickly by the administration of a drug (e.g., propranolol) that blocks β-adrenergic receptors. The specific orbital disorder occurring in Graves' disease produces some or all of the following signs: forward protrusion of the globe (exophthalmos, synonymous with proptosis), bulging of the eyelids around the globe, dilation of conjunctival blood vessels, edema of the conjunctiva (chemosis), and weakness of one or more extraocular muscles, causing diplopia (ophthalmoplegia). The term malignant exophthalmos is used to describe exceptionally severe cases, always with ophthalmoplegia.

Treatment with parenteral adrenal steroids in a dosage of about 20 mg of prednisolone daily cures chemosis and has a prophylactic effect on exophthalmos, but little curative effect. A daily dosage of 40 mg can be used safely for a few weeks. A dosage of 5 mg twice daily can be used safely for many months and appears to play a significant role in preventing malignant exophthalmos. Conversely, treatment of thyrotoxicosis with radioiodine or subtotal thyroidectomy has a severe, exacerbating effect in some cases. Cases of thyrotoxicosis presenting with exophthalmos are best treated with low dosage steroids and carbimazole.

2. *The Studies of Rundle and Pochin*

Exophthalmos is a distressing condition for patients and used to be frightening for doctors because, before steroid treatment was available, it sometimes caused loss of sight through an infective panophthalmitis. It was difficult to understand and difficult to study. However, much of the mystery was lost as a result of ingenious studies of the mechanics of orbital filling and overflow by F. F. Rundle and E. E. Pochin (Rundle and Pochin, 1944; Rundle, 1964). Working with cadavers of thyrotoxic patients with varying degrees of exophthalmos (but no case of malignant exophthalmos) and with nonthyrotoxic, control cadavers, these investigators first noted that exophthalmos persists postmortem, indicating that it is not due to a locally raised vascular pressure. Next, Rundle and Pochin devised a means of measuring degree of orbital filling. Orbital contents (excluding the globe and optic nerve, which are not involved in exophthalmos) were measured by weight. Orbital capacity was measured by plugging the cavity with plasticine, then determining the volume of plasticine so used by water displacement. Degree of orbital filling was expressed as milligrams of orbital contents per milliliter of orbital capacity. Rundle and Pochin showed that there is a linear relationship between Hertel exophthalmometer measurements of exophthalmos and degree of orbital filling. This was a major clarification, but another was to follow, when Rundle and Pochin set out to determine the nature of the bulk increase in the orbital contents. They measured water, fat, and dry fat-free components of the individual orbital constituents. It was found that 70% of the increase in the bulk of the orbital tissues in exophthalmos was due to fat. Most of this excess fat was in the fibro-fatty residue of the orbit, and this increase was chiefly responsible for the total bulk increase in exophthalmos. The lachrymal glands also showed increase in fat content, but the tissue showing the greatest percentage increase was the extraocular musculature. Rundle and Pochin concluded that all thyrotoxic patients have a proliferation of adipose tissue cells in the eye muscles. In exophthalmos this is associated with an increased fat content of the lachrymal glands and the residual tissues of the orbit, there appearing to be a "proliferation of adipose tissue cells throughout the orbit" (Rundle, 1964).

3. *Malignant Exophthalmos*

In this condition there is ophthalmoplegia, and the protrusion of the optic globe is sufficiently great to threaten loss of sight through corneal exposure, leading to ulceration and panophthalmitis. Prior to the advent of steriod therapy, tarsorrhaphy or orbital decompression was frequently required. The striking pathological feature is a gross increase in bulk of the extraocular muscles, easily seen on computerized axial tomography scan. Naffziger (1933), who invented the first surgical procedure for orbital decompression, observed the muscular enlargement and reported histological findings from biopsy, namely loss of striation, interstitial edema, and round cell infiltration. In a more detailed study, Kroll and Kuwabara (1966) performed surgical biopsy on 10 cases of exophthalmos and 13 control cases. In all the exophthalmic cases, but in none of the controls, the extraocular muscles showed interstitial edema and infiltration with lymphocytes, plasma cells, macrophages, and mast cells. However, the muscle cells were unaffected in 9 of the cases, the remaining case showing some muscle cell disorganization and loss of striation. The authors concluded that the primary change in the muscles was an interstitial inflammatory edema and that any alteration of muscle cells seemed to be secondary to the inflammatory change.

The death, from coronary artery occlusion, of a man with malignant exophthalmos enabled Rundle *et al.* (1953) to make a postmortem study, comparable to the previous study of ordinary exophthalmos by Rundle and Pochin. This time there was striking enlargement of the extraocular muscles, which were fusiform, up to 1 cm in diameter, and of rubbery consistency. On light microscopy, it was seen that swelling of individual muscle fibers caused the enlargement. There was a patchy degeneration of muscle tissue, with loss of transverse striations and occurrence of fibrosis, together with edema and infiltration with lymphocytes and plasma cells. Adipose tissue was present in the muscles. The fibro-fatty residual tissue of the orbit also showed infiltration with lymphocytes and plasma cells. The central retinal vein was congested.

As before, Rundle and his colleagues made precise measurements of the various orbital components, this time finding that the excess bulk was solely due to the enlargement of the orbital muscles, which weighed 12.78 gm compared to a mean of 4.2 gm in thyrotoxic patients with ordinary exophthalmos and 3.3 gm in control subjects. The composition of the muscle, as regards proportion of water (81%), and dry, fat-free material (15%) was essentially normal, suggesting that "the actual muscle substance enlarges" (Rundle et al., 1953).

4. Cross-Tissue Reactivity of TSaab as the Cause of Exophthalmos and Pretibial Myxedema

The great majority of patients with exophthalmos show LATS in their blood, frequently at high levels. The correlation is much closer than that between thyrotoxicosis and LATS, which caused Kriss et al., in 1964, to postulate a causal relationship. However, occasional, severe cases of exophthalmos lack LATS, although they invariably have LATS protector if they are thyrotoxic. Pretibial myxedema is even more closely associated with high LATS levels than is exophthalmos (Kriss et al., 1964).

How could thyroid-stimulating autoantibodies, particularly those cross-reacting with the mouse thyroid (LATS), be related to exophthalmos and pretibial myxedema? In 1971, Dandona et al. aroused little interest when they reported that LATS has a stimulatory effect on the adrenal gland of the mouse, similar to that of the pituitary adrenocortical-stimulating hormone (ACTH) (see also Dandona and El Kabir (1980). More recently, Davies et al. (1978) demonstrated binding of TSaab to cellular receptors in the testis of the guinea pig. These findings suggest that cell receptors for anterior pituitary hormones have similarities of specificity, as well as differences, and that in conjunction with the differences in receptors between species, this can lead to cross-reaction between certain TSaab variants and certain non-thyroidal hormone receptors. Furthermore, bovine TSH is known to react with receptors on adipocytes from epididymal tissue of the rat and guinea pig; LATS has a similar action (Hart and McKenzie, 1971).

Although the pathogenesis of exophthalmos remains entirely unestablished, there is suggestive evidence, therefore, that certain variants of TSaab may cause the usual form of the disorder by cross-reacting with a receptor on orbital adipocytes to cause a hypertrophy of orbital adipose tissue. The finding by Rundle and Pochin that the greatest percentage increase in fat content occurs in the extraocular musculature suggests that the adipocytes in this tissue may be particularly affected. These adipocytes may have the function of providing a local source of free fatty acid for the metabolism of the extraocular muscles, whose constant, rapid activity may necessitate the use of a fuel with greater calorific value than glucose, as in the case of the musculature working the wings of a bird.

The mechanism by which TSaab variants could be involved in pretibial myxedema is more obscure. The lesions are reputed to be composed mostly of extracellular mucopolysaccharide, but reinvestigation with modern techniques, including quantitative analysis of constituents and in the light of modern concepts, is indicated.

In malignant exophthalmos the essential feature is enlargement of the extraocular muscles, which appears to be a hypertrophy, from the histological and compositional evidence. As mentioned previously, the water content and dry, fat-free content were entirely normal in the case of Rundle et al. (1953), but the fat content was reduced to 3% compared with 8% in control subjects and 16% in thyrotoxic subjects. It is tempting to speculate that an autoantibody that blocks an adipocyte receptor may indirectly cause a compensatory muscular hypertrophy by depriving the tissue of its usual supply of free fatty acid fuel. Alternatively, a muscle autoantigen could be involved.

To conclude, it seems likely that both malignant and ordinary exophthalmos are based on autoimmune reactions against orbital antigens, yet to be identified. The field invites fresh research approaches.

D. Cross-Tissue Reactivity of Forbidden Clones as the Cause of Complications in Other Autoimmune Diseases

1. Rheumatic Chorea

A highly significant recent discovery is that of Husby et al. (1976), who have demonstrated autoantibodies against corpus striatum neurons in children with chorea. These autoantibodies, or related T cells, are likely to be the cause of rheumatic chorea. They are probably products of variants of the clones that cause the heart lesions (Kaplan and Frengley, 1969).

2. Systemic Lupus Erythematosus (SLE)

Soluble immune complexes presumably form during immune response to every infection, but SLE does not usually supervene because immune complexes are not pathogenic unless they are present in excessively large amounts (Unanue and Dixon, 1967). A characteristic feature of patients who develop SLE is the possession of clones reactive with intracellular components, such as nuclear materials, that can be released into the circulation in large quantity by various agents causing cell lysis. These autoantibodies show variety in their specificity (Tan *et al.*, 1976) which could be related to the variation seen in the clinical spectrum.

3. *Ankylosing Spondylitis*

Several features suggest that this is an autoimmune disease, although the forbidden clones have not yet been identified. The disorder is now recognized as being one member of a genetically related clinical spectrum that includes peripheral arthritis, anterior uveitis, Reiter's disease, psoriasis, ulcerative colitis, and Crohn's disease (Leader, 1977). Variation in the specificity of genetically related forbidden clones could readily account for this clinical diversity.

4. *Diabetic Retinopathy and Nephropathy*

There is now strong evidence that "juvenile-onset" diabetes is based on destruction of the islet beta cells by forbidden clones (Bottazzo *et al.*, 1978). Diabetic retinopathy and Kimmelstiel–Wilson lesions of the kidney are specific for diabetes and occur in a proportion of the patients, in a manner analogous to the occurrence of exophthalmos and pretibial myxedema in thyrotoxicosis. It is possible that variants of the anti-beta cell clones are responsible for these complications.

5. *A Therapeutic Test for a Suspected Autoimmune Pathogenesis*

In distressing or fatal diseases that lack effective therapy at present, it is proper, in my opinion, to submit volunteer patients, knowingly, to experimental procedures carrying a slight risk, if the procedure is likely to provide fundamentally important information. An effective procedure for testing for involvement of autoimmunity in the pathogenesis of a disease is to submit a patient to plasmapheresis and immunosuppression. This has been done with Goodpasture's syndrome (Lockwood *et al.*, 1976) and myasthenia gravis (Pinching *et al.*, 1976) with convincing improvement, confirming the autoimmune basis of these conditions. Dandona *et al.* (1979) have reported improvement in a single case of exophthalmos. Further, more thorough trials would seem warranted in malignant exophthalmos and also in severe schizophrenia, a disorder in which several features suggest an autoimmune basis.

IX. THE PATHOGENESIS OF AUTOIMMUNE DISEASE

A. THE FORBIDDEN CLONE THEORY

1. *Origins*

A famous conceptual achievement was that of Nils Jerne (1955), when he proposed that antibody molecules are not fashioned on a template formed by an invading antigen, but are preformed, waiting to be selected by the antigen. Accepting this radical suggestion, MacFarlane Burnet introduced the concept of the immunological *clone,* a subset of immunocytes, all having identical paratopes (receptors for antigen, see Section VIII,A). Burnet's clonal selection theory of acquired immunity (Burnet, 1959) proposed that virgin clones of immunocytes circulate in the body, awaiting contact with their specific antigens, whereupon they undergo blast transformation and divide repeatedly to produce thousands of descendant cells of the same specificity. Each time a cell division occurs there is a small chance of a DNA copying error (somatic mutation), and if this occurs in a V gene (immunoglobulin variable region gene) it may cause a slight alteration in specificity. In this manner, clonal diversification occurs under pressure of antigenic stimulus.

Burnet (1959) proposed that autoimmune disease is based on the emergence, by somatic mutation, of *forbidden clones* of immunocytes with specificity for a host antigen.

2. *Tolerance Mechanism*

a. Clonal Abortion. Additionally, Burnet (1959) proposed that immune tolerance to self antigens is subserved by a mechanism that causes fetal immunocytes to be deleted by contact with their specific antigens. Subsequently, a differentiation occurs, so that, instead of deletion, contact with specific antigen causes cell division and antibody secretion.

This theory, for which Nossal has coined the apt name, "clonal abortion," has received strong support from ingenious recent work. Nossal and Pike (1975) observed that bone marrow cells from adult mice, cultured *in vitro* for 3 days, produce 5 times more plaque-forming cells against small haptens (e.g., dinitrophenol) when tested in syngeneic, irradiated animals than do the same number of cells that have not been cultured. This is explained by the inability of maturing B cells to escape from the culture, in contrast to their ability to migrate from the bone marrow *in vivo*. If the hapten, conjugated to a carrier protein, is present during the culture, at a concentration of about 3×10^{-8} *M*, there is no increase in the number of plaque-forming cells. The effect is antigen-specific and does not occur with spleen cells. It suggests strongly that immature B cells are inhibited or deleted by contact with antigen.

Other studies with further ingenious *in vitro* techniques have confirmed the resistance of adult spleen cells to clonal abortion (Metcalf and Klinman, 1976; Cambier *et al.*, 1976) but have shown that spleen cells from neonatal animals are susceptible if exposed to the antigen in the absence of helper T cells. Significantly, Teale *et al.* (1979), using a fluorescence-activated cell sorter, have shown that spleens from adult animals contain a subset of immature cells that lack surface immunoglobulin and can be tolerized by contact with antigen.

The finding that bone marrow cells from adult animals are susceptible to clonal abortion seems to indicate that host antigens circulating through the bone marrow continue to exercise deletion or inhibition of nascent reactive clones throughout life. This would explain why autoimmunity does not involve the major histocompatibility antigens, or the A and B erythrocyte alloantigens, and would also explain how Ia antigens could exert a continuing effect. Most host antigens involved in autoimmunity are surface components of fixed cells or relatively sequestered proteins, such as thyroglobulin or brain proteins. In contrast to circulating host components, invading microbial pathogens are normally sucked up lymphatic vessels and passed through a succession of lymph nodes. This provides optimal opportunity for meeting a reactive clone that is in a state of maturity and has the assistance of helper T cells and macrophages, thus facilitating a stimulatory reaction. The change from tolerogenic to reactive state may be a continuing function of location (bone marrow versus lymph node or spleen) rather than an event in chronology. Thus, the work of Nossal and other investigators on clonal abortion has immensely clarified Burnet's original, brilliant, groping concept.

b. Imperfections of Actively Acquired Tolerance. The tolerance achieved by the injection of foreign spleen cells into fetal mice in the classic experiment of Billingham, Brent, and Medawar (1953) was imperfect and inconstant, in contrast to natural tolerance (see discussion in Adams, 1978c). With some mouse strain combinations, the neonatal injections of foreign spleen cells achieves no tolerance at all (Billingham and Brent, 1957). Furthermore, actively acquired tolerance has been shown to depend on serum blocking factors (Viosin *et al.*, 1968) that are present also in chimeric animals produced by embryo fusion

(Phillips and Wegmann, 1973). These findings have cast doubt on clonal abortion as the mechanism for natural tolerance, prompting the proposal that regulator genes, acting intracellularly between parental chromosomes, may be involved (Adams, 1978c). However, the recent experimental evidence for clonal abortion (Section IX,A,2,a) is convincing. The author agrees with Teale and Mackay (1979) that clonal abortion is likely to be the predominant mechanism, but that ancillary mechanisms also exist. The most probable of these is Jerne's network of paratope-idiotope reactions (Section IX,C,4), but it is conceivable that some role is played by regulator genes.

Complete or partial failure of tolerance induction in the experiment of Billingham, Brent, and Medawar may have been due to failure of the injected cells to survive, which is now seen to be a necessary condition for continuing clonal abortion. Such survival could well depend on interclonal reactions that make certain deletions and/or provide certain blocking antibodies, as observed by Voisin.

3. Evidence from Thyroid Autoimmune Disease

The discovery of autoimmune thyroiditis (Doniach and Roitt, 1957; Witebsky et al., 1957) was of especial importance, in that it gained acceptance for the concept of autoimmunity, previously considered invalid (see Section I,E). The first autoantibodies discovered were against thyroglobulin (thyroglobulin autoantibodies, TGaab). They are noncomplement fixing and are now seen to be nonpathogenic, but at the time of their discovery they appeared to be the cause of autoimmune thyroiditis. The anatomical sequestration of thyroglobulin within the spheres of cells forming the thyroid acini provided an explanation for its antigenicity, in that it was thought to be inaccessible to developing immunocytes in the fetus. This was thought to circumvent Burnet's postulated mechanism for tolerance by clonal deletion by antigenic contact in fetal life (Fig. 20), permitting the survival of clones reactive with thyroglobulin. Subsequent onset of autoimmune disease was thought to be consequent on thyroid damage with exposure of thyroglobulin. The finding that small amounts of thyroglobulin are present in the circulation discredited this hypothesis (Roitt and Torrigiani, 1967), but it now seems likely that sequestration is one factor favoring autoimmune reaction.

Meanwhile, Trotter et al. (1957) had discovered a second type of thyroid autoantibodies, which have specificity for a microsomal component of the thyroid cell and are complement-fixing (thyroid microsomal autoantibodies, TMaab). These autoantibodies, or ones not yet discovered of closely related specificity, or cytotoxic T cells of the same

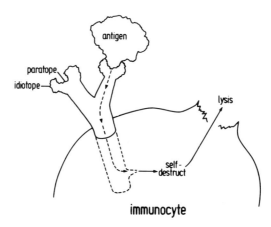

FIG. 20. The concept of clonal deletion by antigenic contact in fetal life (Burnet, 1959). An immature immunocyte is undergoing self-lysis on contact with its complementary antigen. Reproduced, with permission, from Adams and Knight (1980).

specificity, are the probable cause of autoimmune thyroiditis, which has myxedema as an inconstant long-term consequence. W. J. Irvine (1964), treating cases of thyrotoxicosis with therapeutic doses of ^{131}I, observed that titers of TGaab and TMaab regularly rose in apparent response to the increased antigenic stimulus caused by the release of antigen resulting from the damaging effect of the irradiation on the thyroid cells. This was to be expected, but Irvine noticed that in some patients one of the two autoantibodies was absent and that repeated doses of ^{131}I failed to elicit it. From this observation he concluded that autoimmunity was based on an inherited defect of immunological tolerance, present in certain people only.

At about the same time, I encountered a small epidemic of viral thyroiditis, many cases having severe thyroid damage, and waited expectantly for thyroid autoantibodies to appear. None did, from which I realized that the occurrence of autoimmunity requires a predisposition. R. Volpé, a powerful thinker, drew the same conclusion from a similar experience with viral thyroiditis and additionally observed that the thyroid damage had an aggravating effect on thyroid autoimmunity, if it were already present (Volpé et al., 1967; Volpé, 1978) (see also Section II,D,6,c and Figs. 5–7).

4. General Evidence

The consistent finding that autoantibodies occur in only some persons and that they react with normal autoantigens present in everyone (i.e., diseased or autologous tissue is not needed for the demonstration of autoantibodies) indicates that persons who develop autoimmunity have an *abnormality of immune specificity*. The abnormality is specific for each disease and is well described as being the presence of the requisite forbidden clones of immunocytes (see also Section II,D,5,b). The absence of autoimmune disease at birth and its increasing prevalence and variety with advancing age supports the concept that forbidden clones are usually absent at birth, but develop subsequently owing to the occurrence of certain series of somatic mutations in the V genes of dividing immunocytes (Adams, 1977).

B. LESS LIKELY CONCEPTS OF AUTOIMMUNITY

1. Defect of a Tolerance Mechanism

The concept that autoimmunity is caused by a generalized weakness of a hypothetical tolerance mechanism is not tenable in the face of detailed evidence of the highly specific nature of the autoantigen for any individual autoimmune disease (e.g., the TSH receptor in Graves' disease, the acetylcholine receptor of the neuromuscular junction in myasthenia gravis, cell nuclei in SLE, etc.)

Knight *et al.* (1980a) have shown that old NZB mice that have autoantibodies against normal mouse erythrocyte antigens are still tolerant of other self antigens, such as their liver F antigen.

2. Loss of Suppressor T Cells

Some years ago it became reasonable to speculate that the immune system might possess a surveillant mechanism that normally destroys forbidden clones as they arise, autoimmunity representing a failure of this mechanism. The concept received support from studies that appeared to show that the onset of autoimmune anemia and lupus nephritis in the New Zealand mice could be delayed by transfer of thymus cells from young, healthy, syngeneic animals in whom the disorder had not yet developed (Gershwin and Steinberg, 1975). However, more stringent studies with much larger numbers of animals have shown no such effect (Knight and Adams, 1978b). Furthermore, a recent study by Gershwin *et al.* (1979) has revealed that if the asplenia (Dh) gene is transferred to the NZB strain, then the resulting asplenic NZB mice still develop hemolytic anemia but do not have the suppressor cell defect that these authors had earlier contended was responsible for autoimmunity in these mice.

Volpé (1978) continues to espouse the defect of immune surveillance concept, postulating specific suppressor T cells as the deficient agents.

However, suppressor T cells appear to be concerned with quantitative regulation of an immune response, not control of specificity (Taussig, 1974a,b; Nachtigal *et al.*, 1975). A forbidden clone is distinguished only by the specificity of its paratope and its epitope, so any control mechanism with clonal specificity must involve a reaction with one of these two structures. As a paratope cannot react with another paratope (see Section IX,C,4) any surveillance of specificity by the immune system would seem to require not suppressor T cell activity, but paratope-idiotope interaction, as postulated by Jerne (see Section IX,C,4).

3. *B Cell Clones for Autoimmunity Are Universal*

It has been observed that thyroglobulin labeled with ^{125}I adheres to an occasional lymphocyte from the blood of normal people (Bankhurst *et al.*, 1973; Roberts, *et al.*, 1973). From this, it has been deduced that all people have clones of B cells with specificity for thyroglobulin. This deduction is unwarranted because credible evidence of the specificity of the thyroglobulin-binding reaction was not provided. Roberts *et al.* (1973) showed that some patients with thyroid autoimmune diseases have larger numbers of lymphocytes that bind to labeled thyroglobulin than do control subjects, and they also showed that the binding by cells from these patients can be inhibited by the addition of excess unlabeled thyroglobulin. The work deserves wider recognition as a demonstration of antithyroglobulin clones in a proportion of patients with thyroid autoimmune disease. The smaller incidence of binding in the control subjects was not shown to be inhibited by excess unlabeled thyroglobulin and is likely to be nonspecific, in the light of careful studies of such reactions by Byrt and Ada (1969), including observations suggesting involvement of small phagocytic cells, which could be monocytes. Demonstration of a functional reaction induced by thyroglobulin, such as blast transformation or increased uptake of tritiated thymidine would be needed to show the presence of specifically reactive B cells in people who lack the autoantibodies.

C. THE GENETIC PREDISPOSITION TO AUTOIMMUNE DISEASE

1. *Patterns of Inheritance in Man*

The genetic predisposition to thyrotoxicosis, which is familar to every clinical thyroidologist, was studied in over 200 families by Bartels (1941), who concluded that the mode of inheritance was recessive, because the incidence in siblings of the probands was higher than in the parents of the probands. A similar observation led to a similar conclusion by Simpson (1964), working with diabetes mellitus. However, these conclusions were unwarranted because, although the observation indicates the involvement of two genes, these need not necessarily be at the same locus. Thus, involvement of multiple codominant genes is an equally valid interpretation and one that accords better with the regular occurrence of thyroid and islet autoimmune disease in three successive generations (Adams, 1978a). On perusal of McKusick's (1978) catalogs of "Mendelian Inheritance in Man," one finds consistently that with established or suspected autoimmune diseases there is difficulty in deciding whether the mode of inheritance is dominant or recessive, which suggests involvement of multiple codominant genes in the genetic predisposition to all autoimmune disease (Adams, 1978a).

2. Animal Models of Inherited Autoimmune Disease

The New Zealand black (NZB) inbred strain of mice, developed by Franz and Marianne Bielschowsky, show autoimmune hemolytic anemia (Howie and Helyer, 1968). The genetics of this disorder is not yet established. However, hybrids between the NZB and the New Zealand white (NZW) strains show lupus nephritis, which is based on production of copious amounts of complement-fixing immune complexes of autoantibody and a copiously available intracellular antigen (Knight *et al.*, 1977). The disorder has been shown to be based on three codominant genes, one in the NZB strain and two in the NZW strain, including a gene in the *H-2* complex (Knight and Adams (1978a).

3. The V Gene Theory of Inherited Autoimmune Disease

This theory (Adams, 1978a) postulates that the genetic predisposition to autoimmune disease lies in the specificity of the germline immunoglobulin variable region genes (V genes), which code for the amino acid sequences of the heavy and light polypeptide chains that determine the specificity of immunoglobulin paratopes. It is envisaged that species of paratopes occur, not readily interconvertible by somatic mutation, just as species of animals occur and are not interconvertible by germline mutation. Germline V genes are postulated to vary in the proximity of their base sequences to those required for various autoantibodies, and so to vary in the number of somatic mutations they must undergo to reach the autoreactive specificity.

Studies suggesting that LATS invariably contains both κ and λ light chains (Kriss, 1968; Maisey, 1972), if correct, would indicate that the germline light-chain V genes required for TSaab are ubiquitous. However, as anti-κ and anti-λ sera each precipitate about half of the entire

immunoglobulins, nonspecific coprecipitation of the LATS may have
occurred. More recent studies (Zakarija and McKenzie, 1980) have
thrown doubt on the original observations.

Germline V genes could be implicated in the predisposition to autoimmunity in a second manner, by coding for paratopes involved in
anti-idiotope network reactions relevant to occurrence of the forbidden
clones (see Sections IX,C,4 and 5).

4. *Jerne's Immune Networks Theory*

An antibody paratope is now known to be a molecular cleft. It follows
that one paratope cannot combine with another, as a cleft cannot fit a
cleft. However, the lips of paratopes can be antigenic, being known as
idiotopes or variable region antigens (Fig. 20). As an idiotope is coded
for by the same two intertwined polypeptide chains that code for its
adjacent paratope, there is a relationship between paratope specificity
and idiotope specificity. In animal studies, it has proved to be possible
to delete clones bearing certain idiotopes by injecting complement-
fixing antisera with specificity for those idiotopes (Fig. 21) (Eichmann,
1975; Cosenza, 1976).

Jerne (1974) has proposed that clonal deletions by anti-idiotope
reaction are a frequent happening in all animals, both in fetal life
where various combinations of parental V genes will produce interacting clones and in adult life where new clones arise by somatic muta-

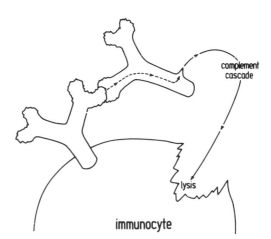

FIG. 21. Clonal deletion by anti-idiotope reaction (Jerne, 1974) An immunocyte is
being lysed by a complement-fixing antibody that has specificity for its idiotope (variable
region antigen). Reproduced, with permission, from Adams and Knight (1980).

tion. Jerne envisages a network of paratope–idiotope reactions, influencing the immune response repertoire of each individual.

5. *The H Gene Theory*

Sex has long been known to have an influence on the incidence of various established or suspected autoimmune diseases, but patterns of inheritance show that the effect is not caused by genes on the X chromosome (McKusick, 1978). More recently, after the discovery by Vladutiu and Rose (1971) that genes in the major histocompatibility region code for autoimmune disease in mice, histocompatibility status has been found to influence the incidence of many diseases in man, including most established or suspected autoimmune diseases (Dausset and Svejgaard, 1977).

Finding tentative evidence to suggest that genes coding for minor histocompatibility antigens might be determinant for autoimmune disease in the New Zealand mice, in addition to the major histocompatibility antigen gene previously mentioned (Section IX,C,2), the author and J. G. Knight have put forward the H (histocompatibility) gene theory, a hypothesis of how histocompatibility antigen genes influence the incidence of autoimmune diseases (Adams and Knight, 1980). The H gene theory accepts Burnet's (1959) theory that nascent clones in fetal life are deleted by contact with their complementary antigens (Fig. 20), this mechanism being important for securing absence of reaction to parental histocompatibility antigens. Jerne's concept of clonal deletion by anti-idiotope reaction is also accepted (Fig. 21). It follows that histocompatibility antigen genes will influence the immune response repertoire positively as well as negatively because certain deletions will eliminate anti-idiotype clones and so permit the occurrence of immune responses that would otherwise be absent.

According to the H gene theory, the effect of sex on the incidence of an autoimmune disease is mediated by male sex antigens, coded for by genes on the Y chromosome. These antigens impose certain clonal deletions, like other histocompatibility antigens, and so have positive (e.g., ankylosing spondylitis, deletion of clones reactive with the idiotopes of the presumptive pathogenic clones) and negative (e.g., thyrotoxicosis, deletion of certain potential precursors of TSaab clones) effects on the incidence of autoimmune diseases.

6. *Conclusions*

Burnet's (1959) forbidden clone hypothesis remains the most likely explanation for the occurrence of TSaab and other autoantibodies, which appear to arise by somatic mutations occurring in V genes. The genetic predisposition to thyrotoxicosis and other autoimmune diseases appears to be mediated by multiple codominant genes, which have both positive and negative influence. Such genes, appropriately designated immune response (Ir) genes, are often linked to the major or a minor histocompatibility locus. The H gene theory postulates that histocompatibility-linked Ir genes (including Ia genes) predispose to autoimmunity by influencing the immune response repertoire through the effect of their clonal deletions on the network of paratope–idiotope clonal deletions envisaged by Jerne. Immunoglobulin V genes have been shown to influence the immune response to certain antigens, but whether they are involved in the genetic predisposition to autoimmunity is not yet known.

D. Toward a General Principle of Therapy for Autoimmune Disease

If, as seems probable, autoimmunity is not based on a remediable defect of a tolerance mechanism, then the best prospect for improved therapy would seem to lie in the development of methods for the selective destruction of forbidden clones (Adams, 1978a). Since it has proved to be possible in animal studies to delete selectively clones bearing certain idiotopes, and since idiotope specificity has a relationship to paratope specificity (see Section IX,C,4), administration of appropriately specific, complement-fixing anti-idiotope sera seems to be a possible way of deleting forbidden clones. A huge amount of work is needed to find the pathogenic clones for each disease, to isolate the cells or autoantibodies by affinity chromatography with the appropriate autoantigen, to compare the relationship of paratope repertoire to idiotope repertoire, and to make appropriately specific anti-idiotope sera. Another approach, which might be easier, though not without hazard of exacerbation, is the attachment of a radioactive or poisonous agent to a preparation of the autoantigen, to destroy forbidden clones through reactions that use the specificity of their paratopes. Ada and Byrt (1969) have pioneered this approach, but it has not yet been applied to destruction of forbidden clones.

X. Summary

The thyroid-stimulating autoantibodies link together a fascinating diversity of fields of knowledge, including endocrinology, pathology, immunology, genetics, and chemistry. This chapter recounts some of the intellectual adventures involved in the acquisition of our present understanding of the nature of these molecules, of the manner in which they act, and of the reasons for their occurrence. Furthermore, the clear insight into the pathogenesis of autoimmune disease that has been provided by study of the TSaab appears to have revealed the principle on which improved therapy of autoimmune disease in general will depend, namely, *selective destruction of forbidden clones of immunocytes*. Methods for achieving this are already apparent, but their realization as practicable therapy will require an immense scientific effort. In the last two decades of the nineteenth century, medicine advanced at an unparalleled rate as the causes of a score of diseases were revealed through application of Pasteur's germ theory. At present there is a similar rate of progress as a succession of long-familiar diseases are being shown to be based on autoimmunity. We are poised for a second great therapeutic harvest, comparable to that which came from immunization and antibiotics, when we succeed in devising comparable prophylaxis and therapy for the autoimmune diseases.

REFERENCES

Ada, G., and Byrt, P. (1969). *Nature (London)* 222, 1291–1292.
Adams, D. D. (1958). *J. Clin. Endocrinol. Metab.* 18, 699–712.
Adams, D. D. (1960). *Endocrinology* 66, 658–664.
Adams, D. D. (1961). *J. Clin. Endocrinol Metab.* 21, 799–805.
Adams, D. D. (1965). *Br. Med. J.* 1, 1015–1019.
Adams, D. D. (1975). *N. Z. Med. J.* 81, 15–17.
Adams, D. D. (1977). *In* "Immunology in Medicine" (E. J. Holborow and W. G. Reeves, eds.), pp. 373–430. Academic Press, New York.
Adams, D. D. (1978a). *J. Clin. Lab. Immunol.* 1, 17–24.
Adams, D. D. (1978b). *Patient Management* 7, No. 11, 11–24.
Adams, D. D. (1978c). *J. Clin. Lab. Immunol.* 1, 87–90.
Adams, D. D., and Kennedy, T. H. (1962). *Proc. Univ. Otago Med. Sch.* 40, 6.
Adams, D. D., and Kennedy, T. H. (1965). *J. Clin. Endocrinol. Metab.* 25, 571–576.
Adams, D. D., and Kennedy, T. H. (1967). *J. Clin. Endocrinol. Metab.* 27, 173–177.
Adams, D. D., and Kennedy, T. H. (1968). *J. Clin. Endocrinol. Metab.* 28, 325–331.
Adams, D. D., and Kennedy, T. H. (1971). *J. Clin. Endocrinol. Metab.* 33, 47–51.
Adams, D. D., and Knight, J. G. (1980). *Lancet* 1, 396–398.
Adams, D. D., and Purves, H. D. (1951). *Proc. Univ. Otago Med Sch.* 29, 24–25.
Adams, D. D., and Purves, H. D. (1956). *Proc. Univ. Otago Med. Sch.* 34, 11–12.
Adams, D. D., and Purves, H. D. (1955). *Endocrinology* 57, 17–24.
Adams, D. D., and Purves, H. D. (1957). *Can. J. Biochem. Physiol.* 35, 993–1004.
Adams, D. D., and Sharard, A. (1965). *Australas. Ann. Med.* 14, 192–194.
Adams, D. D., Purves, H. D., and Sirett, N. E. (1961). *Endocrinology* 68, 154–155.

Adams, D. D., Kennedy T. M., Purves, H. D., and Sirett, N. E. (1962a). *Endocrinology* **70**, 801–805.

Adams, D. D., Purves, H. D., Sirett, N. E., and Beaven, D. W. (1962b). *J. Clin. Endocrinol. Metab.* **22**, 623–626.

Adams, D. D., Lord, J. M., and Stevely, H. A. A. (1964). *Lancet* **2**, 497–498.

Adams, D. D., Kennedy, T. H., and Purves, H. D. (1966). *Aust. J. Exp. Biol. Med. Sci.* **44**, 355–364.

Adams, D. D., Kennedy, T. H., Choufoer, J. C., and Querido, A. (1968). *J. Clin. Endocrinol. Metab.* **28**, 685–692.

Adams, D. D., Kennedy, T. H., and Purves, H. D. (1969). *J. Clin. Endocrinol. Metab.* **29**, 900–903.

Adams, D. D., Kennedy, T. H., and Utiger, R. D. (1971). *In* "Further Advances in Thyroid Research" (K. Fellinger and R. Hofer, eds.), pp. 1049–1056. Vienna Medical Academy, Vienna.

Adams, D. D., Kennedy, T. H., and Utiger, R. D. (1972). *J. Clin. Endocrinol. Metab.* **34**, 1074–1079.

Adams, D. D., Kennedy, T. H., and Stewart, R. D. H. (1974a). *Br. Med. J.* **1**, 199–201.

Adams, D. D., Kennedy, T. H., and Stewart R. D. H. (1974b). *Ann. Acad. Med.* (*Singapore*) **3**, 212–217.

Adams, D. D., Fastier, F. N., Howie, J. B., Kennedy, T. H., Kilpatrick, J. A., and Stewart, R. D. H. (1974c). *J. Clin. Endocrinol. Metab.* **39** 826–832.

Adams, D. D., Kennedy, T. H., Stewart, J. C., Utiger, R. D., and Vidor, G. I. (1975). *J. Clin. Endocrinol. Metab.* **41**, 221–228.

Adams, D. D., Kennedy, T. H., and Stewart R. D. H. (1976). *Aust. N. Z. J. Med.* **6**, 300–304.

Arnaud, C. D., Kneubuhler, H. A. Seiling, V. L., Wightman, B. K., and Engbring, N. H. (1965). *J. Clin. Invest.* **44**, 1287–1294.

Aron, M. (1931). *C. R. Soc. Biol.* **106**, 609–611.

Astwood, E. B. (1949). *Adv. Intern. Med.* **3**, 237–274.

Bankhurst, A. D., Torrigiani, G., and Allison, A. C. (1973). *Lancet* **1**, 226–230.

Bartels, E. D. (1941). "Heredity in Graves' Disease." Munksgaard, Copenhagen.

Bastomsky, C. H., and McKenzie, J. M. (1968). *Endocrinology* **83**, 309–313.

Bates, R. W., Garrison, M. M., and Howard, T. B. (1959). *Endocrinology* **65**, 7–17.

Beall, G. N., and Solomon, D. H. (1965). *Clin. Res.* **13**, 240.

Beall, G. N., and Solomon, D. H. (1966). *J. Clin. Endocrinol. Metab.* **26**, 1382–1388.

Berson, S. A., Yalow, R. S., Bauman, A., Rothschild, M. A., and Newerly, K. (1956). *J. Clin. Invest.* **35**, 170–190.

Billingham, R. E., and Brent, L. (1957). *Transplant. Bull.* **4**, 67–71.

Billingham, R. E., Brent, L., and Medawar, P. B. (1953). *Nature* (*London*) **172**, 603–606.

Bottazzo, G. F., Mann, J. I., Thorogood, M., Baum, J. D., and Doniach, D. (1978). *Br. Med. J.* **2**, 165–168.

Brown, J., and Munro, D. S. (1967). *J. Endocrinol.* **38**, 439–449.

Burke, G., (1968). *Endocrinology* **83**, 1210–1216.

Burnet, F. M. (1959). "The Clonal Selection Theory of Acquired Immunity." Cambridge Univ. Press, London and New York.

Byrt, P., and Ada, G. L. (1969). *Immunology* **17**, 503–516.

Cambier, J. C., Kettman, J. R., Vitetta, E. S., and Uhr, J. W. (1976). *J. Exp. Med.* **144**, 293–297.

Cameron, H. C. (1948). "Joseph Lister." Heinemann, London.

Carneiro, L., Dorrington, K. J., and Munro, D. S. (1966). *Lancet* **2**, 878–881.

Choufoer, J. C., van Rhijn, M., Kassenaar, A. A. H., and Querido, A. (1963). *J. Clin. Endocrinol. Metab.* **23**, 1203-1216.

Choufoer, J. C., van Rhijn, M., and Querido, A. (1965). *J. Clin. Endocrinol. Metab.* **25**, 385-402.

Ciereszko, L. S. (1945). *J. Biol. Chem.* **160**, 585-592.

Clark, F., and Horn, D. B. (1965). *J. Clin. Endocrinol. Metab.* **25**, 39-45.

Coindet, J. R. (1821). *Ann. Chim. Phys.* **16**, 252.

Connolly, R. J., Vidor, G. I., and Stewart, J. C. (1970). *Lancet* **1**, 500-502.

Cope, O., Rawson, R. W., and McArthur, J. W. (1947). *Surg. Gynecol. Obstet.* **84**, 415-426.

Cosenza, H. (1976). *Eur. J. Immunol.* **6**, 114-116.

Crigler, J. F. (1960). *In* "Hormones in Human Plasma" (H. N. Antoniades, ed.), pp. 201-223. Little, Brown, Boston, Massachusetts.

Dameshek, W. (1965). *Ann. N. Y. Acad. Sci.* **124**, 6-28.

Dameshek, W., and Schwartz, S. O. (1938). *Am. J. Med. Sci.* **196**, 769-792.

Dandona, P., and El Kabir, D. J. (1980). *Clin. Endocrinol.* **12**, 379-383.

Dandona, P., Mitchell, P., and El Kabir, D. J. (1971). *Clin. Sci.* **40**, 21 p.

Dandona, P., Marshall, N. J., Bidey, S. P., Nathan, A., and Harvard, C. W. H. (1979). *Br. Med. J.* **1**, 374-376.

D'Angelo, S. A., Paschkis, K. E., Gordon, A. S., and Cantarow, A. (1951). *J. Clin. Endocrinol.* **11**, 1237-1253.

Dausset, J., and Svejgaard, A. (1977). "HLA and Disease." Munksgaard, Copenhagen.

Davies, T. F., Smith, B. R., and Hall, R. (1978). *Endocrinology* **103**, 6-10.

De Robertis, E. (1948). *J. Clin. Endocrinol Metab.* **8** 956-966.

Dirmikis, S. (1974). *J. Endocrinol.* **63**, 427-438.

Dirmikis, S. M., and Munro, D. S. (1975). *Br. Med. J.* **2**, 665-666.

Dobyns, B. M., and Lennon, B. (1948). *J. Clin. Endocrinol. Metab.* **8**, 732-748.

Doniach, D., and Marshall, N. J. (1977). *In* "Autoimmunity" (N. Talal, ed.), pp. 621-642. Academic Press, New York.

Doniach, D., and Roitt, I. M. (1957). *J. Clin. Endocrinol. Metab.* **17**, 1293-1304.

Dorrington, K. J., Carneiro, L., and Munro, D. S. (1965). *In* "Current Topics in Thyroid Research" (C. Cassano and M. Andreoli, eds.), pp. 455-463. Academic Press, New York.

Dorrington, K. J., Carneiro, L., and Munro, D. S. (1966) *J. Endocrinol* **34** 133-134.

Dubos, R. J. (1951). "Louis Pasteur," Gollancz, London.

Dumont, J. E. (1971). *Vitam. Horm. (N. Y.)* **29**, 287-412.

Edelman, G. M., and Poulik, M. D. (1961). *J. Exp. Med.* **113**, 861-884.

Ehrlich, P., and Morgenroth, J. (1900; republished 1956). *In* "The Collected Papers of Paul Ehrlich" (F. Himmelweit, ed.), pp. 205-212. Pergamon, Oxford.

Ehrlich, P., and Morgenroth, J. (1901; republished 1956). *In* "The Collected Papers of Paul Ehrlich" (F. Himmelweit, ed.), pp 246-255. Pergamon, Oxford.

Eichmann, K. (1975). *Eur. J. Immunol.* **5**, 511-517.

Fleischman, J. B., Pain, R. H., and Porter, R. R. (1962). *Arch. Biochem. Biophys., Suppl.* **1**, 144-174.

Florsheim, W. H., Williams, A. D., and Schoenbaum, E. (1970) *Endocrinology* **87**, 881-888.

Freund, J., Thomson, K. J., Hough, H. B., Sommer, H. E., and Pisani, T. M. (1948). *J. Immunol.* **60**, 383-398.

Gaddum, J. H. (1953). *Pharmacol. Rev.* **5**, 87-132.

Gershwin, M. E., and Steinberg, A. D. (1975). *Clin. Immunol. Immunopathol.* **4**, 38-45.

Gershwin, M. E., Castles, J. J., Ikeda, R. M., Erickson, K., and Montero, J. (1979). *J. Immunol.* **122**, 710–717.

Goldsmith, R. E., Herber, C., and Lutsch, G. (1958). *J. Clin. Endocrinol. Metab.* **18**, 367–378.

Graves, R. J. (1838). "Clinical Lectures," pp. 134–136. Adam Waldie, Philadelphia, Pennsylvania.

Greenwood, F. C., Hunter, W. M., and Glover, J. S. (1963). *Biochem. J.* **89**, 114–123.

Greer, M. A., and DeGroot, L. J. (1956). *Metabolism* **5**, 682–696.

Gross, J., and Pitt-Rivers, R. (1953). *Biochem. J.* **53**, 652–657.

Gudernatsch, J. F. (1914). *Am. J. Anat.* **15**, 431–476.

Harington, C. R. (1933). "The Thyroid Gland." Oxford Univ. Press, London and New York.

Hart, I. R., and McKenzie, J. M. (1971). *Endocrinology* **88**, 26–30.

Hartsock, C. L. (1926). *J. Am. Med. Assoc.* **86** 1334–1338.

Hertz, S., and Oastler, E. G. (1936). *Endocrinology* **20**, 520–525.

Hetzel, B. S. (1970). *Med. J. Aust.* **2**, 615–622.

Howie, J. B., and Helyer, B. J. (1968). *Ad. Immunol.* **9**, 215–264.

Husby, G., Van de Rijn, I., Zabriskie, J. B., Abdin, Z. M., and Williams, R. C. (1976). *J. Exp. Med.* **144**, 1094–1110.

Ibbertson, H. K. (1979). *Clin. Endocrinol. Metab.* **8**, 97–128.

Irvine, W. J. (1964). *Quart. J. Exp. Physiol.* **49**, 324–337.

Jerne, N. K. (1955). *Proc. Natl. Acad. Sci. U.S.A.* **41**, 849–853.

Jerne, N. K. (1974). *Ann. Immunol. (Inst. Pasteur)* **125C**, 373–389.

Kaneko, T., Zor, U., and Field, J. B. (1970). *Metab. Clin. Exp.* **19**, 430–438.

Kaplan, M. H., and Frengley, J. D. (1969). *Am. J. Cardiol.* **24**, 459–473.

Kendall-Taylor, P. (1972). *J. Endocrinol.* **52**, 533–540.

Kennedy, T. H., and Purves, H. D. (1956). *Aust. J. Biol. Sci.* **9** 586–592.

Kilpatrick, J. A. (1974). *N. Z. Med. J.* **80**, 495–496.

Kimball, O. P. (1925). *J. Am. Med. Assoc.* **85**, 1709–1710.

Kirkham, K. E. (1962). *J. Endocrinol.* **25**, 259–269.

Klainer, L. M., Chi, Y. M., Friedberg, S. L., Rall, T. W., and Sutherland, E. W. (1962). *J. Biol. Chem.* **237**, 1239–1343.

Knight, A. (1977). Studies on the Thyroid-Stimulating Autoantibodies. Ph.D. Thesis University of Otago, Dunedin, New Zealand.

Knight, A., and Adams, D. D. (1973a). *Proc. Univ. Otago Med. Sch.* **51**, 11–13.

Knight, A., and Adams, D. D. (1973b). *Proc. Univ. Otago Med. Sch.* **51**, 49–50.

Knight , A., and Adams, D. D. (1976). *Proc. Univ. Otago Med. Sch.* **54**, 79–80.

Knight, J. G., and Adams, D. D. (1978a). *J. Exp. Med.* **147**, 1653–1660.

Knight, J. G., and Adams, D. D. (1978b). *J. Clin. Lab. Immunol.* **1**, 151–158.

Knight, A., and Adams, D. D. (1980). *Hormone Res.* **13**, 69–80.

Knight, J. G., Adams, D. D., and Purves, H. D. (1977). *Clin. Exp. Immunol.* **28**, 352–358.

Knight, J. G., Knight, A., and Winchester, G. (1980a). *Cell. Immunol.* **56** (in press).

Knight, A., Cague, W. S., and Adams, D. D. (1980b) *In* "Manual of Clinical Immunology" (N. R. Rose and H. Friedman, eds.), 2nd ed., pp. 391–402. American Society for Microbiology, Washington, D.C.

Knox, A. J. S., von Westarp, C., Row, V. V., and Volpé, R. (1976a). *Metabolism* **25**, 1217–1223.

Knox, A. J. S., von Westarp, C., Row, V. V., and Volpé, R. (1976b). *J. Clin. Endocrinol. Metab.* **43**, 330–337.

Kocher, T. (1910). *Arch. Klin. Chir.* **96**, 403.

Kohler, P. O., Mardineg, M. R., and Ross, G. T. (1967). *Endocrinology* **81**, 671–672.

Kohn, L. D. (1978). *In* Receptors and Recognition" (P. Cuatrecasas and M. F. Greaves, eds.), Ser. A, Vol. 5, pp. 133–212.

Kriss, J. P. (1968). *J. Clin. Endocrinol. Metab.* **28**, 1440–1444.

Kriss, J. P., Pleshakov, V., and Chien, J. R. (1964). *J. Clin. Endocrinol. Metab.* **24**, 1005–1028.

Kriss, J. P., Pleshakov, V., Rosenblum, A. L., Holderness, M., Sharp, G., and Utiger, R. (1967). *J. Clin. Endocrinol. Metab.* **27**, 582–593.

Kroll, A. J., and Kuwabara, T. (1966). *Arch. Ophthalmol.* **76**, 244–257.

Leader (1977). *Lancet* **2**, 591–595.

Levey, G. S., and Pastan, I. (1970). *Life Sci.* **9**, 67–73.

Lockwood, C. M., Rees, A. J., Pearson, T. A., Evans, D. J., and Peters, D. K. (1976). *Lancet* **1**, 711–715.

Loeb, H. A., and Bassett, R. B. (1930). *Proc. Soc. Exp. Biol. Med.* **27**, 490–492.

McGiven, A. R., Adams, D. D., and Purves, H. D. (1965). *J. Endocrinol.* **32**, 29–33.

McKenzie, J. M. (1958a). *Endocrinology* **62**, 865–868.

McKenzie, J. M. (1958b). *Endocrinology* **63**, 372–382.

McKenzie, J. M. (1959). *Trans. Assoc. Am. Physicians* **72**, 122–130.

McKenzie, J. M. (1960). *J. Clin. Endocrinol. Metab.* **20**, 380–388.

McKenzie, J. M. (1961). *J. Clin. Endocrinol. Metab.* **21**, 635–647.

McKenzie, J. M. (1962a). *Proc. R. Soc. Med.* **55**, 539–544.

McKenzie, J. M. (1962b). *J. Biol. Chem.* **237**, PC3571–3572.

McKenzie, J. M. (1964). *J. Clin. Endocrinol. Metab.* **24**, 660–668.

McKenzie, J. M., and Fishman, J. (1960). *Proc. Soc. Exp. Biol. Med.* **105**, 126–128.

McKenzie, J. M., and Gordon, J. (1965). *In* "Current Topics in Thyroid Research" (C. Cassano and M. Andreoli, eds.), pp. 445–454. Academic Press, New York.

McKenzie, J. M., and McCullagh, E. P. (1968). *J. Clin. Endocrinol. Metab.* **28**, 1177–1182.

McKenzie, J. M., and Zakarija, M. (1977). *Recent Prog. Horm. Res.* **33**, 29–53.

McKenzie, J. M., Zakarija, M., and Sato, A. (1978). *Clin. Endocrinol. Metab.* **7**, 31–45.

McKusick, V. A. (1978). "Mendelian Inheritance in Man," 5th ed. Johns Hopkins Press, Baltimore, Maryland.

Maisey, M. N. (1972). *Clin. Endocrinol* **1**, 189–198.

Major, P. W., and Munro, D. S. (1960). *J. Endocrinol.* **20**, XIX–XX.

Major, P. W., and Munro, D. S. (1962). *Clin. Sci.* **23**, 463–475.

Manley, S. W., Bourke, J. R., and Hawker, R. W. (1972). *J. Endocrinol.* **55**, 555–563.

Manley, S. W., Bourke, J. R., and Hawker, R. W. J. (1974a). *J. Endocrinol.* **61**, 419–436.

Manley, S. W., Bourke, J. R., and Hawker, R. W. J. (1974b). *J. Endocrinol.* **61**, 437–445.

Marine, D., and Kimball, O. P. (1921). *J. Am. Med. Assoc.* **77**, 1068–1070.

Marine, D., and Lenhart, C. H. (1909). *Arch. Int. Med.* **4**, 253–270.

Meek, J. C., Jones, A. E., Lewis, V. J., and Vanderlaan, W. P. (1964). *Proc. Natl. Acad. Sci. U.S.A.* **52**, 342–349.

Mehdi, S. Q., and Nussey, S. S. (1975). *Biochem. J.* **145**, 105–111.

Mercer, C. J., Sharard, A., Westerink, C. J. M., and Adams, D. D. (1960). *Lancet* **2**, 19–21.

Metcalf, E. S., and Klinman, N. R. (1976). *J. Exp. Med.* **143**, 1327–1340.

Miyai, K., Fukuchi, M., Kumahara, V., and Abe, H. (1967). *J. Clin. Endocrinol. Metab.* **27**, 855–860.

Möbius, P. J. (1886). *Arch. Psychiat.* **17**, 301.

Muggeo, M. Kahn, C. R., Bar, R. S., Rechler, M., Flier, J. S., and Rothe, J. (1979). *J. Clin. Endocrinol. Metab.* **49**, 110–119.

Mukhtar, E. D., Smith, B. R., Pyle, G. A., Hall, R., and Vice, P. (1975). *Lancet* **1**, 713–715.

Munro, D. S. (1959). *J. Endocrinol.* **19**, 64–73.

Murray, S., and Ezrin, C. (1966). *J. Clin. Endocrinol. Metab.* **26**, 287.

Nachtigal, D., Zan-Bar, I., and Feldman, M. (1975). *Transplant. Rev.* **26**, 87–93.

Naffziger, H. C. (1933). *Arch. Ophthalmol.* **9**, 1–7.

Nossal, G. J. V., and Pike, B. L. (1975). *J. Exp. Med.* **141**, 904–917.

Nowell, P. C. (1960). *Cancer Res.* **20**, 462–466.

Oddie, T. H., Meschan, I., and Wotham, J. (1955). *J. Clin. Invest.* **34**, 106–114.

Odell, W. D., Wilber, J. F., and Paul, W. E. (1965). *J. Clin. Endocrinol. Metab.* **25**, 1179–1188.

Onaya, T., and Solomon, D. H. (1969). *Endocrinology* **85**, 1010–1017.

Onaya, T., Tokani, M., Yamada, T., and Ochi, Y. (1973). *J. Clin. Endocrinol. Metab.* **36**, 859–866.

Origiazzi, J., Williams, D. E., Chopra, I. J., and Solomon, D. H. (1976). *J. Clin. Endocrinol. Metab.* **42**, 341–355.

Ozawa, Y., Maciel, R. M. B., Chopra, I. J., Solomon, D. H., and Beall, G. N. (1979). *J. Clin. Endocrinol. Metab.* **48**, 381–387.

Patel, Y. C., Burger, H. G., and Hudson, B. (1971). *J. Clin. Endocrinol. Metab.* **33**, 768–774.

Phillips, S. M., and Wegmann, T. G. (1973). J. Exp. Med. **137**, 291–300.

Pinchera, A., Liberti, P., Martino, E., Fenzi, G. F., Grasso, L., Rovis, L., and Baschieri, L. (1969). *J. Clin. Endocrinol. Metab.* **29**, 231–238.

Pinching, A. J., Peters, D. K., and Newsom Davis, J. (1976). *Lancet* **2**, 1373–1376.

Pitt-Rivers, R., and Cavalieri, R. R. (1964). *in* "The Thyroid Gland" (R. Pitt-Rivers and W. R. Trotter, eds.), Vol. 1, pp. 87–112. Butterworth, London.

Plummer, H. S. (1913). *Trans. Assoc. Am. Physicians* **28**, 587–591.

Purves, H. D. (1964). *In* "The Thyroid Gland" (R. Pitt-Rivers and W. R. Trotter, eds.), Vol. 2, pp. 1–38. Butterworth, London.

Purves, H. D., (1966) *In* "The Pituitary Gland" (G. W. Harris and B. T. Donovan, eds.), Vol. 1, pp. 147–232. Butterworth, London.

Purves, H. D. (1974). *N. Z. Med. J.* **80**, 477–479.

Purves, H. D., and Adams, D. D. (1961). *In* "Advances in Thyroid Research" (R. Pitt-Rivers, ed.), pp. 184–188. Pergamon, Oxford.

Purves, H. D., and Griesbach, W. E. (1949). *Br. J. Exp. Pathol.* **30**, 23–30.

Rawson, R. W., and Starr, P. (1938). *Arch. Intern. Med.* **61**, 726–738.

Roberts, I. M., Whittingham, S., and Mackay, I. R. (1973). *Lancet* **2**, 936–940.

Roitt, I. M., and Torrigiani, G. (1967). *Endocrinology* **81**, 421–429.

Rundle, F. F. (1964). *In* "The Thyroid Gland" (R. Pitt-Rivers and W. R. Trotter, eds.), Vol. 2, pp. 171–197. Butterworth, London.

Rundle, F. F., and Pochin, E. E. (1944). *Clin. Sci.* **5**, 51–74.

Rundle, F. F., Finlay-Jones, L. R., and Noad, K. B. (1953). *Australas. Ann. Med.* **2**, 128–135.

Scanlon, M. F., Smith, B. R., and Hall, R. (1978). *Clin. Sci. Mol. Med.* **55**, 1–10.

Schell-Frederick, E., and Dumont, J. E. (1970). *In* "Biochemical Actions of Hormones" (G. Litwack, ed.), Vol. 1, pp. 415–463. Academic Press, New York.

Schockaert, J. A. (1931). *Proc. Soc. Exp. Biol. Med.* **29**, 306–308.

Sclare, G. (1960). *Biol. Neonatorum* **2**, 132–146.

Scott, T. W., Good, B. F., and Ferguson, K. A. (1962). *Endocrinology* **71**, 120–129.

Sharard, A., and Adams, D. D. (1965). *Proc. Univ. Otago Med. Sch.* **43**, 25.

Sharard, A., Purves, H. D., and Cague, W. S. (1970). *Proc. Univ. Otago Med. Sch.* **48**, 77–78.

Shishiba, Y., Solomon, D. H., and Davidson, W. D. (1970). *Endocrinology* **86**, 183–190.
Shishiba, Y., Shimizu, T., Shizuko, Y., and Shizuma, K. (1973). *J. Clin. Endocrinol. Metab.* **36**, 517–521.
Shishiba, Y., Yoshimura, S., and Shimizu, T. (1974). *Endocrinology* **95**, 922–925.
Shishiba, Y., Miyachi, Y., Takaishi, M., and Ozawa, Y. (1978). *J. Clin. Endocrinol. Metab.* **46**, 841–848.
Simpson, N. E. (1964). *Diabetes* **13**, 462–471.
Smith, B. R., and Hall, R. (1974a). *Lancet* **2**, 427–431.
Smith, B. R., and Hall, R. (1974b). *FEBS Lett.* **42**, 301–304.
Smith, B. R., Dorrington, K. J., and Munro, D. S. (1969). *Biochim. Biophys. Acta* **192**, 277–285.
Smith, P. E. (1926). *Anat. Rec.* **32**, 221.
Smith, P. E., and Smith, I. P. (1922). *J. Med. Res.* **43**, 267–284.
Solomon, D. H. (1954). *J. Clin. Endocrinol. Metab.* **14**, 772.
Stanbury, J. B. (1969). "Endemic Goiter." Pan-American Health Organisation Scientific Publication, No. 193, pp. 1–447.
Stanbury, J. B., Brownell, G. L., Riggs, D. S., Perinetti, H., Itoiz, J., and del Castillo, E. B. (1954). "Endemic Goitre," Harvard Univ. Press, Cambridge, Massachusetts.
Sunshine, P., Kusumoto, H., Kriss, J. P., Pleshakov, V., and Chien, J. R. (1965). *Pediatrics* **36**, 869–876.
Sutherland, E. W., and G. A. Robinson (1966). *Pharmacol Rev.* **18**, 145–162.
Tan, E. M., Robinson, J., and Robitaille, P. (1976). *Scand. J. Immunol.* **5**, 811–818.
Taussig, M. J. (1974a). *Nature (London)* **248**, 234–236.
Taussig, M. J. (1974b). *Nature (London)* **248**, 236–238.
Teale, J. M., and Mackay, I. R. (1979). *Lancet* **2**, 284–287.
Teale, J. M., Layton, J. E., and Nossal, G. J. V. (1979). *J. Exp. Med.* **150**, 205–217.
Trotter, W. R., Belyavin, G., and Waddams, A. (1957). *Proc. R. Soc. Med.* **50**, 961–962.
Unanue, E. R., and Dixon, F. J. (1967). *Adv. Immunol.* **6**, 1–90.
Utiger, R. D. (1965). *J. Clin. Invest.* **44**, 1277–1286.
Vladutiu, A. O., and Rose, N. R. (1971). *Science* **174**, 1137–1138.
Voisin, G. A., Kinsky, R. G., and Maillard, J. (1968). *Ann. Inst. Pasteur (Paris)* **115**, 855–879.
Volpé, R. (1978). *Clin. Endocrinol. Metab.* **7**, 3–29.
Volpé, R., Row, V. V., and Ezrin, C. (1967). *J. Clin. Endocrinol. Metab.* **27**, 1275–1284.
Wall, J. R., Good, B. F., Forbes, I. J., and Hetzel, B. S. (1973). *Clin. Exp. Immunol.* **14**, 555–563.
Werner, S. C., Otero-Ruiz, E., Seegal, B. C., and Bates, R. W. (1960) *Nature (London)* **185**, 472–473.
Witebsky, E., Rose, N. R., Terplan, K., Paine, J. R., and Egan, R. W. (1957). *J. Am. Med. Assoc.* **164**, 1439–1447.
Wolff, J. (1969). *Am. J. Med.* **47**, 101–124.
Wolff, J., Chaikoff, I. L., Goldberg, R. C., and Meier, J. R. (1949). *Endocrinology* **45**, 504–513.
Yamazaki, E., Noguchi, A., Sato, S., and Slingerland, D. W. (1961). *J. Clin. Endocrinol. Metab.* **21**, 1127–1138.
Zakarija, M., and McKenzie, J. M. (1978). *J. Clin. Endocrinol. Metab.* **47**, 249–254.
Zakarija, M., and McKenzie, J. M. (1980). *In* "Thyroid Research VIII" (J. R. Stockigt and S. Nagataki, eds.), pp. 669–672. Australian Academy of Science, Canberra.

Role of Cyclic Nucleotides in Secretory Mechanisms and Actions of Parathyroid Hormone and Calcitonin

E. M. BROWN

Division of Endocrinology, Peter Bent Brigham Hospital, Boston, Massachusetts

G. D. AURBACH

Metabolic Diseases Branch, National Institute of Arthritis, Metabolism, and Digestive Diseases, National Institutes of Health, Bethesda, Maryland

I. Introduction

Advances in the past 5 years have considerably furthered knowledge of the role of cyclic nucleotides in the regulation of the secretion and action of parathyroid hormone (PTH) and calcitonin (CT). The development of more purified preparations of PTH-secreting cells has made it feasible to assess directly intracellular cyclic nucleotide content and its relationship to hormonal secretion. Likewise, the separation of distinct functional and morphologic classes of bone cells has made possible more detailed analyses of the sites of action and mechanistic basis of hormonal effects on bone. Labeled ligands are being used to analyze by direct binding methods for hormone receptors on the several isolated cell types. Finally, elegant microdissection techniques and the application of ultrasensitive histochemical bioassays have furthered our understanding of the action of PTH and CT on the kidney. In the present chapter* we review progress in these areas with emphasis on advances in methods, regulation of cyclic nucleotides by hormones and other agents, and mechanisms for cyclic nucleotide control of cellular functions.

II. Role of Cyclic Nucleotides in PTH Secretion

A. Parathyroid Anatomy and Physiology

A brief summary of parathyroid anatomy and physiology as well as the biosynthesis of PTH will serve as a basis for subsequent discussion of possible sites of action of various secretagogues and the role of cyclic nucleotides. For a more complete treatment of these areas, the interested reader is referred to the excellent reviews of Roth and Schiller (1976) and Habener and Potts (1978).

1. Anatomy

The chief cell (Fig. 1) is the major cell type responsible for biosynthesis and secretion of PTH. As with other cells actively engaged in the synthesis of polypeptide hormones, the cell contains abundant rough endoplasmic reticulum (RER), a prominent Golgi apparatus, and dense membrane-bound secretory vesicles containing PTH. Microtubules and

---

*The authors have not attempted to present in this review an exhaustive citation of the literature in this field. To do so would expand the review beyond reasonable limits. We have, however, made an effort to cite representative recent works, and often classic or index papers as well, on particular topics.

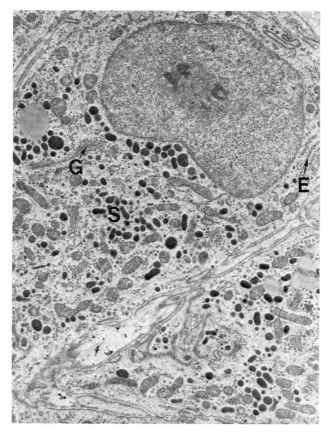

FIG. 1. Active chief cell in bovine parathyroid gland showing numerous secretory granules (S). Arrays of endoplasmic reticulum (E) and Golgi apparatuses (G) are also visible in the cytoplasm. Lipid bodies (L) are infrequent. × 9275.

microfilaments, possibly involved in the secretory process, are located in the periphery of the cell. Inactive chief cells contain a more dispersed RER and less prominent Golgi structure and have abundant glycogen and lipofuscin. In has been suggested that there is a continuous cycle of active to inactive chief cells (Roth and Raisz, 1966). The temporal aspects of this cycle, however, and the functional capacity of the inactive chief cells are unknown.

2. *PTH Biosynthesis*

Recent elegant studies on the biosynthesis of parathyroid hormone and other polypeptides destined for cellular export have demonstrated the general existence of larger precursor peptides that are progressively cleaved to yield the principal secretory product. The initial biosynthetic product (preproparathyroid hormone) contains 115 amino acids (Kemper *et al.*, 1974, 1976). The amino-terminal 25 residues, the highly hydrophobic "leader" or "signal" sequence, are rapidly cleaved off during or shortly after synthesis of the nascent polypeptide. The function of the "pre" sequence appears to be to direct the newly synthesized polypeptide into the cisternae of the RER where the membrane-bound enzyme that removes this segment of the molecule resides. The remaining 90 amino acid segment [proparathyroid hormone (Kemper *et al.*, 1972; Hamilton *et al.*, 1971)] is transported to the Golgi apparatus by uncertain mechanisms, possibly involving microtubules (Kemper *et al.*, 1975). The cleavage of the highly basic six amino acid "pro" sequence of PTH takes place at or near the Golgi. Evidence has been presented for a particulate trypsin-like enzyme that converts pro-PTH to PTH within the parathyroid gland (MacGregor *et al.*, 1976; Habener *et al.*, 1977a). It has recently been suggested from studies with pancreatic beta cells that the dibasic amino acid linkage between the "pro" sequence of several polypeptides and the native sequence is recognized and cleaved by glandular kallikrein(s) (Ole-Moiyoi *et al.*, 1979).

After processing of the prohormone, native 1–84 PTH and parathyroid secretory protein (PSP), a glycoprotein of unknown function (Kemper *et al.*, 1974), are packaged into secretory vesicles. Recent evidence suggests localization of these two molecules in the same vesicle (Ravazzola *et al.*, 1978). Further processing of the native hormone, however, may take place prior to secretion. Direct secretion of C-terminal fragments of PTH as well as 1–84 PTH has been shown in several *in vivo* (Mayer *et al.*, 1979b; Flueck *et al.*, 1977) and *in vitro* (Hanley *et al.*, 1978) systems. It has been assumed, primarily through analogy with other secretory systems, that PTH release occurs by exocytosis (fusion of the secretory granule with the plasma membrane, with subsequent release of granule contents into the extracellular space).

3. Parathyroid Physiology

The development of a radioimmunoassay for PTH (Berson *et al.*, 1963) made it feasible to determine directly the effects of diverse secretagogues on PTH secretion. Studies *in vivo* (Sherwood *et al.*, 1966, 1968) as well as *in vitro* (Sherwood *et al.*, 1970; Targovnik *et al.*, 1971) demonstrated an inverse relationship between extracellular calcium or magnesium concentrations and PTH release. Phosphate, on the other hand, caused no independent effect on PTH secretion (Sherwood *et al.*,

1968). Since two of the principal functions of PTH are to regulate calcium resorption from bone and reabsorption from the renal tubule, the inhibitory effect of calcium on secretion afforded a simple, closed negative feedback loop to control calcium in the extracellular fluid.

More recently, it has been shown that β-adrenergic catecholamines also enhance PTH secretion *in vivo* (Fischer *et al.*, 1973) and *in vitro* (Williams *et al.*, 1973), although the physiologic significance of this effect remains uncertain. The direct demonstration of adenylate cyclase activity in homogenates of parathyroid gland (Dufresne *et al.*, 1971; Matsuzaki and Dumont, 1972) implicated this enzyme in the regulation of PTH secretion by calcium and other agents known to stimulate enzymic activity (i.e., β-adrenergic agonists). The remainder of this section will be devoted to exploring the role of cyclic nucleotides in the control of PTH release by calcium, β-adrenergic catecholamines, and other agents subsequently found to modulate hormone secretion. This subject is also treated in a review by Peck and Klahr (1979).

B. Early Evidence for the Involvement of Cyclic Nucleotides in PTH Secretion

The development of *in vitro* parathyroid slice and fragment preparations made it possible to explore indirectly cyclic nucleotide involvement in secretion. Williams *et al.* (1973) showed that phosphodiesterase inhibitors and dibutyryl cyclic AMP (cAMP) stimulated PTH release from bovine parathyroid slices. This observation suggested that increases in cellular cAMP content might be linked to enhanced secretion. Abe and Sherwood (1972) demonstrated that elevated calcium concentrations decreased cAMP release from bovine parathyroid slices in direct proportion to the decrease in PTH secretion. These workers suggested that modulation of cAMP synthesis by adenylate cyclase might regulate hormone secretion.

C. Limitations of Intact Organ Preparations

The parathyroid gland, in addition to parathyroid cells, contains a number of other cell types, including variable numbers of fat cells, endothelial cells, fibroblasts, and mast cells (Roth and Schiller, 1976). In addition, large numbers of red blood cells are invariably trapped in tissue fragments. Thus, it is not possible to quantitate directly parathyroid cell cyclic nucleotides in intact organ preparations. Moreover, release of cyclic nucleotides from tissue fragments may represent contributions from several different cell types. Finally, it is unlikely that all cells in a macroscopic fragment receive equal exposure to extracellular hormones, ions, or nutrients. Thus, while intact organ preparations have been useful in studying regulation of PTH secretion by various secretagogues, direct evaluation of the relationship of parathyroid cellular cAMP to PTH secretion requires a more purified cell preparation. Such dispersed or isolated cell preparations have been employed by a number of workers with other tissues.

D. DEVELOPMENT OF DISPERSED PARATHYROID CELL PREPARATIONS

Several workers have developed dispersed parathyroid cell preparations in different species. Brown et al. prepared dispersed bovine (Brown et al., 1976a) and human (Brown et al., 1978a) cell systems. Okano et al. (1976) have reported studies with monolayer cultures of bovine parathyroid cells. Morrissey and Cohn (1978) have developed a dispersed porcine parathyroid cell preparation. All these systems employed enzymic digestion of minced parathyroid tissue. In the bovine system (Brown et al., 1976a), fat cells liberated during the digestion float during sedimentation and washing of the parathyroid cells. Red blood cells sediment more slowly than the small clumps of parathyroid cells and may be largely eliminated by repeated washes. The final preparation contains 90-95% parathyroid cells by light and electron microscopy (H. Hargraves and E. M. Brown, unpublished observations).

To employ such dispersed cell preparations for studying the role of cyclic nucleotides in secretion requires that the in vitro systems accurately reflect parathyroid function in vivo. The appearance of dispersed bovine parathyroid cells on electron microscopy (Brown et al., 1976a) is essentially identical to that of parathyroid cells in the gland in situ. Moreover, direct comparison of parathyroid function in vivo and in vitro has been carried out with human parathyroid tissue (Brown et al., 1979a). Calcium infusion was carried out preoperatively in patients with primary hyperparathyroidism. Dispersed cells were prepared from pathologic parathyroid tissue, and the effects of increased calcium concentration of PTH release were assessed. When in vivo and in vitro results were compared, there was close agreement regardless of the absolute degree of suppressibility of the tissue. There likewise is good agreement between in vivo and in vitro studies of parathyroid secretory function in the cow, although such studies have not been carried out in the same laboratory. The inhibition of secretion by calcium as well as the stimulation by epinephrine are qualitatively very similar in studies with dispersed cells (Brown et al., 1978c) and in studies of the venous effluent of bovine parathyroid glands (Mayer *et al.*, 1976, 1979b). With such cell preparations, the possibility exists that receptors might be damaged by the enzymic digestion procedure. Moreover, small numbers of contaminating cell types could contribute to the effects of various secretagogues on cAMP accumulation. Comparison with changes in PTH secretion provides additional evidence that the parathyroid cell is the source of the cyclic nucleotide.

E. AGENTS THAT MODIFY CYCLIC NUCLEOTIDES AND SECRETION

The recent development (Harper and Brooker, 1975) of highly sensitive radioimmunoassays for cyclic nucleotides employing acetylation of tissue extracts has made it possible to measure cellular cAMP and cGMP in small amounts of tissue. With this cAMP assay and radioimmunoassay for PTH, it is possible to determine hormone secretion and cellular cAMP with several hundred thousand cells.

1. *Agents That Elevate cAMP in Bovine Parathyroid Cells*

a. β-Adrenergic Catecholamines. β-Adrenergic actions in a variety of tissues are mediated through activation of adenylate cyclase. It was not surprising, therefore, the β-adrenergic agonists enhanced cAMP accumulation (Brown *et al.*, 1977a) as well as adenylate cyclase activity (Brown *et al.*, 1977b) in dispersed bovine parathyroid cells. The increased cAMP was due to increases in both intracellular as well as extracellular cAMP (Brown *et al.*, 1978c). Intracellular cAMP increases rapidly (less than 1 minute) up to 60-fold, reaches a maximum within 5–10 minutes, and slowly decreases to control levels over the ensuing 30–60 minutes (Fig. 2). Extracellular cAMP increases progressively as long as intracellular cAMP remains elevated. With agents that cause smaller increases in intracellular cAMP, such as the phosphodiesterase inhibitor methylisobutylxanthine (MIX) (see later), there is a correspondingly smaller increase in extracellular cAMP (Fig. 2). Without agonists, there is virtually no release of cAMP into the medium (Fig. 2). Thus, while there is a general correspondence between intra- and extracellular cAMP, the latter may not be an adequate measure of intracellular cAMP, particularly with a heterogeneous cell population.

The time course for increases in PTH secretion with isoproterenol is also very rapid ($\leq$ 2.5 minutes), consistent with a mediatory role for cAMP (Brown *et al.*, 1978c). The addition of ($-$)-propranolol, a potent β-adrenergic blocker, to cells stimulated with ($-$)-isoproterenol causes a rapid decrease in the rate of PTH release as well as intracellular

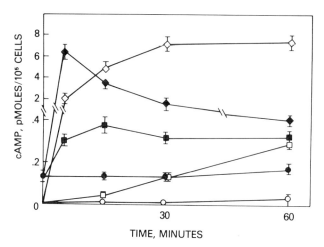

FIG. 2. Effects of agonists on intra- and extracellular cyclic AMP (cAMP). Dispersed cells were incubated with 1.0 mM calcium alone (circles), 1.0 mM Ca^{2+} plus 2×10^{-4} M MIX (squares), or 1.0 mM Ca^{2+} plus 10^{-6} M $(-)$-isoproterenol (diamonds). Intracellular (filled symbols) and extracellular (open symbols) cAMP were determined by radioimmunoassay at the times indicated. Note the break in the scale on the ordinate. From Brown et al. (1978c) with permission.

cAMP levels. This observation is consistent with the hypothesis that increases in cAMP are causally related to an enhanced rate of secretion.

The bovine parathyroid β-adrenergic receptor may also be directly identified with the iodinated β blocker [^{125}I]iodohydroxybenzylpindolol (Brown et al., 1976b). Studies with this ligand suggest the presence of 5000–10,000 receptors per cell that show saturability and stereospecificity for β-adrenergic agonists and antagonists that would be expected of this receptor (Brown et al., 1977b).

The order of potency of the β-adrenergic agonists $(-)$-isoproterenol, $(-)$-epinephrine, and $(-)$-norepinephrine in direct binding studies, as well as in stimulation of cAMP content and secretion, indicate the presence of a β_2 adrenergic receptor (Lands et al., 1967). Studies with the selective β_1 antagonist practolol ($K_i \cong 3 \times 10^{-5}$) and the β_2 antagonist butoxamine ($K_i \cong 3 \times 10^{-6}$) (E. M. Brown et al., unpublished observations) are also consistent with a β_2 receptor. Kukreja et al. (1976), on the other hand, have suggested that bovine parathyroid tissue slices contain a β_1 receptor based on the inhibition of isoproterenol-stimulated secretion by butoxamine and practolol. These authors, however, have not reported data for the agonists employed above or for cAMP accumulation in a homogeneous cell preparation.

The function of the bovine parathyroid β-adrenergic receptors is uncertain. Bovine parathyroid glands, unlike human glands (Norberg *et al.*, 1975), do not appear to have noradrenergic nerve endings terminating on parathyroid cells (Jacobowitz and Brown, 1980). Nevertheless, *in vivo* evidence suggests that the parathyroid is capable of responding to changes in circulating catecholamines within the physiologic range (Mayer *et al.*, 1979a; Blum *et al.*, 1978a,b).

b. *Dopaminergic Catecholamines.* Dopaminergic agonists, such as dopamine and epinine, cause a dose-dependent, 20- to 30-fold increase in cAMP accumulation and a 2- to 4-fold stimulation of PTH release from dispersed bovine parathyroid cells (Brown *et al.*, 1977c). These effects are blocked by dopaminergic antagonists such as flupenthixol or fluphenazine, but not by β-adrenergic or α-adrenergic inhibitors. Recent studies (Attie *et al.*, 1980) indicate that the parathyroid dopaminergic receptor is a D_1 receptor, acting through stimulation of adenylate cyclase. The presence of a bovine parathyroid dopamine receptor has also been confirmed *in vivo* (Blum *et al.*, 1979).

The functional role of these dopaminergic receptors is also uncertain. It is of interest, however, that while no dopaminergic nerve endings have been found in the bovine parathyroid gland, there are abundant mast cells containing large amounts of dopamine (Jacobowitz and Brown, 1980). The physiologic significance of these cells is unknown.

c. *Secretin.* Secretin (10^{-7} M) causes a 4- to 6-fold increase in cAMP content and a 1.5- to 2-fold stimulation of PTH release (Windeck *et al.*, 1978). Other gastrointestinal hormones, such as vasoactive intestinal peptide (VIP), glucagon, gastrin or pentagastrin, and cholecystokinin, have no such effects. While there are known interactions between gastrointestinal hormones and calcitonin secretion (see below), it is not yet known whether similar relationships exist for the parathyroid gland *in vivo*.

d. *Prostaglandin E_2 (PGE$_2$).* Prostaglandin E_2 causes modest increases in cAMP accumulation (2-fold) and PTH release (1.5-fold) from dispersed bovine parathyroid cells (Gardner *et al.*, 1978). There was no effect of indomethacin, a prostaglandin synthesis inhibitor, on calcium-regulated PTH release, which suggests that endogenous prostaglandin production by such cell preparations did not have a major effect on hormone secretion. A similar effect of prostaglandins of the E series has been noted in monolayer cultures of bovine parathyroid cells (Okano *et al.*, 1976).

e. *Cholera Toxin.* Cholera toxin activates adenylate cyclase in essentially all tissues in which it has been tested. In dispersed bovine parathyroid cells, after a 30-minute lag time, cholera toxin alone enhanced cAMP accumulation and PTH secretion (Brown *et al.*, 1979b). In the presence of agents that raise cAMP content, such as dopamine or secretin, the cells were rendered more sensitive to the effects of the agonists on cAMP content and secretion. No such change was noted with agents that lower cAMP content, such as α-adrenergic agonists or $PGF_{2\alpha}$ (Gardner *et al.*, 1979a) (see Section II, E, 3,b).

f. Phosphodiesterase Inhibitors. Inhibitors of phosphodiesterase, such as MIX, enhanced cAMP accumulation 3-fold or more and PTH release 2-fold in dispersed bovine parathyroid cells (Brown *et al.*, 1978c). Moreover, cAMP content in response to other agonists was also increased about 3-fold.

2. Relationship of cAMP Accumulation to PTH Release in Dispersed Bovine Parathyroid Cells

Comparisons were carried out between effects of increasing concentrations of agonists or antagonists on cAMP accumulation and PTH release under identical experimental conditions (Brown *et al.*, 1978c) (Fig. 3). PTH release was enhanced half-maximally by significantly lower concentrations of agonist than cAMP accumulation, suggesting that secretion could be maximally stimulated by submaximal concentrations of cAMP. Plots of the increase in rate of hormone secretion as a function of the logarithm of the increment in cAMP over control at any concentration of agonist give a straight line up to concentrations of cAMP maximally stimulating secretion (Fig. 4). Moreover, the same relationship was observed regardless of whether the agonist employed was isoproterenol, dopamine, secretin, or MIX. This observation makes it unlikely that different "pools" of cAMP mediate the effects of different agonists on secretion.

3. Agents That Decrease cAMP Content and Secretion in Dispersed Bovine Parathyroid Cells

a. α-Adrenergic Catecholamines. Mixed α- and β-adrenergic agonists such as $(-)$-epinephrine or $(-)$-norepinephrine cause 50% or less of the maximal increase in cAMP content observed with $(-)$-isoproterenol in dispersed bovine parathyroid cells (Brown *et al.*, 1978b). This difference is largely obviated in the presence of the α-adrenergic inhibitor phentolamine. An inhibitory effect of α-adrenergic agents on cAMP accumulation was also suggested by a direct inhibition of isoproterenol- or dopamine-stimulated cAMP accumulation by $(-)$-epinephrine. The effects of mixed α- and β-adrenergic agonists in this system, therefore, represent the sum of stimulatory β properties and inhibitory α properties.

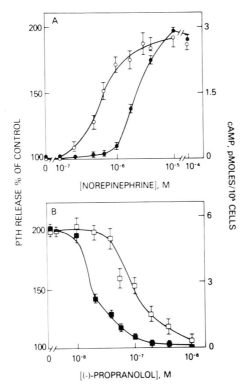

FIG. 3. Effects of β-adrenergic agonists and antagonists on cyclic AMP (cAMP) content of, and PTH release from, bovine parathyroid cells. In panel A, increases in cAMP content (●) and PTH release (○) are plotted as a function of increasing concentrations of norepinephrine. In panel B, cells were incubated with $10^{-6}M$ (−)-isoproterenol, and the effects of increasing concentrations of (−)-propranolol on cAMP (■) and PTH release (□) are indicated. In both panels, the incubation time was 5 minutes. From Brown *et al.* (1978c) with permission.

b. Prostaglandin $F_{2\alpha}$ ($PGF_{2\alpha}$). Prostaglandins of the F series inhibit basal as well as agonist-stimulated cAMP accumulation and PTH secretion. This effect did not appear to be mediated through any of the adrenergic receptors discussed previously, since α-adrenergic, β-adrenergic, and dopaminergic antagonists did not affect the response of either cAMP or PTH to $PGF_{2\alpha}$. Studies on the relationship of agonist-stimulated cAMP accumulation to PTH release with or without $PGF_{2\alpha}$ suggest that the effects of the prostaglandin on secretion could be explained on a quantitative basis by the decrease in cellular cAMP (Brown *et al.*, 1978c). Similar observations were made for the α-adrenergic inhibition of cAMP accumulation and PTH release. The physiologic significance of this receptor is uncertain, since prostaglan-

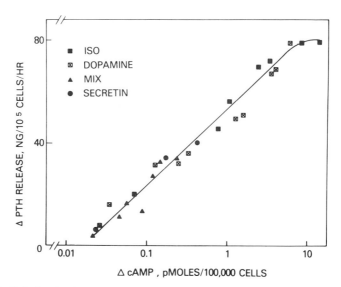

Fig. 4. Relationship between increases in agonist-stimulated cyclic AMP (cAMP) accumulation and PTH release. Each point represents the increase in cAMP content and PTH release rate over control at a given concentration of the agonists shown. iso, isoproterenol; MIX, methylisobutylxanthine. Incubation time was 5 minutes at a calcium concentration of 1.0 mM. From Brown et al. (1978c) with permission.

din synthesis inhibitors did not alter the inhibition of PTH release by calcium (Gardner et al., 1979a).

c. *Nitroprusside.* The vasodilator nitroprusside is a potent inhibitor of both cAMP accumulation and PTH release from dispersed bovine parathyroid cells (Gardner et al., 1979b). As with $PGF_{2\alpha}$, studies with selective antagonists suggest that this, inhibition is not mediated through the adrenergic receptors on the bovine parathyroid cells.

d. *Divalent Cations.* Calcium and magnesium ions each lower cAMP content and PTH release from dispersed bovine parathyroid cells, although magnesium is 3-fold less potent on a molar basis (Brown et al., 1978c; Habener and Potts, 1976). The general correspondence between decreases in cAMP content and secretion with these different agents suggests that cAMP may mediate the effects of agents that lower, as well as of agents that elevate intracellular cAMP. Studies of the interaction of calcium with agents that elevate cAMP, however, suggest that calcium does not act solely by decreasing cAMP accumulation.

Dispersed bovine parathyroid cells incubated with increasing concentrations of dopamine at either high (1.5 mM) or low (0.5 mM) am-

bient calcium concentration (Brown *et al.*, 1978c) show a dispropor-
tionate inhibition of secretion relative to cAMP accumulation (Fig. 5).
Dopamine-stimulated cAMP accumulation plotted as a function of
change in rate of secretion at two different calcium concentrations
(Fig. 5) reveals two parallel log-linear relationships. At the higher
calcium concentration, a given increase in secretory rate was associated with a 10-fold or higher increase in intracellular cAMP content. That is, elevated extracellular calcium appeared to alter not only
cAMP content per se, but also the secretory response to a given intracellular cAMP level.

From studies with the calcium ionophore A23187 (Habener *et al.*,
1977a; Brown *et al.*, 1980), it seems likely that the parathyroid cell
responds to changes in extracellular calcium concentration through an
alteration in intracellular calcium. A23187 increases the sensitivity of

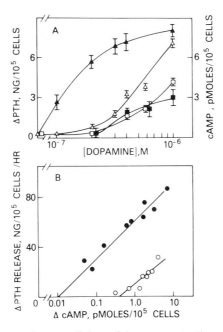

FIG. 5. Effect of increased extracellular calcium concentration on the relationship
between cyclic AMP (cAMP) accumulation and PTH release in response to dopamine.
Panel A shows the effect of increasing dopamine concentrations on cAMP (open symbols)
or PTH release (filled symbols) at 0.5 mM calcium (triangles) or 1.5 mM calcium (squares).
In panel B, the results (0.5 mM Ca^{2+}, ●; 1.5 mM calcium, ○) are plotted as in Fig. 4. Note
the shift in the log-linear relationship to the right at 1.5 mM Ca^{2+}. Incubation time was
5 minutes. From Brown *et al.* (1978c) with permission.

the bovine parathyroid cell to extracellular calcium concentration. This effect is observed for calcium-regulated secretion in the absence of agonists as well as for agonist-stimulated cAMP generation. Moreover, at a given extracellular calcium concentration, the addition of ionophore inhibits agonist-stimulated secretion more than cAMP accumulation. Thus, plots as illustrated in Fig. 5 show shifts toward higher cAMP concentrations by ionophore in the relationship between cAMP and secretion (Brown et al., 1980), just as observed with an increase in extracellular calcium concentration. Studies of ^{45}Ca flux in dispersed bovine parathyroid cells suggest that the ionophore acts, at least in part, through mobilization of intracellular calcium stores (Brown et al., 1980). Ramp et al. (1979) suggest that some minimal quantity of calcium transfer across the parathyroid cell membrane is required for hormone secretion. At zero added calcium there was no detectable release of hormone from isolated thyroparathyroid gland complexes in vitro. Verapamil, which inhibits calcium entry into cells, inhibited hormone release with 1 mM calcium in the medium, conditions normally favoring secretion. Verapamil enhanced release at 2.5 mM calcium, which normally suppresses secretion. Calcium fluxes have not been carried out to determine the nature of verapamil action on parathyroid preparations.

It should be noted that, unlike most secretory cell systems, the calcium ionophore does not stimulate PTH secretion. The enhanced secretion observed with A23187 in other cells has been taken as evidence in support of the concept of "stimulus-secretion coupling" (agonist-induced stimulation of secretion through increases in intracellular calcium concentration) (Douglas, 1968; Rubin, 1970). "Stimulus-secretion coupling," therefore, may not contribute to the regulation of PTH secretion. In fact, Bruce and Anderson (1979) have recently shown that conditions associated with enhanced PTH secretion from mouse parathyroid glands (e.g., hypocalcemia) cause hyperpolarization of the gland. In other secretory cells, stimulation of secretion is frequently accompanied by depolarization of the cell membrane.

4. Agents That Increase Cyclic GMP (cGMP)

Nitroprusside. Nitroprusside increases cGMP accumulation and guanylate cyclase activity in dispersed parathyroid cells in parallel with inhibition of cAMP accumulation and secretion (D. G. Gardner et al., unpublished observations). Since neither exogenous cGMP nor dibutyryl cGMP inhibited cAMP content or secretion, it seems unlikely that the effects of nitroprusside on these parameters were mediated by the changes in cGMP metabolism.

5. Agents That Modulate Cyclic Nucleotides and PTH Secretion in Human Parathyroid Cells

The difficulties inherent in obtaining supplies of fresh, normal human parathyroid tissue have so far precluded detailed studies of the regulation of cAMP and PTH secretion with normal human cells. A number of agents, however, have been defined that alter cAMP accumulation and hormone release from cells prepared from pathologic parathyroid tissue (adenomas and primary parathyroid hyperplasia) (Brown *et al.*, 1979c). A comparison of the agents that modify cAMP and secretion in the human and bovine cell systems is shown in Table I, and a summary follows.

a. β-adrenergic Catecholamines. Cell preparations from nearly all pathologic parathyroid glands show an increase in cAMP content in response to β-adrenergic agonists (Brown, *et al.*, 1979c). The responses vary, however, from small (less than 2-fold) to a magnitude approaching that of bovine parathyroid cells (30-fold). In addition, the subtype of receptor varies among cell preparations from different pathologic glands. In nearly half the cases, the receptor was β_1, and in the remainder it was of the β_2 subtype as defined by the relative potency of $(-)$-isoproterenol, $(-)$-epinephrine, and $(-)$-norepinephrine. The significance of this finding is uncertain. It might indicate that in the normal population the parathyroid β receptor is not invariably of one subtype. Alternatively, one or the other receptor subtype might repre-

TABLE I

COMPARISON OF THE EFFECTS OF AGONISTS ON cAMP
ACCUMULATION IN BOVINE OR HUMAN PARATHYROID
CELLS[a,b]

Agonist	Bovine	Human
β-Adrenergic	↑↑↑↑	− to ↑↑↑
Dopamine	↑↑↑	−
Histamine	−	↑ to ↑↑↑↑
Secretin	↑↑	−
Glucagon	−	↑↑ to ↑↑↑
PGE$_2$	↑	↑ to ↑↑↑
α-Adrenergic	↓↓	NT
PGF$_{2\alpha}$	↓↓↓	− to ↑

[a] Human cells were prepared from pathologic human parathyroid tissue (see text).

[b] −, Indicates no effect; ↑, ↓, indicate stimulation or inhibition of cAMP content, respectively. NT, not tested.

sent a neoplastic transformation of the normal parathyroid β receptor. In other tissues, ectopic β receptors in tumors have been described (L. T. Williams *et al.*, 1977) as well as a change in receptor subtype attendant upon cellular transformation (Sheppard, 1977).

The secretory response to β-adrenergic catecholamines varied considerably, as well as the magnitude of cAMP response and receptor subtype (Brown *et al.*, 1979c). Inhibition of the secretory response was observed at high calcium concentrations as with bovine tissue; in addition, there was also a wide variation in responsiveness to $(-)$-isoproterenol at 1.0 mM calcium concentration. The basis for this variability has not been determined.

It was also possible to demonstrate β-adrenergic receptors directly with [^{125}I]iodohydroxybenzylpindolol (Brown *et al.*, 1979c). The receptor had the characteristics of saturability, high affinity, and stereospecificity for $(-)$- and $(+)$-propranolol observed with the bovine parathyroid receptor. Derenoncourt *et al.* (1977) have also demonstrated β-adrenergic receptors on homogenates of fragments of pathologic parathyroid tissue in organ culture.

As with the bovine parathyroid gland, the physiological significance of the response to β-adrenergic catecholamines is uncertain. Shah *et al.* (1975) have demonstrated an increase in peripheral PTH after insulin-induced hypoglycemia. Caro *et al.* (1979) have also reported that propranolol lowers immunoreactive PTH and serum calcium in patients with primary hyperparathyroidism. These effects are small and may reflect in part changes in circulating catecholamines and hemodynamics. It is also possible that adrenergic nerve endings are involved, since histofluorescent studies have shown nerves terminating on human parathyroid cells (Norberg *et al.*, 1975).

b. Histamine. Histamine stimulates cAMP accumulation and PTH release from dispersed cells prepared from tissue of patients with adenomas and primary parathyroid hyperplasia (Brown *et al.*, 1979c). Accumulation of cAMP is enhanced from 2- to 100-fold and is inhibited by the histamine antagonists promethazine and cimetidine; secretion is stimulated up to 2-fold by 10^{-5} M histamine (Brown, 1980). The physiologic significance of human parathyroid histamine receptors is unknown. It is of interest, however, that human cells respond to histamine but not to dopamine, while the reverse is true for dispersed bovine parathyroid cells. As with bovine parathyroid tissue, human parathyroid glands also contain mast cells, which, in analogy to other human tissues, would be expected to store histamine but not dopamine.

c. Glucagon. Glucagon also enhances cAMP accumulation and secretion in dispersed parathyroid cells from pathologic tissue (Brown *et al.*, 1979c). Content of cAMP is increased up to 20-fold, and maximal increases in PTH release (2-fold) are similar to those observed with isoproterenol and histamine in these cell preparations (E. M. Brown, unpublished observations). The concentration of glucagon half-maximally stimulating cAMP accumulation is similar to that observed in other tissues (Rodbell *et al.*, 1971). Unlike bovine parathyroid cells, human parathyroid cells are not stimulated by secretin. It is not yet clear whether normal human parathyroid cells have a receptor for glucagon or other gastrointestinal hormones. It is possible that enteroparathyroid relationships exist in man. Alternatively, glucagon as well as histamine responsiveness may represent examples of "ectopic" hormone receptors not present in normal cells.

d. Prostaglandin E_2 (PGE$_2$). Prostaglandins of the E series consistently stimulate cAMP accumulation and PTH release in cell preparations from pathologic human parathyroid tissue. PGE_2 is most effective; PGE_1 causes less response; and $PGF_{2\alpha}$ stimulates cAMP accumulation only in some cell preparations at high concentrations (Gardner *et al.*, 1980). Unlike bovine parathyroid cells, however, $PGF_{2\alpha}$ has no inhibitory actions in these cells. Whether normal human parathyroid cells have inhibitory $PGF_{2\alpha}$ receptors or whether the absence of these inhibitory receptors is related to the abnormal inhibition of PTH release by calcium (see below) with pathologic parathyroid tissue is not known.

e. Effects of Divalent Cations. Brown *et al.* (1978a, 1979d) have shown abnormal regulation of PTH release by calcium in dispersed cells prepared from abnormal human parathyroid tissue. In most cell preparations from parathyroid adenomas, maximal inhibition of PTH release is similar to that observed with normal human parathyroid cells, but the sensitivity to calcium is diminished. That is, the "set-point" (calcium concentration half-maximally inhibiting PTH release) is increased. In the remaining adenomatous glands, maximal suppressibility is 50% or less. It is not yet clear whether there are corresponding changes in the responsiveness of cAMP to elevated calcium concentrations.

6. *Agents That Modulate Release of Cyclic Nucleotides and PTH from Porcine Parathyroid Cells*

Relatively few data are available as yet on the effects of various secretagogues on cyclic nucleotides and secretion with porcine parathyroid cells. Isoproterenol appears to enhance cAMP content whereas increased extracellular calcium concentrations decrease cellular cAMP with parallel changes in PTH secretion (Morrissey and Cohn, 1979a). The effects of other agents on these parameters in porcine parathyroid cells are awaited with interest.

7. *Agents with Uncertain Effects on Intracellular Cyclic Nucleotides*

A number of additional agents have been defined that modify PTH secretion *in vivo* or *in vitro*. In many instances, these have not been tested in dispersed cell systems in which effects on cyclic nucleotides could be quantitated. In some cases, the same secretagogues tested in other systems have been associated with changes in cyclic nucleotides, suggesting cyclic nucleotide-mediated actions in the parathyroid. In others, the agent in question has not caused changes in cyclic nucleotides in other tissues.

a. Vitamin D Metabolites. Several vitamin D metabolites have been reported to alter PTH secretion *in vivo* and *in vitro*. In several instances, contradictory effects have been observed (for review, see Golden *et al.*, 1979), and the physiologic significance of these observations is uncertain. For example, 1,25-dihydroxyvitamin D has been reported to stimulate (Oldham *et al.*, 1974; Canterbury *et al.*, 1978), inhibit (Chertow *et al.*, 1975a) or have no effect (Tanaka *et al.*, 1979) on PTH secretion. The effects of this metabolite, however, have not been evaluated on intracellular cAMP in a purified cell preparation. Recently, Dietel *et al.* (1979) have reported 1,25-dihydroxyvitamin D-induced inhibition of cAMP release into the medium from parathyroid tissue slices in association with inhibition of PTH release. As discussed above, however, changes in the release of cyclic nucleotides from tissue fragments must be interpreted with caution. This interesting observation will require confirmation in a more purified cell preparation.

b. Anion Transport Inhibitors. Probenecid and disodium 4–acetamido-4′–isothiocyanostilbene-2,2′–disulfonate (SITS) which inhibit anion transport in other systems, have been found to lower basal and stimulated PTH release from dispersed bovine parathyroid cells by 70% or more (Brown *et al.*, 1978d). At high concentrations, these agents reduce isoproterenol-stimulated cAMP accumulation by 50–60%. On a quantitative basis, however, this decrease in cAMP could not account for the degree of inhibition of secretion (Brown *et al.*, 1978c). It has been suggested that anion transport blockers inhibit the secretion of PTH and other hormones and neurotransmitters by an action on the exocytotic process per se (Pollard *et al.*, 1977).

c. Other Factors That Modify PTH Secretion. Vitamin A has been reported to stimulate PTH release *in vitro* (Chertow *et al.*, 1975b). The mechanisms underlying this effect, however, and the possible involvement of cyclic nucleotides are uncertain. Calcitonin enhanced PTH secretion from porcine parathyroid tissue slices *in vitro* (Fischer *et al.*, 1971). Since calcitonin stimulates adenylate cyclase activity and cAMP accumulation in other tissues (see Section VI,B), it seems probable that this effect is mediated through similar mechanisms in the porcine parathyroid. The secretion of PTH from rat parathyroid glands in organ culture was stimulated by cortisol (Au, 1976). The potential role of cAMP in this action has not been investigated.

G. A. Williams *et al.* (1978) found that ethanol increases serum iPTH in normal subjects and enhances PTH secretion from bovine parathyroid tissue slices. The mechanisms by which ethanol augments parathyroid secretion are unknown, but ethanol has been shown to stimulate cAMP accumulation in other tissues (Vesely *et al.*, 1978). Somatostatin was found by Hargis *et al.* (1978) to inhibit PTH secretion from normal bovine and adenomatous human parathyroid tissue *in vitro* and to lower serum PTH in rat and monkey. Other investigators, on the other hand, found no effects of somatostatin infusion on basal or stimulated PTH concentration *in vivo* in man (Deftos *et al.*, 1976). While somatostatin caused modest inhibition of cAMP accumulation in some tissues (Borgeat *et al.*, 1974; Efandic *et al.*, 1975), the mechanism by which it produced its effects on the parathyroid gland remain unknown. Microtubule and microfilament inhibitors decrease PTH release *in vitro* (Reaven and Reaven, 1975; Chertow *et al.*, 1977). While this effect suggests a role for these structures in PTH secretion, an action on other cellular processes has not been excluded. Alterations in cAMP metabolism were not investigated.

F. Mechanisms That Regulate Cellular Cyclic Nucleotides

1. *Adenylate Cyclase*

A number of cell surface hormone receptors activate adenylate cyclase through a GTP dependent process discussed in Section IV,B. The actions of cholera toxin on the adenylate cyclase system appear to be mediated through the inhibition of a specific GTPase that normally inactivates the catalytic form of adenylate cyclase (Cassel and Selinger, 1977). β-Adrenergic (Brown *et al.*, 1977b) and dopaminergic (Attie *et al.*, 1980) catecholamines and PGE_2 (D. G. Gardner, E. M. Brown *et al.*, unpublished observations) cause receptor-mediated activation of adenylate cyclase in bovine parathyroid cell membrane preparations. Histamine (Simon and Kather, 1977; Nakajima *et al.*, 1971), secretin (Rodbell *et al.*, 1970; Desbuquois, 1974), and glucagon (Rodbell *et al.*, 1971) also activate the enzyme in other systems, although this action has not yet been shown in membrane preparations from purified parathyroid cells. The effects of agonists that cause large increases in parathyroid cell cAMP content, such as isoproterenol or dopamine, are not additive, which suggests that these hormone-receptor complexes may activate a common pool of adenylate cyclase enzyme.

The effects of cholera toxin on basal- and agonist-stimulated cAMP accumulation in dispersed parathyroid cells are also consistent with the postulated mechanism of action of this agent. With agonists that maximally increase cAMP content, such as isoproterenol, the predominant effect of cholera toxin is to enhance the effect of a given degree of receptor occupancy (Brown *et al.*, 1979b). That is, the sensitivity to the agonist is increased. With agents that cause a submaximal effect, such as secretin, both maximal cAMP accumulation and apparent potency are increased.

The mechanistic basis of the inhibitory effects of α-adrenergic agonists and PGF$_{2\alpha}$ are not yet understood in detail. In some cases, such as the platelet, α-adrenergic receptors are coupled to inhibition of adenylate cyclase (Jakobs *et al.*, 1976). The α-adrenergic-mediated decrease in agonist-stimulated cAMP accumulation in dispersed bovine parathyroid cells (Brown *et al.*, 1978b) is consistent with an inhibition of adenylate cyclase, as shown in Fig. 6. Direct evidence for this hypothesis in parathyroid membrane preparations, however, is lacking.

PGF$_{2\alpha}$ causes a modest inhibition of adenylate cyclase activity in luteal cells (Thomas *et al.*, 1978). Whether a similar mechanism is operative in bovine parathyroid cells is not known. In any event, the close coupling between effects on cAMP accumulation and PTH release in this system makes it an excellent experimental model for studying the mechanism of action of various hormonal agents that cause receptor-mediated changes in parathyroid secretion.

There are several possible bases for the inhibitory effects of calcium on cAMP content and secretion in dispersed bovine parathyroid cells. Calcium inhibits adenylate cyclase in a variety of tissues, including equine (Matsuzaki and Dumont, 1972), canine (Dufresne *et al.*, 1971), bovine (Attie *et al.*, 1980), and human (Rodriquez *et al.*, 1978) parathyroid gland. Reported K_i values for this effect vary from 10^{-6} to 10^{-3} M. Cytosolic calcium concentrations have been measured in only a few instances (Scarpa *et al.*, 1978), and are 10^{-8} to 10^{-7} M under basal conditions. The physiologic relevance, therefore, of inhibitory effects of calcium in the range of 10^{-6} to 10^{-3} M is uncertain.

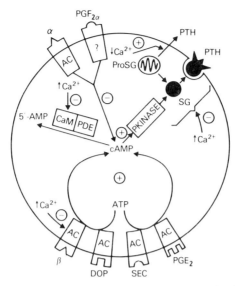

Fig. 6. Schematic diagram for regulation by calcium and cyclic AMP (cAMP) of PTH secretion. β, DOP, SEC, and PGE$_2$ represent the receptors for β-adrenergic catecholamines, dopaminergic catecholamines, secretin, and prostaglandin E$_2$, respectively, stimulating cAMP accumulation through activation of adenylate cyclase (AC). α and PGF$_{2\alpha}$ are the receptors for α-adrenergic catecholamines and prostaglandin F$_{2\alpha}$, which lower cAMP content. cAMP is hydrolyzed by phosphodiesterase (PDE), one form of which is activated by calmodulin (CaM). The effects of cAMP are presumably mediated by protein kinase (PKINASE), leading to activation of exocytosis of secretory granules (SG) containing PTH. Possible sites of action of calcium are indicated: inhibiting adenylate cyclase, activating phosphodiesterase, inhibiting PTH release distal to cAMP generation, or stimulating (low calcium) the release of immature secretory granules (ProSG). (+), Positive effect on secretion of PTH; (−), inhibitory effect on secretion.

2. Phosphodiesterase

It has also been found that calcium activates cyclic nucleotide phosphodiesterase through a calcium-dependent regulatory protein, calmodulin (Cheung, 1970; Kakiuchi and Yamazaki, 1970; Teo and Wang, 1973). This small, acidic, polyfunctional protein is probably present in all tissues (for comprehensive reviews, see Cheung, 1979; Wolff and Brostrom, 1979). In addition to its effects on phosphodiesterase, it also causes a calcium-dependent activation of adenylate cyclase in some tissues, as well as phospholipase A$_2$, myosin light-chain kinase, glycogen phosphorylase kinase, Ca-Mg ATPase, and probably other proteins (Cheung, 1979). This activation occurs at 1–10 μM Ca, above resting cytosolic [Ca^{2+}], but within the range observed in activated cells (during muscle contraction, for example).

Calmodulin and a calmodulin-activated phosphodiesterase have recently been found in dispersed bovine parathyroid cells (E. M. Brown, 1980). The relationship of calmodulin to a previously described porcine parathyroid calcium-binding protein (Oldham *et al.*, 1974) is uncertain. Thus, in this sytem, increased extracellular calcium might inhibit the formation as well as enhance the degradation of cAMP.

Cyclic AMP appears to be removed from the cell through a specific transport process that is blocked by probenecid (Davoren and Sutherland, 1963). This process may also be inhibited by PGA_1 (Brunton and Mayer, 1979). It has not been ruled out that calcium lowers cAMP by increased cellular efflux of cAMP.

G. Mechanisms That Mediate the Effects of cAMP

1. *Role of Protein Kinase*

It is generally accepted that the effects of cAMP are mediated through alterations in the activity of protein kinase(s). In the inactive state, the enzyme is a tetramer, consisting of two regulatory or cAMP binding subunits and two catalytic subunits (R_2C_2). After interaction of the holoenzyme with cAMP, the R–cAMP complex dissociates, activating the catalytic subunit. The free catalytic moiety then is thought to phosphorylate various cellular substrates to produce characteristic physiologic alterations.

Techniques have been developed for assessing the degree of activation of protein kinase in intact cells. With the sensitive acetylated radioimmunoassay described above, it is possible to measure directly cyclic nucleotides bound to the regulatory subunit of protein kinase (Dufau *et al.*, 1977; Terasaki and Brooker, 1977). Thus, after hormonal perturbation of an intact cell preparation, an indirect measurement of changes in the degree of kinase activation may be made. A second approach is to assay directly the content of free catalytic subunit (c) in extracts of cells (Corbin *et al.*, 1973). Under appropriate conditions, there is relatively slow dissociation or association of protein kinase after homogenization of a tissue, and changes in the content of catalytic subunit may be made after manipulation by secretagogues.

Although these techniques have not yet been applied to dispersed parathyroid cells, it seems likely that, as in other tissues, increases in intracellular cAMP will correlate with changes in the activity of cAMP-dependent protein kinase. Indeed, the log-linear relationship between intracellular cAMP and increased secretion rate in dispersed bovine parathyroid cells may reflect, in part, interactions of cAMP with protein kinase. With bovine parathyroid cells, as with other cell types (e.g., Dufau *et al.*, 1977), agonist-stimulated cAMP accumulation may be in excess of that required to enhance maximally the biologic response (see Fig. 3). The plateau in the log-linear relationship in Fig. 4 might represent, therefore, activation of protein kinase sufficient to achieve a maximal secretory rate.

As noted above, it has recently become clear that changes in calcium concentration may modulate the activity of various protein kinases through calmodulin-mediated mechanisms. Thus, parathyroid cell calmodulin might alter the response to cAMP as well as change cAMP content per se.

2. Possible Secretory Mechanisms Modulated by Calcium, Cyclic Nucleotides, and Protein Kinase

The anatomic sites of action of calcium and other secretagogues on the biosynthesis and secretion of parathyroid hormone have not been established. Calcium and cyclic nucleotides have not been shown to have major effects on the rate of formation of proparathyroid hormone or the conversion of the prohormone to native PTH (Habener *et al.*, 1974, 1975). Present evidence, therefore, suggests that these agents affect secretion at more distal loci.

MacGregor *et al.* (1975), in studies of bovine parathyroid tissue, and more recently Morrissey and Cohn (1979a,b), with dispersed porcine parathyroid cells, have presented evidence for distinct pools of PTH differentially affected by calcium or by agents elevating cyclic nucleotide content. Their data are consistent with an effect of low calcium predominantly on the mobilization of newly synthesized PTH. Whether this hormone is not in secretory granules [the "bypass" pathway (MacGregor *et al.*, 1975)] or is located in immature secretory granules is not yet clear. β-Adrenergic agonists or dibutyryl cAMP, on the other hand, appear to stimulate the release of PTH synthesized more than 60 minutes previously, perhaps located within the dense secretory granules seen in Fig. 1.

The molecular mechanisms whereby reduced concentrations of calcium and increased concentrations of cAMP induce exocytosis in the parathyroid cell remain obscure. Studies in a number of secretory cell types have suggested that microtubules and microfilaments may be involved in the secretory process (Lacy *et al.*, 1968; Wolff and Williams, 1973; Hoffstein and Weisman, 1978). It has been shown that cAMP enhances phosphorylation of microtubules (Goodman *et al.*, 1970) and microtubule associated proteins (Sloboda *et al.*, 1975).

Microfilaments contain a variety of proteins, at least one of which [filamen (Davies *et al.*, 1977)] may be phosphorylated by a cAMP-dependent protein kinase. Moreover, non-muscle cell myosin, which has been postulated to be involved in cell motility or movement of cellular organelles, as in exocytosis, may be phosphorylated by a calcium-dependent kinase (Pires and Perry, 1977). The calcium-regulatory protein associated with this kinase appears to be identical to calmodulin (Yagi et al., 1978). Myosin has recently been demonstrated in the human parathyroid by immunofluorescence (Amenta and Cavallotti, 1979).

Thus it is conceivable that a series of phosphorylations, regulated by cAMP as well as cytosolic calcium, might be involved in parathyroid hormone secretion. It is also possible that entirely distinct events, such as the calcium-enhanced intracellular degradation of PTH (Fischer et al., 1972; Habener et al., 1975; MacGregor et al., 1975), modulate the secretory process.

III. Role of Cyclic Nucleotides in Calcitonin Secretion

Suitable experimental systems have become available only recently for evaluating directly the role of cyclic nucleotides in calcitonin (CT) secretion. Because of the limited data on intracellular cAMP and CT release, this topic will be discussed only briefly.

A. C-Cell Anatomy and Physiology

The thyroid C cells or parafollicular cells in mammals and cells of the ultimobranchial body in birds and fish produce CT, a 32 amino acid peptide with hypocalcemic properties. Like the chief cells of the parathyroid gland, the C cell possesses an abundant biosynthetic apparatus and secretory vesicles. In response to hypercalcemia or secretagogues (see below), CT is released, having its principal actions on bone cells and renal tubules. Its hypocalcemic effects are mediated by inhibition of bone resorption as well as calciuria and phosphaturia (discussed further in Sections V and VI). The finding of CT-like immunoreactivity in the pituitary (Deftos et al., 1978) raises the possibility of as yet unrecognized actions of the hormone.

Early in vivo studies showed that calcitonin was present in the thyroid gland (Hirsch et al., 1963) and that it could be released by local perfusion with hypercalcemic blood (Copp et al., 1963). It was subsequently found that several gastrointestinal peptides, such as pancreozymin-cholecystokinin (Care, 1970) or pentagastrin (Care et al., 1971a; Cooper et al., 1971), were also CT secretagogues. These observations suggested the possibility of a gastrointestinal C-cell feedback system (Care et al., 1971c).

B. Experimental Systems for Studying Cyclic Nucleotides and Calcitonin Secretion

Progress in elucidating the role of cAMP in regulating CT secretion has been hindered by the lack of a suitable purified CT-secreting cell system. In the thyroid gland, C cells account for only a small fraction of the total cell population. The ultimobranchial gland contains a higher fraction of CT-secreting cells; the development of a monolayer culture from this tissue (Roos *et al.*, 1974) may allow a more direct assessment of cyclic nucleotide metabolism and its regulation. The relevance of observations with this sytem to human and other mammalian systems, however, still must be evaluated.

Calcitonin-secreting cell lines from medullary thyroid carcinomas have been established (Gagel *et al.*, 1980; Epstein *et al.*, 1980). These systems should also facilitate direct determination of cellular cAMP and its relationship to CT release.

C. Indirect Evidence for a Role of cAMP in Regulating Calcitonin Release

There is considerable indirect evidence suggesting that increases in cAMP content enhance CT secretion. Cyclic AMP analogs, such as dibutyryl cAMP, and phosphodiesterase inhibitors increase CT release both *in vivo* (Care *et al.*, 1970a, 1971a; Avioli *et al.*, 1971) and *in vitro* (Bell, 1970; Cooper *et al.*, 1977; Feinblatt and Raisz, 1971; Feinblatt *et al.*, 1973). Cyclic GMP derivatives, on the other hand, are not effective (Bell, 1973; Roos *et al.*, 1974; Care *et al.*, 1970a; Avioli *et al.*, 1971). Agents known to stimulate adenylate cyclase in other tissues, such as PGE_2, glucagon, and β-adrenergic agonists, also stimulate CT secretion (Care *et al.*, 1970a,b, 1971b; Avioli *et al.*, 1971; Bell, 1970; Roos *et al.*, 1974). Stimulation by the nucleotides GTP, ITP, and UTP (Bell, 1973) might reflect enhancement of adenylate cyclase activity, since these compounds have been shown to stimulate adenylate cyclase in homogenates of parathyroid cells (Attie *et al.*, 1980) and other cell types (Bilezikian and Aurbach, 1974; Rodbell *et al.*, 1971). Such nucleotide triphosphates, however, are generally thought to penetrate intact cell membranes poorly.

Enhancement of CT secretion *in vivo* by epinephrine requires coadministration of an α-adrenergic blocker (Avioli *et al.*, 1971; Care *et al.*, 1971a). Thus, it is possible that α-adrenergic agonists mediate inhibitory effects on cAMP metabolism similar to those observed in dispersed bovine parathyroid cells.

Other agents that stimulate CT release *in vivo*, such as gastrin and cholecystokinin-pancreozymin (Care, 1970b; Care *et al.*, 1971c; Cooper *et al.,* 1971; Roos and Deftos, 1976; Roos, 1977), are believed to act independently of cAMP in other tissues. It is likely, therefore, that CT secretion can be modulated by mechanisms other than changes in this cyclic nucleotide.

D. DIRECT EVIDENCE FOR A ROLE OF cAMP IN REGULATING CALCITONIN RELEASE

Recently, rat medullary carcinomas have been employed to evaluate directly the role of cAMP in regulating CT secretion. Epstein *et al.* (1980) found that adenylate cyclase activity was enhanced by glucagon and isoproterenol in extracts of CT-secreting medullary carcinomas of WAG/rij rats. These same agonists enhanced CT release in intact animals, whereas calcium and pentagastrin, which stimulated CT secretion *in vivo,* inhibited or had no effect, respectively, on adenylate cyclase activity *in vitro.* Gagel *et al.* (1980), in the 6-23 and 44-2 rat medullary thyroid carcinoma cell lines, found that glucagon enhanced both cAMP accumulation and CT release, while K^+- or Ca^{2+}-stimulated CT secretion were not associated with changes in cellular cAMP. These results suggest at least two mechanisms for CT secretion, one involving activation of adenylate cyclase (i.e., glucagon and isoproterenol), the second acting independently of cAMP (K^+, Ca^{2+}, and pentagastrin). The nature of the latter mechanism(s) is uncertain, but both calcium and potassium might augment secretion through stimulus–secretion coupling (Douglas, 1968; Rubin, 1970). Further studies on the role of cAMP and other mechanisms in regulating CT secretion in normal and abnormal cells will be awaited with interest.

IV. MECHANISM OF ACTION OF PARATHYROID HORMONE IN THE KIDNEY

A. RECEPTORS

1. *Identification with Adenylate Cyclase Measurements*

The initial studies of Chase and Aurbach (1968, 1970) indicated that parathyroid hormone caused activation of adenylate cyclase in kidney and bone. This constituted indirect evidence that receptors for the hormone must exist in these tissues and that in the kidney PTH receptors, found principally in the cortex, appear to be distinct anatomically from those for vasopressin, principally located in the renal medulla. The work of Rosenblatt *et al.* (1977) showing that certain synthetic

PTH analogs inhibit PTH specific activation of adenylate cyclase constituted further proof that receptors for the hormone must exist. The studies cited above (Chase and Aurbach, 1968) suggested the possibility that PTH receptors were localized in the proximal tubule. Chabardes *et al.* (1978, 1977) have utilized adenylate cyclase measurements on microdissected tubule preparations as a means to analyze for hormone receptors along the course of the nephron. They find that PTH receptors are distributed in cortical regions of both the proximal and the distal tubule. Two areas of the proximal cortical tubule, the early convoluted and the straight portion, respond to PTH. In the distal cortical tubule parathyroid-sensitive enzyme is found in the granular portion. (In the mouse, the cortical ascending limb also responds to PTH.) Distinct sites segregated at least partially from the parathyroid-responsive regions are found for CT (primarily cortical ascending limb), vasopressin (collecting tubule), and catecholamines. The latter act also in the distal convoluted tubule, but at a site just proximal to the site for PTH. A schematic illustration of the several hormone-sensitive sites is given in Fig. 7. The distribution found for PTH-sensitive adenylate cyclase agrees remarkably well with the physiological findings and micropuncture studies suggesting that PTH influences phosphate transport at distal as well as proximal tubular sites (Puschett, 1978). Shlatz *et al.* (1975) further have separated renal plasma membranes into preparations representing the brush border on the one hand and the plasma front on the other. Membranes

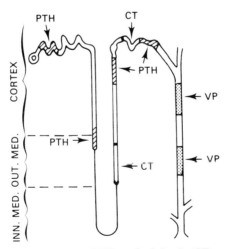

FIG. 7. Schematic diagram depicting PTH- and calcitonin (CT)-sensitive regions of the nephron of the rabbit. VP, vasopressin. Modified from Chabardes *et al.* (1978).

representing the plasma front respond to PTH, indicating that receptors for the hormone are located at the basal portion of the cell. Chambers *et al.* (1978) have developed extremely sensitive cytochemical assays for enzymes activated in response to PTH in the kidney. Their studies lend still further support for two separate regions of the nephron sensitive to PTH. In the proximal convoluted tubule PTH causes activation of alkaline phosphatase and carbonic anhydrase. In the distal convoluted tubule PTH at extremely low concentration (1–1000 femtograms/ml) causes activation of glucose-6-dehydrogenase. The exquisitely sensitive response of this latter enzyme forms the basis for an ultrasensitive biological assay for PTH (Chambers *et al.*, 1978; Fenton *et al.*, 1978; Goltzman *et al.*, 1980).

2. *PTH Receptors—Direct Identification*

Direct identification of putative receptors for PTH in the kidney has been reported by Sutcliffe *et al.* (1973), Nissenson and Arnaud (1979), Segre *et al.* (1979), Dibella *et al.* (1974), Malbon and Zull (1974), and Heath and Aurbach (1975). Radioactive ligands utilized include bPTH 1–34, norleucine-substituted bPTH 1–34 amide with tyrosine at position 34 (Segre *et al.*, 1979), iodinated bPTH 1–84, a tritiated bPTH 1–84 derivative (Malbon and Zull, 1974) and ^{75}Se-Met-PTH obtained biosynthetically (Sutcliffe *et al.*, 1973). Definitive validation of receptor binding studies for PTH has been difficult. Most of the studies show an apparent affinity of labeled PTH for the receptor that approximates reasonably well the half-maximal concentrations required for activation of adenylate cyclase in renal membranes. Studies on reversibility of binding and parallelism of apparent affinities in receptor binding versus adenylate cyclase studies are not complete. Unfortunately, few laboratories have available arrays of PTH analogs of sufficiently diverse K_m values for specificity testing in concomitant adenylate cyclase and binding assays. Definitive receptor binding studies must take into account general knowledge of the structure–activity relationships for PTH. Full agonist activity requires the amino terminal 1–34 peptide sequence of PTH. Progressive shortening of the carboxyl terminus, e.g., peptide sequences 1–28 or 1–30, show reduced biopotencies. Shortening at the amino terminus virtually completely destroys biological activity, but the peptide sequences 3–34 (or modified congeners of it) are competitive inhibitors (Segre *et al.*, 1979). Such competitive inhibitors were shown by Segre *et al.* (1979) and Rosenblatt *et al.* (1980) to compete against ^{125}I-labeled PTH ligand binding to canine renal membrane receptors. Significantly shorter chains, although of much lower affinity, can inhibit binding to the receptor. A decapeptide representing residues 25–34 showed a K_i on binding of 3 to 5 × $10^{-4}M$ (Rosenblatt et al., 1980). The latter authors concluded that the 25–34 region of parathyroid peptides is the minimum essential for receptor binding activity.

Heath and Aurbach (1975) found that oxycel preparations of porcine ACTH inhibited apparent receptor binding of PTH without comparable inhibition of adenylate cyclase activity. This finding raised serious concern about the biological specificity of iodinated PTH binding studies. In more recent studies (Segre et al., 1979; Nissenson and Arnaud, 1978; Malbon and Zull, 1974), ACTH did not seem to impair PTH binding or, if so, only at high concentrations that also inhibited PTH activation of adenylate cyclase (Nissenson and Arnaud, 1978). However, in some studies lower concentrations of ACTH were used than necessary for adequate control. Rosenblatt et al. (1980) note, moreover, that ACTH sequence 1–11 has significant homologies with PTH sequence 15–25. This finding may account for some of the ACTH interactions with presumed PTH receptors. Overall, the studies on direct identification of PTH receptors using radioactive ligands are highly suggestive. On the other hand, the several discrepancies cited indicate that definitive validation of PTH receptor binding requires still further work.

Desensitization ("down-regulation") has been described in several hormone receptor systems (Kahn, 1976). This is a phenomenon wherein receptors undergo apparent loss upon exposure to hormone and may reflect aggregates (patching and capping of surface receptors) of receptors containing bound hormone that are subsequently internalized within the cell. Forte and his associates (Forte et al., 1976, 1978; Carnes et al., 1978; Nickols et al., 1979) have described decreased responsiveness in vivo (cAMP excretion) and in vitro (adenylate cyclase activation and cAMP accumulation) of kidney tissue after exposure to high concentrations of exogenous or endogenous PTH. Endogenous hormone hypersecretion was induced via vitamin D depletion. Similarly, Tomlinson et al. (1974) have shown apparent loss of sensitivity of urinary cAMP excretion in man after injection of large amounts of PTH. In the vitamin D-depleted rat, hormone responsiveness was restored after correction of hypocalcemia via calcium injection or administration of vitamin D (Forte et al., 1976). Heersche et al. (1978) showed that exposure of bone in vitro to certain hormones led to refractoriness of the tissue to subsequent addition of the hormone in generation of cAMP. In their system, desensitization was specific. Bone preincubated with prostaglandin E_1 or salmon CT lost responsiveness to subsequent addition of the same agent, but not to heterologous agent. Thus, preincubation with PTH caused desensitization only to that hormone, but not to PGE_1 or salmon CT; the PGE_1 and salmon CT desensitizations similarly were specific for the homologous agents. Desensitization to CT is described further in Section VI,B.

B. ADENYLATE CYCLASE, MECHANISM OF COUPLING AND ACTIVATION

Current research indicates that activation of adenylate cyclase is not a function solely dependent upon hormone-receptor interactions. In particular, studies with β-adrenergic systems show that hormonal activation of adenylate cyclase is dependent upon at least three or four interacting proteins or enzymes: (a) hormone receptor; (b) guanine nucleotide and guanine nucleotide regulatory protein; (c) adenylate cyclase catalytic unit; (d) GTPase enzyme (Cassel and Selinger, 1978; Pfeuffer, 1977; Ross et al., 1978; Spiegel et al., 1979; Limbird et al., 1980). The interaction of hormone with receptor facilitates binding of an endogenous guanine nucleotide (most likely guanosine triphosphate, GTP) with a guanine nucleotide-binding regulatory protein. Recent studies suggest that this regulatory protein is deficient in pseudohypoparathyroidism (see Section VII). The activity of adenylate cyclase is dependent upon interaction with the guanine nucleotide binding protein and GTP (Spiegel et al., 1979). With GTP bound to it, the regulatory protein–adenylate cyclase complex is active. A guanosine triphosphatase (GTPase) activity is responsible for deactivating adenylate cyclase (Cassel and Selinger, 1978). Guanosine triphosphate as well as the nonhydrolyzable guanine nucleotide analog, guanylylimidodiphosphate, facilitate activation of parathyroid hormone-stimulatable adenylate cyclase (Hunt et al., 1976). Unlike certain of the β-adrenergic systems, however, guanine nucleotide interaction with the system in the kidney is not totally dependent upon hormonal occupation of the PTH receptor. Presumably this phenomenon represents more facile receptor-independent guanine nucleotide interaction with the regulatory unit as well as heterogeneity of receptor systems in the kidney, which respond to a number of hormones and ligands in addition to PTH.

C. CYCLIC AMP ACCUMULATION IN THE KIDNEY AND EFFECTS ON PROTEIN KINASE

Activation of adenylate cyclase in the kidney leads to accumulation of cyclic 3′,5′-AMP in renal tissue. Accumulation of cAMP in response to parathyroid hormone has been observed in vivo (Nagata and Rasmussen, 1968) and *in vitro* with renal slices (Steiner *et al.*, 1972), isolated cells (Michelakis, 1970), or isolated renal tubules (Melson *et al.*, 1970). In general, these studies also confirm the observations with adenylate cyclase activation that effects of PTH are localized primarily to the renal cortex (see Section IV,A,1).

Cyclic AMP accumulated within receptor-bearing cells causes activation of enzymes or ion transport systems that respond physiologically to PTH. These cAMP-mediated phenomena are activated presumably through phosphorylation of proteins that are substrates for protein kinases. Biochemical interactions with protein kinases are discussed in Section II,G,1. Kinase activation by cAMP has been implicated in the activation of diverse systems under control of hormones in a variety of tissues including activation of ion transport in avian erythrocytes, toad bladder, and mammalian kidney. PTH stimulation of protein kinase via cAMP production has been identified in renal tissue (DeRubertis and Craven, 1976; Ausiello *et al.*, 1976; Kinne *et al.*, 1975). Of particular interest is the apparent polarity of distribution of cAMP-dependent protein kinase in the renal cell. In the identification of cAMP by immunofluorescent techniques, Dousa and Steiner (1978) found, after injection of PTH, aggregation of fluorescent granules at the luminal surface of tubular cells. Moreover, separation of luminal brush border membranes from basal lateral membranes in the renal cortical tubule indicates that cAMP protein kinase is located at the luminal (brush border microvilli) region (Kinne *et al.*, 1975; Insel and Saktor, 1970). Thus, it is implied that cAMP, generated at the plasma membrane as a function of PTH-activated adenylate cyclase, migrates through the cell, binds to the cAMP receptor–kinase complex, and activates the kinase at the luminal surface. The concentration of cAMP at the luminal surface may explain the ready access of cAMP to the luminal fluid and thus the appearance in the urine of large amounts of nephrogenously generated cAMP under the influence of circulating PTH.

D. ACTIVATION OF ENZYME AND TRANSPORT PROCESSES IN THE RENAL TUBULE

A number of systems are activated within the renal tubule in response to PTH: alkaline phosphatase, glucose-6-phosphate dehydrogenase (Chambers *et al.*, 1978), gluconeogenesis (Nagata and Rasmussen, 1970), and transport of sodium and phosphate (Agus *et al.*, 1971, 1973) and calcium (Agus *et al.*, 1973; Biddulph and Wrenn, 1977; Bourdeau and Burg, 1980). Activation of transport processes and gluconeogenesis seem clearly dependent upon the intermediation of cAMP in that addition of exogenous dibutyryl cAMP stimulates each of these processes (Biddulph and Wrenn, 1977; Bell *et al.*, 1972; Nagata and Rasmussen, 1970). Since cAMP-dependent protein kinases are concentrated at the luminal brush border of the renal tubule itself, one might assume that activation of the protein kinase system with phosphorylation of a specific protein involved in transport mediate these cAMP-dependent actions of parathyroid hormone. There is, however, no direct evidence to support this assumption, and indeed the PTH activation of glucose-6-phosphate dehydrogenase and alkaline phosphatase (Chambers *et al.*, 1978) are yet to be established, as is likely as cAMP-dependent processes. The localization of cAMP-dependent protein kinase at the luminal brush border of the renal tubular cell makes it possible that the transport phenomena activated thereby also exist in polar distribution along the luminal border of the cell. The facts that cAMP is found in the tubular fluid and that cAMP-dependent kinases are located in the luminal border of the cells raise the possibility that cAMP might be a mediator of cell-to-cell communication along the course of the nephron. This phenomenon would allow for the possibility of activation of enzymes within the nephron at a site distant from the cell immediately activated by PTH interaction with specific hormone receptors. There is evidence that cAMP can be a mediator of cell-to-cell communication in microorganisms (Konijn *et al.*, 1969). Such a possibility in the nephron has yet to be tested, however.

V. Mechanism of Action— Calcitonin

Identification of Receptors

Among the hormonal receptor systems identified via direct binding studies with radioactive ligands the calcitonin (CT) receptor system shows one of the highest correlations between affinity for the receptor and biological activities. Salmon CT-I can be radioiodinated with little modification of standard procedures to high specific activities (Marx *et al.*, 1972). This radioactive ligand binds rapidly to sites on plasma membranes prepared from kidney or bone. Salmon CT-I, among the most, if not the most, potent molecule biologically, is also the most efficacious in inhibiting binding (a measure of affinity for receptor) of iodinated CT. Once bound, [^{125}I]SCT dissociates very slowly from the receptor (Marx *et al.*, 1973). The radioiodinated ligand shows the same affinity as unlabeled salmon CT itself. It has been established as well that iodinated CT (salmon) is fully active biologically *in vitro* as well as *in vivo* (Marx *et al.*, 1973). Tests that utilize adenylate cyclase as a parameter of biological activity provide an index of biological potency for a series of CT congeners. In these adenylate cyclase assays the CT analogs show the same relative apparent affinities for binding to receptors as found *in vivo* for biological activity. These several observations all substantiate the biological significance of receptor activity determined with [^{125}I]SCT.

1. *Biological Function of Calcitonin Receptors and Linkage through Adenylate Cyclase*

Activation of adenylate cyclase enzyme in kidney and bone appears to be dependent upon guanine nucleotides in that addition of guanylylimidodiphosphate enhances the apparent affinity of CT in activating adenylate cyclase (Marx and Aurbach, 1975; Loreau *et al.*, 1978). Loreau *et al.* found a modest increase in rate of dissociation of labeled calcitonin from renal receptors in the presence of guanylylimidodiphosphate, whereas Marx and Aurbach (1975) did not observe such a change. The reason for this discrepancy is not clear. The significance of CT receptors, identified as [^{125}I]SCT binding sites, for biological activity also is supported by experiments showing that detergents cause parallel loss of receptor binding activity and CT-stimulatable adenylate cyclcase activity (Marx and Aurbach, 1975). The concentration curve for detergent-induced loss of receptor from the membrane was the same as for loss of CT-stimulated adenylate cyclase. Fluoride-sensitive cyclase persisted in the membrane after detergent treatment that caused loss of CT-stimulated adenylate cyclase. The effects of guanine nucleotides on CT-stimulated adenylate cyclase activity as well as the reported effects on iodinated CT binding to receptor imply that receptor binding of agonist is coupled to activation of the adenylate cyclase enzyme.

Tashjian *et al.* (1978) have studied the "escape" phenomenon wherein skeletal tissue cultured *in vitro* loses responsiveness to CT. They found that there is a progressive loss of detectable binding sites for CT throughout 36–48 hours of culture, at which time there remained only 10–30% of the original apparent receptor concentration. The loss of receptor sites was more rapid with salmon CT than with the less potent porcine CT. Receptor activity is recovered upon subsequent incubation of tissue with CT-free media. It is not totally clear whether receptor loss in the bone culture system represents complete loss of receptors from the cell surface after interaction with CT or whether the apparent receptor loss reflects persistent occupancy of the receptor.

The phenomenon of receptor loss discussed above may represent a type of control ("down-regulation") that has been observed in several hormone receptor systems, i.e., receptor loss induced by homologous agonists. Heterologous control of CT receptors may also exist. Sraer *et al.* (1974) have described an increase in number of CT receptors in kidneys taken from parathyroidectomized rats. Their finding of an apparent increase in specific activity of CT receptors (sites per milligram of renal tissue protein) might reflect reduced circulating concentrations of CT associated with hypocalcemia. (Calcitonin might regulate tissue content of CT receptors; see preceding discussion on "escape" phenomenon.) Other interpretations of this are possible, however. Indeed, the effect on CT receptors may not be specific, since 5'-nucleotidase (marker for brush border) specific activity was also higher in the parathyroidectomized rats.

2. *General Distribution of Calcitonin Receptors*

Receptors for CT have been found not only in skeletal and renal tissue, but also in certain lymphocyte cell lines (Marx *et al.*, 1974). Appearance of CT-sensitive adenylate cyclase in intestinal macrophages also has been described (Minkin *et al.*, 1977). As more and more cell systems are tested, it may become apparent that CT receptors are rather widely distributed in nature. It is of interest to note that although CT polypeptides have undergone remarkable structural changes during the course of evolution, there is little or no evidence suggesting phylogenetic modification in the nature of CT receptors. The receptors found on human lymphocytes show kinetic characteristics similar to those found in rat tissues, and human CT, which is remarkably less potent than salmon CT in rat tissues, also shows the same low potency ratio with human lymphocyte receptors. It would be important to extend these studies to CT receptors in submammalian species, particularly fish, to substantiate the hypothesis that there has been little evolutionary change in receptors.

3. *Distribution of Calcitonin Receptors in Kidney*

Chabardes and collaborators (Chabardes *et al.*, 1978) have analyzed microdissected segments of renal tubules for distribution of CT-sensitive adenylate cyclase. They found that CT activates adenylate cyclase in medullary ascending thick limb of the nephron as well as an area of the distal cortical tubule (see Fig. 7). In the mouse and rabbit, tubule CT activates adenylate cyclase in segments distinctly proximal to those affected by parathyroid hormone in the distal convoluted tubule. Although there is a high degree of overlap between CT- and parathyroid hormone-sensitive segments in the distal convoluted tubule of the human kidney (Chabardes *et al.*, 1980), results with rabbit and mouse kidney show that receptors for CT are clearly distinct from those sensitive to parathyroid hormone. Their observations (Chabardes *et al.*, 1978) that the medullary ascending limb of the rabbit kidney contains high concentrations of CT-sensitive adenylate cyclase fit with the observations of Marx *et al.* (1972), which showed relatively high concentrations of CT-sensitive adenylate cyclase in the outer medullary zone of the rat kidney.

4. *Physiological Significance of Calcitonin Receptors in the Kidney*

The physiological importance of CT receptors in the nephron is not clearly apparent. The fact that CT causes natriuresis (Haas *et al.*, 1971; Bijvoet *et al.*, 1971; Keeler *et al.*, 1970), calciuria [Bijvoet *et al.*, 1971; Haas *et al.*, 1971; and others (see review of Peck and Klahr, 1979)], and phosphaturia (Nielsen *et al.*, 1971; Robinson *et al.*, 1966; Sorensen *et al.*, 1972) suggests that cAMP generated in the nephron in response to CT can influence ion transport. Calcitonin influences on ion transport presumably also are mediated through cAMP activation of protein kinase in analogy to induction of sodium and potassium transport *in vitro* by cAMP in avian erythrocytes (Gardner *et al.*, 1974). [See Strewler and Orloff (1977) for a general review on the role of cAMP in the transport of electrolytes.] Most studies of renal transport of solutes in response to CT have utilized high doses of the hormone. A striking effect of CT on calcium transport in fish has been reported by Milhaud *et al.* (1977). They found that salmon CT at a concentration of 10^{-7} M caused a decrease in the entry of calcium from seawater across the gill of the salmon. Norepinephrine produced the opposite effect—an eight-fold increase in influx of calcium from seawater. This may prove to be a useful preparation in which to test further cAMP-mediated transport phenomena.

VI. Mechanism of Action of Parathyroid Hormone and Calcitonin in Bone

The studies of Chase and Aurbach (1970) showed that PTH as well as CT caused an increase in cAMP content of bone, and Vaes (1968) showed that dibutyryl cAMP added to bone *in vitro* caused release of lysozomal enzymes. These studies, as well as those of Klein and Raisz (1971) showing that dibutyryl cAMP caused bone resorption *in vitro,* all implied that cAMP was involved in the PTH-mediated demineralization of bone and release of calcium therefrom. The increase in cAMP in response to CT was an apparent paradox in that calcitonin is a physiological antagonist *in vivo* and *in vitro* to the bone-resorbing effects of PTH. The separation of a class of cells (osteoclasts) responding predominantly to calcitonin may help to resolve this paradox.

A. Cell Types Involved

Early observations suggested that the population of osteoclasts in bone were increased after administration of PTH to animals or in clinical hyperparathyroidism. This led to the concept that osteoclasts represent selectively the target cells for PTH action in bone. It is now apparent that parathyroid hormone influences all three bone cell types—osteoclasts, osteoblasts, and osteocytes. Recent work with separated distinct cell types establishes direct PTH effect on osteoblastic as well as osteoclastic function and shows that there are specific receptors for PTH on each cell type (Wong and Cohn, 1974, 1978; Luben *et al.,* 1976; Rao *et al.,* 1977). During the course of incubation of fetal calvaria with collagenase there is differential release of cells sensitive to CT on the one hand and PTH on the other. Cells released early respond

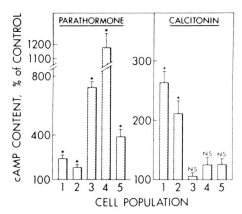

FIG. 8. Distinct bone cell populations sensitive to parathyroid hormone and calcitonin, respectively. Cells are released at different rates from bone treated with collagenase *in vitro.* Cells bearing receptors for calcitonin (osteoclast-like) are released early in the course of digestion. Another group of cells (osteoblast-like), released later in the course of digestion, are sensitive to parathyroid hormone but not calcitonin. From Cohn and Wong (1978).

markedly to CT and less strikingly to PTH. Cells released later respond strikingly to PTH but not to CT (Fig. 8). The calcitonin-sensitive cells resemble osteoclasts whereas the cells most sensitive to PTH and lacking calcitonin responsiveness resemble osteoblasts.*

B. CALCITONIN RECEPTORS IN BONE

The effects of PTH and CT on adenylate cyclase in skeletal tissue establish that receptors for these hormones exist in bone. Direct identification of receptors by radioligand binding studies, however, has been definitively established only for CT (Marx *et al.*, 1972; Tashjian, 1978). [^{125}I]Calcitonin (salmon) shows high affinity for CT receptors in bone and affinities for diverse CT congeners parallel those found with receptors in the kidney (see Section V). There is a close correlation between affinity of congeners as inhibitors of iodinated CT binding with the apparent affinity of these congeners in stimulating production of cAMP in bone *in vitro* (Marx *et al.*, 1972). These findings imply biological relevance for the direct receptor binding experiments. Bone incubated with CT *in vitro* loses responsiveness to the hormone during the course of incubation. This phenomenon has been termed "escape" (Raisz *et al.*, 1972; Tashjian *et al.*, 1978). Tashjian *et al.* (1978) have studied the escape phenomenon (also discussed above) in terms of receptor function and cAMP generation. There is progressive loss of detectable receptor in bone incubated *in vitro* with CT. However, receptor loss accounts only in part for the escape mechanism since 10–30% of initial receptors are still intact when escape is total. Whether receptor destruction, cell internalization of receptors, or irreversible occupancy by agonists account for the loss in detectable receptors has not been established.

C. ADENYLATE CYCLASE ACTIVITY IN BONE AND BONE CELLS

Membrane preparations from fetal bones contain adenylate cyclase enzyme, which can be activated by PTH or CT (Chase *et al.*, 1969a; Heersche *et al.*, 1974). This direct activation of the enzyme by these

---

*Osteoblasts and osteoclasts not only show distinct hormonal responsiveness but appear to arise from distinct progenitor cells (Hall, 1975; Walker, 1978; Marks, 1973). Osteopetrotic mice and rats show defective or absent osteoclastic function in bone. The defect can be corrected by injection of monocyte cell lines or thymic tissue from normal animals (Walker, 1978; Milhaud, 1978). Moreover, macrophages have been shown to contain parathyroid hormone receptors (Minkin *et al.*, 1977). These several observations suggest the possibility that osteoclasts may not find origin in skeletal tissue per se.

hormones accounts for the increase in cAMP content of skeletal tissue or cells derived from it upon exposure to PTH or CT. Populations of freshly isolated bone cells are highly sensitive to the PTH effect on cAMP accumulation (Rodan and Rodan, 1974). Direct stimulation by PTH of adenylate cyclase in membrane preparations has been observed with several isolated cell systems including osteoblast- and osteoclast-like cells (Wong and Cohn, 1974; Rao *et al.*, 1977; Zull *et al.*, 1978; Smith and Johnson, 1974), murine osteogenic sarcoma cells (Martin *et al.*, 1976; Majeska *et al.*, 1978) and human foreskin fibroblasts (Goldring *et al.*, 1978). These isolated cell systems may prove useful for future explorations into the mechanisms of adenylate cyclase activation by PTH.

D. Protein Kinases

The metabolic effects of cAMP generation in cells generally appear to be mediated through activation of cyclic nucleotide-sensitive protein kinases. The latter proteins are involved in mediating the cellular actions of cAMP (see discussion on cAMP accumulation in the kidney in Section IV,C). The amount of cAMP bound to its receptor determines the degree of activation of kinase and the degree of tissue response upon interaction of an agonist with receptors at the cell surface. The concentration of bound cAMP correlates better than total cAMP content with tissue response. Marcus *et al.* (1979) have identified cAMP receptor sites in bone cells and have shown that receptor occupancy by cAMP parallels closely cAMP accumulation in such cells.

E. Cyclic AMP Responses in Skeletal Tissue

In general, reagents that cause enhanced accumulation of cAMP in bone also cause bone resorption *in vitro* as well as *in vivo*. The exception is CT, which, although it enhances accumulation of cAMP in bone, is a physiological inhibitor of the bone resorption induced by other agents that act through cAMP. This apparent paradox is explained in part by the fact that CT may act on a different class of cells than those responding to bone-resorbing agents. Also compatible with this hypothesis is the observation that dibutyryl cAMP in one concentration range stimulates bone resorption *in vitro*. At a higher concentration range its effect is to inhibit bone resorption (Raisz *et al.*, 1968). Dibutyryl cAMP also causes release of lysozomal enzymes from bone *in vitro* (Vaes, 1968), and it is believed that these enzymes are involved in the process of hormonally induced bone resorption. Other functions influenced by cAMP in cells include phosphorylation of microtubule assemblies (see review by Dedman *et al.*, 1979), change in cell shape and morphology (Jones and Boyde, 1978), and alterations in ion transport (see discussion under kidney). These processes also might be intermediate in hormonally induced bone resorption. Indeed, colchicine and vinblastine, agents that interrupt microtubular function, inhibit bone resorption *in vitro* (Raisz *et al.*, 1973), and ionophores that promote cell calcium uptake also induce bone resorption *in vitro* (Dziak and Stern, 1975). However, the major functions influenced by cAMP and responsible for physiological resorption of bone have yet to be identified with certainty.

F. Cyclic Nucleotide Phosphodiesterase in Bone and Bone Cells

Cyclic nucleotide phosphodiesterase has been identified in bone (Heersche *et al.*, 1974; Marcus, 1975; Chen and Feldman, 1978), and addition of cyclic nucleotide phosphodiesterase inhibitors causes an increase in basal cAMP content of bone tissue and enhances the effects of PTH, CT, and other effectors in increasing cAMP content of bone. Dibutyryl cAMP increases bone cAMP content through inhibition of endogenous phosphodiesterase activity (Heersche *et al.*, 1971). Glucocortocoids inhibit skeletal phosphodiesterase activity and potentiate the effect of PTH in increasing cAMP content in bone (Chen and Feldman, 1978). Pharmacological concentrations of thyroid hormones also increase skeletal cAMP content through inhibition of cyclic nucleotide phosphodiesterase (Marcus, 1975). In the latter study, both high K_m and low K_m phosphodiesterases were identified. Phosphodiesterases in several other tissues also show heterogeneity of phosphodiesterases in terms of apparent affinity for substrate.

Certain phosphodiesterases (Cheung *et al.*, 1970) are regulated by calmodulin, a calcium-dependent protein that can influence the activity of adenylate cyclase as well (see review by Wolff and Brostrom, 1979). Since hormonal regulation of calcium seems to be important in the control of bone cells (see review by Rasmussen *et al.*, 1976), it would be important to study calcium fluxes under the control of hormones in bone *in vitro* and the relationship of these changes in fluxes in influencing calmodulin activity and the control of phosphodiesterase and adenylate cyclase activity in bone. Several fetal murine bone systems used *in vitro* and cells derived therefrom might prove to be useful in such studies on skeletal tissue-calmodulin activity.

VII. Cyclic Nucleotides in the Extracellular Fluids

A. Effects of Parathyroid Hormone

The effects of PTH on adenylate cyclase and generation of cAMP within the renal tubule are reflected in the rate of urinary excretion of cAMP. Part of cAMP excreted in the urine is accounted for by clearance from plasma by glomerular filtration, and the rest represents cAMP generated in the kidney itself (nephrogenous cAMP, NcAMP). Cyclic AMP and cyclic GMP (cGMP) show similar half-times, approximately 20 minutes, in the circulation (Broadus et al., 1970a). Part of the loss from the plasma compartment is accounted for by glomerular filtration and the rest by destruction through cyclic nucleotide phosphodiesterase in diverse tissues. Although several nonparathyroid factors have been shown to increase cAMP in various portions of the nephron, e.g., CT, β-adrenergic catecholamines, vasopressin, and prostaglandins of the E series, none is a significant influence on urinary cAMP under normal physiological circumstances. In normal subjects PTH represents the major renotropic factor influencing nephrogenous cAMP under basal conditions. Broadus et al. (1977) have carried out extensive analyses of cAMP clearance in normal subjects and those with parathyroid disorders. Determination of nephrogenous cAMP allowed sharp differentiation of hypoparathyroid, normal, and hyperparathyroid groups (Fig. 9). Discrimination almost as good was afforded by expressing total urinary cAMP as a function of (GFR)—nanomoles glomerular filtration rate of cAMP per 100 ml GF. The latter parameter is simply constructed from urinary cAMP determinations with simultaneous determination of plasma and urine creatinine. Recent studies indicate that parathyroid gland responses in vivo reflected as nephrogenous cAMP correlate well with results for parathyroid secretion from cells isolated from glands taken from subjects tested in vivo (Brown et al., 1979a).

An abnormal calcium challenge test also may be elicited in primary hyperparathyroidism. Nephrogenous cAMP remains abnormally high even with administration of an oral calcium test dose that suppresses NcAMP in normal subjects or those with secondary hyperparathyroidism (Broadus et al., 1978a). Nephrogenous cAMP determinations also appear useful in evaluating subjects with renal lithiasis. One form of renal lithiasis is characterized by hyperabsorption of calcium from the gut. Administration of an oral calcium challenge in these subjects causes a significant 54% decrease in nephrogenous cAMP. Another form of renal lithiasis is associated with a renal loss of

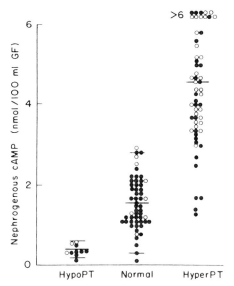

FIG. 9. Nephrogenous urinary cyclic AMP (cAMP) as a function of parathyroid (PT) status. Notice that this parameter affords differentiation of parathyroid hypofunction as well as hyperfunction. Open symbols represent subjects with renal impairment. Nephrogenous cAMP/100 ml GF = urinary cAMP/100 ml GF –plasma cAMP.

calcium, increased PTH in plasma by radioimmunoassay, and increased basal NcAMP. Administration of a calcium load to these subjects causes only a modest fall in nephrogenous cAMP (Broadus *et al.*, 1978b). Some of the latter may represent cases of primary hyperparathyroidism superimposed on a renal "calcium leak" defect.

B. PSEUDOHYPOPARATHYROIDISM

Pseudohypoparathyroidism, originally described by Albright and his associates (1942), represents a type of parathyroid hypofunction caused not by lack of secretion but by lack of response of receptor tissue to endogenously secreted PTH. Hypocalcemia results from lack of renal responsiveness to PTH with the ultimate consequence of reduced synthesis of 1,25-dihydroxycholecalciferol in the kidney (Drezner *et al.*, 1976). The skeletal response to PTH may be relatively better preserved. Chase *et al.* (1969a) showed that this disorder is associated with a deficient response in terms of urinary cAMP excretion to exogenously administered PTH. It was thus postulated that pseudohypoparathyroidism might be caused by a defective receptor-adenylate cyclase unit in the kidney (and possibly bones) of subjects

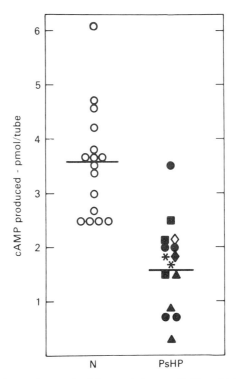

FIG. 10. Deficient guanine nucleotide regulatory unit (G unit) in pseudohypopara-thyroidism (PsHP). G unit was extracted from red cell membranes of normal (○) or affected subjects and assayed as enzyme activity after addition to adenylate cyclase catalytic unit of turkey erythrocyte membranes. ●, Unrelated subjects with PsHP; ◇, pseudopseudo hypoparathyroid mother of daughter (◆) with complete syndrome; other like symbols (*, ■, ▲) represent families with multiple affected members. Modified from Levine *et al.* (1980).

with this disorder. The response to cAMP (tested with exogenous di-butyryl cAMP) is usually normal (Bell *et al.*, 1972). An occasional variant, pseudohypoparathyroidism II, shows an apparently normal cAMP response and may reflect a defect in the cell receptor for cAMP itself (Drezner *et al.*, 1973).

The hypothesis of grossly defective receptor-adenylate cyclase in pseudohypoparathyroidism was challenged, however, by the findings of Marcus *et al.* (1971) and Drezner *et al.* (1978), who reported PTH-sensitive adenylate cyclase in renal tissue taken from cases of pseudohypoparathyroidism. The latter group suggested that there was a defect in guanine nucleotide regulation of adenylate cyclase; enzyme activity *in vitro* appeared reduced at low, but not at high, GTP concentrations. Recent evidence from two laboratories indicates that the guanine nucleotide regulatory protein is deficient in classic pseudohypoparathyroidism (Levine *et al.*, 1980; Farfel *et al.*, 1980). Mature human red cell membranes normally contain the regulatory protein, but not significant amounts of adenylate cyclase enzyme activity. The red cell membrane content of the regulatory protein can be assayed by adding membrane extracts to suitable adenylate cyclase containing acceptor systems, e.g., turkey erythrocyte membranes or membranes from S49 lymphoma cell mutants lacking the protein. Red cell membranes from cases of classic pseudohypoparathyroidism (showing the constitutional as well as biochemical features of the disease) contain about half the normal content of the regulatory protein (Fig. 10). This finding may explain the decreased PTH responsiveness as well as some of the more general defects (Wolfsdorf *et al.*, 1978; Carlson *et al.*, 1977; Marx *et al.*, 1971) in hormonal responsiveness found in the disorder. One case (Fig. 10) has repeatedly shown a normal complement of the protein. This suggests that phenotypic expression of the disease could also be brought about by a defect in yet another gene, perhaps one controlling a different protein in the receptor–adenylate cyclase complex.

REFERENCES

Abe, M., and Sherwood, L. M. (1972). *Biochem. Biophys. Res. Commun.* **48**, 396–401.

Agus, Z. S., Puschett, J. B., Senesky, D., and Goldberg, M. (1971). *J. Clin. Invest.* **50**, 617–262.

Agus, Z. S., Gardner, L. B., Bech, L. H., and Goldberg, M. (1973). *Am. J. Physiol.* **224**, 1143–1148.

Albright, F., Burnett, C. H., Smith, P. H., and Parson, W. (1942). *Endocrinology* **30**, 922–932.

Amenta, F., and Cavalotti, C. (1979). *Experientia* **35**, 663–664.

Attie, M. F., Brown, E. M., Gardner, D. G., Spiegel, A. M., and Aurbach, G. D. *Endocrinology* **107**, 1776–1781.

Au, W. Y. (1976). *Science* **193**, 1015–1017.

Aurbach, G. D., and Chase, L. R. (1976). *In* Vitamins & Hormones Vol. 38 Brown & Aurbach "Parathyroid Gland" (G. D. Aurbach, ed.), ["Handbook of Physiology" (R. O. Greep and E. B. Astwood, eds.), Vol. VII], pp. 353–381. Am. Physiol. Soc., Washington, D.C.

Ausiello, D., Handler, J., and Orloff, J. (1976). *Biochim. Biophys. Acta* **451**, 372–381.

Avioli, L. V., Shieber, W., and Kipnis, D. M. (1971). *Endocrinology* **88**, 1337–1340.

Baksi, S. N., and Kenny, A. D. (1979). *Pharmacology* **18**, 169–174.

Baumann, K., Chan, Y.-L, Bode, F., and Papavassiliou, F. (1977). *Kidney Intl.* **11**, 77–85.

Bell, N. H. (1970). *J. Clin. Invest.* **49**, 1368–1373.

Bell, N. H. (1973). *Nature (London)*, *(New Biol.)* **245**, 85–86.

Bell, N. H., Avery, S., Sinha, T., Clark, C. M., Jr., Allen, D. O., and Johnston, C., Jr. (1972). *J. Clin. Invest.* **51**, 816–823.

Berson, S. A., Yalow, R. S., Aurbach, G. D., and Potts, J. T., Jr. (1963). *Proc. Natl. Acad. Sci. U.S.A.* **49**, 613–617.

Biddulph, D. M., and Wrenn, R. W. (1977). *J. Cyclic Nucleotide Res.* **3**, 129–138.

Biddulph, D. M., Currie, M. G., and Wrenn, R. W. (1971). *Endocrinology* **104**, 1164–1171.

Bilezikian, J. P., and Aurbach, G. D. (1974). *J. Biol. Chem.* **249**, 157–161.

Blum, J. W., Bianca, W., Naf, F., Kunz, P., Fischer, J. A., and DaPrada, M. (1978a). *Horm. Metab. Res.* **11**, 246–251.

Blum, J. W., Fischer, J. A., Hunziker, W. H., Binswanger, U., Picotti, G. B., DaPrada, M., and Guillebeau, A. (1978b). *J. Clin. Invest.* **61**, 1113–1122.

Blum, J. W., Fischer, J. A., Kunz, P., Binswanger, U., and Da Prada, M. (1979). *Program 61st Annu. Meet. Endocr. Soc.* Abstract No. 4.

Borgeat, P., Labrile, F., and Brovin, J. (1974). *Biochem. Biophys. Res. Commun.* **56**, 1052–1059.

Borle, A. B., and Uchikawa, T. (1979). *Endocrinology* **104**, 122–129.

Bourdeau, J. E., and Burg, M. B. (1980). *Am. J. Physiol.* (in press).

Bourdeau, J. E., and Burg, M. B. (1980). *Adv. Cyclic Nucleotide Res.* **13**, 133–180.

Breslau, N., and Moses, A. M. (1978). *J. Clin. Endocrinol. Metab.* **46**, 389–395.

Broadus, A. E., Kaminsky, N. I., Hardman, J. G., Sutherland, E. W., and Liddle, G. W. (1970a). *J. Clin. Invest.* **49**, 2222–2236.

Broadus, A. E., Kaminsky, N. I., Northcutt, R. C., Hardman, J. G., Sutherland, E. W., and Liddle, G. W. (1970b). *J. Clin. Invest.* **49**, 2237–2245.

Broadus, A. E., Mahaffey, J. E., Bartter, F. C., and Neer, R. M. (1977). *J. Clin. Invest.* **60**, 771–783.

Broadus, A. E., Deftos, L. J., and Bartter, F. C. (1978a). *J. Clin. Endocrinol. Metab.* **46**, 477.

Broadus, A. E., Dominguez, N., and Bartter, F. C. (1978b). *J. Clin. Endocrinol. Metab.* **47**, 751–760.

Brown, E. M. (1980). *Endocrinology* **107**, 1998–2003.

Brown, E. M., (1980). *J. Clin. Endocrinol. Metab.* **51**, 1325–1329.

Brown, E. M., Hurwitz, S., and Aurbach, G. D. (1976a). *Endocrinology* **99**, 1582–1588.

Brown, E. M., Hauser, D., Troxler, F., and Aurbach, G. D. (1976b). *J. Biol. Chem.* **251**, 1232–1238.

Brown, E. M., Hurwitz, S., and Aurbach, G. D. (1977a). *Endocrinology* **100**, 1696–1702.

Brown, E. M., Hurwitz, S., Woodard, C. J., and Aurbach, G. D. (1977b). *Endocrinology* **100**, 1703–1709.

Brown, E. M., Carroll, R. J., and Aurbach, G. D. (1977c). *Proc. Natl. Acad. Sci. U.S.A.* **74**, 4210–4213.

Brown, E. M., Brennan, M. F., and Hurwitz, S. (1978a). *J. Clin. Endocrinol. Metab.* **46**, 267–276.

Brown, E. M., Hurwitz, S. H., and Aurbach, G. D. (1978b). *Endocrinology* **103**, 893–899.

Brown, E. M., Gardner, D. G., Windeck, R. A., and Aurbach, G. D. (1978c). *Endocrinology* **103**, 2323–2333.

Brown, E. M., Pazoles, C. J., Creutz, C. E., Aurbach, G. D., and Pollard, H. B. (1978d). *Proc. Natl. Acad. Sci. U.S.A.* **75**, 876–880.

Brown, E. M., Broadus, A. E., Brennan, M. F., Gardner, D. G., Marx, S. J., Spiegel, A. M., Downs, R. W., Jr., Attie, M. F., and Aurbach, G. D. (1979a). *J. Clin. Endocrinol. Metab.* **48**, 604–609.

Brown, E. M., Gardner, D. G., Windeck, R. A., and Aurbach, G. D. (1979b). *Endocrinology* **104**, 218–225.

Brown, E. M., Gardner, D. G., Windeck, R. A., Hurwitz, S., Brennan, M. F., and Aurbach, G. D. (1979c). *J. Clin. Endocrinol. Metab.* **48**, 618–626.

Brown, E. M., Gardner, D. G., Brennan, M. F., Marx, S. J., Spiegel, A. M., Attie, M. F., Downs, R. W., Jr., Doppman, J. L., and Aurbach, G. D. (1979d). *Am. J. Med.* **66**, 923-931.

Brown, E. M., Gardner, D. G., and Aurbach, G. D. (1980). *Endocrinology* **106**, 133-138.

Bruce, B. R., and Anderson, N. C., Jr. (1979). *Am. J. Physiol.* **236**, C15-C21.

Brunton, L. L., and Mayer, S. E. (1979). *J. Biol. Chem.* **254**, 9714-9720.

Canterbury, J. M., Lerman, S., Claflin, A. J., Henry, H., Norman, A., and Reiss, E. (1978). *J. Clin. Invest.* **61**, 1375-1383.

Capen, C. C., Koestner, A., and Cole, C. C. (1965). *Lab. Invest.* **14**, 1673-1690.

Care, A. D. (1970). *Fed. Proc., Fed. Am. Soc. Exp. Biol.* **29**, 253.

Care, A. D., Bates, R. F. L., and Gitelman, H. J. (1970a). *J. Endocrinol.* **48**, 1-15.

Care, A. D., Bates, R. F. L., Phillippo, M., Lequin, R. M., Hackeny, W. H. L., Barlet, J. P., and Larvon, P. (1970b). *J. Endocrinol.* **48**, 667-668.

Care, A. D., Bates, R. F. L., and Gitelman, H. J. (1971a). *Ann. N. Y. Acad. Sci.* **185**, 317-326.

Care, A. D., Bates, R. F. L., Swaminathan, R., and Ganguli, P. C. (1971b). *J. Endocrinol.* **51**, 735-744.

Care, A. D., Bruce, J. B., Boelkins, J., Kenny, A. D., Conway, H., and Anast, C. S. (1971c). *Endocrinology* **89**, 262-271.

Carlson, H. E., Brickman, A. S., and Bottazzo, G. F. (1977). *N. Engl. J. Med.* **296**, 150-144.

Carnes, D. L., Anast, C. S., and Forte, L. R. (1978). *Endocrinology* **102**, 45-51.

Caro, J. F., Castro, J. C., and Glennan, J. A. (1979). *Ann. Int. Med.* **91**, 740-741.

Cassel, D., and Selinger, Z. (1978). *Proc. Natl. Acad. Sci. U.S.A.* **74**, 3307-3311.

Chabardes, D., Imbert-Teboul, M., Montègut, M., Clique, A., and Morel, F. (1976). *Proc. Natl. Acad. Sci. U.S.A.* **73**, 3608-3612.

Chabardes, D., Imbert-Teboul, M., Gagnan-Brunette, M., and Morel, F. (1978). *In* "Endocrinology of Calcium Metabolism" (D. H. Copp and R. V. Talmage, eds.), pp. 209-215. Excerpta Med. Found., Amsterdam.

Chabardes, D., Gagnan-Brunette, M., Imbert-Teboul, M., Gontcharevskaia, O., Montegut, M., Clique, A., and Morel, F. (1980). *J. Clin. Invest.* **65**, 439-448.

Chambers, D. J., Schäfer, H., Laugharn, J. A., Jr., Johnstone, J., Zanelli, J. M., Parsons, J. A., Bitensky, L., and Chayen, J. (1978). *In* "Endocrinology of Calcium Metabolism" (D. H. Copp and R. V. Talmage, eds.), pp. 216-220. Excerpta Med. Found., Amsterdam.

Chase, L. R. (1975). *Endocrinology* **96**, 70-76.

Chase, L. R., and Aurbach, G. D. (1967). *Proc. Natl. Acad. Sci. U.S.A.* **58**, 518-525.

Chase, L. R., and Aurbach, G. D. (1968). *Science* **159**, 545-547.

Chase, L. R., and Aurbach, G. D. (1970). *J. Biol. Chem.* **245**, 1520-1526.

Chase, L. R., and Obert, K. A. (1975). *Metabolism* **24**, 1067-1071.

Chase, L. R., Fedak, S. A., and Aurbach, G. D. (1969a). *Endocrinology* **84**, 761-768.

Chase, L. R., Melson, G. L., and Aurbach, G. D. (1969b). *J. Clin. Invest.* **48**, 1832-1844.

Chen, T. L., and Feldman, D. (1978). *Endocrinology* **102**, 589-596.

Chertow, B. S., Baylink, D. J. Wergedal, J. E., Su, M. H. H., and Norman, A. W. (1975a). *J. Clin. Invest.* **56**, 668-678.

Chertow, B. S., Williams, G. A., Baker, G. R., Surbaugh, R. D., and Hargis, G. K. (1975b). *Exp. Cell Res.* **93**, 388-394.

Chertow, B. S., Manke, D. J., Williams, G. A., Baker, G. R., Hargis, G. K., and Buschmann, R. S. (1977). *Lab. Invest.* **36**, 198-205.

Cheung, W. Y. (1970). *Biochem. Biophys. Res. Commun.* **38**, 533-538.

Cheung, W. Y. (1973). *J. Biol. Chem.* **248**, 5950-5955.

Cheung, W. Y. (1979). *Science* **207,** 19–27.

Cohn, D. V., and Wong, G. L. (1978). *In* "Endocrinology of Calcium Metabolism" (D. H. Copp and R. V. Talmage, eds.). Excerpta Med. Found., Amsterdam.

Cooper, C. W., Schwesinger, W. H., Mahgoub, A. M., and Ontjes, D. A. (1971). *Science* **172,** 1238–1240.

Cooper, C. W., Ramp, W. K., Becker, D. I., and Ontjes, D. A. (1977). *Endocrinology* **101,** 304–311.

Copp, D. H., Cameron, E. C., Cheney, B. A., Davidson, A. G. F., and Henge, K. G. (1962). *Endocrinology* **70,** 638–649.

Corbin, J. D., Soderling, T. R., and Park, C. R. (1973). *J. Biol. Chem.* **248,** 1813–1821.

Currie, M. G., and Biddulph, D. M. (1979). *Prostaglandins* **17,** 211–222.

Davies, P., Shizuta, Y., Olden, M., Gallo, J., and Pastan, I. (1977). *Biochem. Biophys. Res. Commun.* **74,** 300–307.

Davoren, P. R., and Sutherland, E. W. (1963). *J. Biol. Chem.* **238,** 3009–3015.

Dedman, J. R., Brinkley, B. R., and Means, A. R. (1979). *Adv. Cyclic Nucleotide Res.* **11,** 131–174.

Deftos, L. J., Lorenzi, J. J., Bohannon, N., Tsalakian, E., Scheider, V., and Gerich, J. E. (1976). *J. Clin. Endocrinol. Metab.* **43,** 205–207.

Deftos, L. J., Burton, D., Bone, H. G., Catherwood, B. D., Parthemore, J. G., Moore, R. Y., Minick, S., and Guellemin, R. (1978). *Life Sci.* **23,** 743–748.

Dennis, V. W. (1976). *Kidney Intl.* **10,** 373–380.

Derenoncourt, F. J., Bilezikian, J. P., Feind, C. R., Weber, C. J., Hardy, M. A., and Reemtsa, K. (1977). *Clin. Res.* **25,** 389 (abstr.).

DeRubertis, F. R., and Craven, P. A. (1976). *J. Clin. Invest.* **57,** 1442–1450.

Desbuquois, B. (1974). *Eur. J. Biochem.* **46,** 439–450.

DiBella, F. P., Dousa, T. P., Miller, S. S., and Arnaud, C. D. (1974). *Proc. Natl. Acad. Sci. U.S.A.* **71,** 723–726.

Dietel, M., Dorn, G., Montz, R., and Altenahr, E. (1979). *Endocrinology* **105,** 237–245.

Douglas, W. W. (1968). *Br. J. Pharmacol.* **34,** 451.

Dousa, T., P., and Steiner, A. L. (1978). *In* "Endocrinology of Calcium Metabolism" (D. H. Copp and R. V. Talmage, eds.), pp. 221–225. Excerpta Med. Found., Amsterdam.

Dousa, T. P., Hui, Y. F. S., and Barnes, L. D. (1975). *Endocrinology* **97,** 802–807.

Dousa, T. P., Hui, Y. F. S., and Barnes, L. D. (1978). *J. Lab. Clin. Med.* **92,** 252–261.

Downs, R. W., Jr., Spiegel, A. M., Singer, M., Reen, S., and Aurbach, G. D. (1980). *J. Biol. Chem.* 949–954.

Drezner, M. K., and Burch, W. M., Jr. (1978). *J. Clin. Invest.* **62,** 1222–1227.

Drezner, M. K., Neelon, F. A., and Lebovitz, H. E. (1973). *N. Engl. J. Med.* **289,** 1056–1060.

Drezner, M. K., Neelon, F. A., Haussler, M., McPherson, H. T., and Lebovitz, H. E. (1976). *J. Clin. Endocrinol. Metab.* **42,** 621–628.

Dufau, M. L., Tsuruhara, T., Horner, K. A., Podesta, E., and Catt, K. J. (1977). *Proc. Natl. Acad. Sci. U.S.A.* **74,** 3419–3423.

Dufresne, L. R., Anderson, R., and Gitelman, H. J. (1971). *Clin. Res.* **19,** 529A.

Dziak, R., and Stern, P. H. (1975). *Endocrinology* **97,** 1281–1287.

Efandic, S., Grill, V., and Luft, R. (1975). *FEBS Lett.* **5S,** 131–133.

Eilon, G., and Raisz, L. G. (1978). *Endocrinology* **103,** 1969–1975.

Epstein, S., Pantzer, E., Queener, S. F., and Bell, N. H. (1980). *Program 2nd Ann. Meet. Am. Soc. Bone Mineral Res.* Abstract No. 8.

Farfel, Z., Brickman, A. S., Kaslow, H. R., Brothers, V. M., and Bourne, H. R. (1980). *N. Engl. J. Med.* **303,** 237–242.

Feinblatt, J. D., and Raisz, L. G. (1971). *Endocrinology* **88,** 797–804.

Feinblatt, J. D., Raisz, L. G., and Kenny, A. D. (1973). *Endocrinology* **93,** 277–284.

Fenton, S., Somers, S., and Heath, D. A. (1978). *Clin. Endocrinol.* **9**, 381–384.

Fischer, J. A., Oldham, S. B., Sizemore, G. W., and Arnaud, C. D. (1971). *Horm. Metab. Res.* **3**, 223–224.

Fischer, J. A., Oldham, S. B., Sizemore, G. W., and Arnaud, C. D. (1972). *Proc. Natl. Acad. Sci. U.S.A.* **69**, 2341–2345.

Fischer, J. A., Blum, J. W., and Binswanger, U. (1973). *J. Clin. Invest.* **52**, 2434–2440.

Flueck, J. A., DiBella, F. P., Edis, A. J., Kehrwald, J. M., and Arnaud, C. D. (1977). *J. Clin. Invest.* **60**, 1367–1375.

Forte, L. R., Nickols, G. A., and Anast, C. S. (1976). *J. Clin. Invest.* **57**, 559–568.

Forte, L. R., Carnes, D. L., Nickols, G. A., and Anast, C. S. (1978). *J. Supramol. Struct.* **9**, 179–188.

Gagel, R. F., Zeytinoglu, F. N., Tashjian, A. H., Hammer, R. A., and Leeman, S. E. (1980). *Program 2nd Annu. Meet. Soc. Bone Mineral Res.* Abstract No. 8.

Gardner, J. D., Klaeveman, H. L., Bilezikian, J. P., and Aurbach, G. D. (1974). *J. Biol. Chem.* **249**, 516–520.

Gardner, D. G., Brown, E. M., Windeck, R. A., and Aurbach, G. D. (1978). *Endocrinology* **103**, 577–582.

Gardner, D. G., Brown, E. M., Windeck, R. A., and Aurbach, G. D. (1979a). *Endocrinology* **104**, 1–7.

Gardner, D. G., Brown, E. M., and Aurbach, G. D. (1979b). *Endocrinology* **105**, 360–366.

Gardner, D. G., Brown, E. M., Attie, M. F., and Aurbach, G. D. (1980). *J. Clin. Endocrinol. Metab.* **51**, 20–25.

Golden, P., Mazey, R., Greenwalt, A., Martin, K., and Slatopolsky, E. (1979). *Mineral Electrolyte Metab.* **2**, 1–6.

Goldring, S. R., Dayer, J.-M., Russell, R. G. G., Mankin, H. J., and Krane, S. M. (1978). *J. Clin. Endocrinol. Metab.* **46**, 425–433.

Goltzman, D. (1978). *Endocrinology* **102**, 1555–1562.

Goltzman, D., Callahan, E. N., Tregear, G. W., and Potts, J. T., Jr. (1978). *Endocrinology* **103**, 1352–1360.

Goltzman, D., Henderson, B., and Loveridge, N. (1980). *J. Clin. Invest.* **65**, 1309–1317.

Goodman, D. B. P., Rasmussen, H., DiBella, S., and Guthrow, C. E., Jr. (1970). *Proc. Natl. Acad. Sci. U.S.A.* **67**, 652–659.

Haas, H. G., Dambacher, M. A., Guncaga, J., and Lauffenburger, T. (1971). In "Calcium, Parathyroid Hormone and the Calcitonins" (R. V. Talmage and P. L. Munson, eds.), pp. 299–301. Excerpta Medica, Amsterdam.

Habener, J. F., and Potts, J. T., Jr. (1976). *Endocrinology* **98**, 197–202.

Habener, J. F., and Potts, J. T., Jr. (1978). In "Metabolic Bone Disease" (L. V. Avioli, and S. M. Krane, eds.), Vol. 2, pp. 1–147. Academic Press, New York.

Habener, J. F., Kemper, B. W., Potts, J. T., Jr., and Rich, A. (1974). *Endocr. Res. Commun.* **1**, 239.–246.

Habener, J. F., Kemper, B. W., and Potts, J. T., Jr. (1975). *Endocrinology* **97**, 431–441.

Habener, J. F., Stevens, T. D., Ravazzola, T., Orci, L., and Potts, J. T., Jr. (1977a). *Endocrinology* **101**, 1524–1537.

Habener, J. F., Change, H. T., and Potts, J. T., Jr. (1977b). *Biochemistry* **16**, 3910–3917.

Hall, B. K. (1975). *Anat. Rec.* **183**, 1–11.

Hamilton, J. W., MacGregor, R. R., Chu, L. L. H., and Cohn, D. V. (1971). *Endocrinology* **89**, 1440–1447.

Hanley, D. A., Takatsuki, K., Sutton, J. M., Schneider, A. B., and Sherwood, L. M. (1978). *J. Clin. Invest.* **62**, 1247–1254.

Hargis, G. K., Williams, G. A., Reynolds, W. A., Chertow, B. S., Kukreja, S. C., Bower, E. N., and Henderson, W. J. (1978). *Endocrinology* **102**, 745–750.

Harper, J. F., and Brooker, G. (1975). *J. Cyclic Nucleotide Res.* **1**, 207–218.

Heath, D. A., and Aurbach, G. D. (1975). *In* "Calcium-Regulating Hormones" (R. V. Talmage, M. Owen, and J. A. Parsons, eds.), pp. 159–162. Excerpta Med. Found., Amsterdam.

Heersche, J. N. M., Fedak, S. A., and Aurbach, G. D. (1971). *J. Biol. Chem.* **246**, 6770–6775.

Heersche, J. N. M., Marcus, R., and Aurbach, G. D. (1974). *Endocrinology* **94**, 241–247.

Heersche, J. N. M., Heyboer, M. P. M., and Ng, B. (1978). *Endocrinology* **103**, 333–340.

Hirsch, P. F., Gauteir, G. F., and Munson, P. L. (1963). *Endocrinology* **73**, 244–252.

Hoffstein, S., and Weisman, G. (1978). *J. Cell Biol.* **78**, 796–781.

Holtrop, M. E., Raisz, L. G., and Simmons, H. A. (1974). *J. Cell Biol.* **60**, 346–355.

Holtrop, M. E., King, G. J., and Raisz, L. G. (1978). *In* "Endocrinology of Metabolism" (D. H. Copp and R. V. Talmage, eds.), pp. 91–96. Excerpta Med. Found., Amsterdam.

Hunt, N. H., Martin, T. J., Michelangeli, V. P., and Eisman, J. A. (1976). *J. Endocrinol.* **69**, 401–412.

Insel, P., Balakir, R., and Sacktor, B. (1975). *J. Cyclic Nucleotide Res.* **1**, 107–122.

Jacobowitz, D., and Brown, E. M. (1980). *Experientia* **36**, 115–116.

Jakobs, K. H., Saur, W., and Schultz, G. (1976). *J. Cyclic Nucleotide Res.* **2**, 381–392.

Jones, S. J., and Boyde, A. (1978). *In* "Scanning Electron Microscopy of Bone Cells in Culture" (D. H. Copp and R. V. Talmage, eds.), pp. 97–104. Excerpta Med. Found., Amsterdam.

Kahn, C. R. (1976). *J. Cell. Biol.* **70**, 261–286.

Kakiuchi, S., and Yamazaki, R. (1970). *Biochem. Biophys. Res. Commun.* **41**, 1104–1110.

Kaminsky, N. I., Broadus, A. E., Hardman, J. G., Jones, D. J., Jr., Ball, J. H., Sutherland, E. W., and Liddle, G. W. (1970). *J. Clin. Invest.* **49**, 2387–2395.

Keeler, R., Walker, V., and Copp, D. H. (1970). *Can. J. Physiol. Pharmacol.* **48**, 838–841.

Kemper, B., Habener, J. F., Potts, J. T., Jr., and Rich, A. (1972). *Proc. Natl. Acad. Sci. U.S.A.* **69**, 643–647.

Kemper, B., Habener, J. F., Mulligan, R. C., Potts, J. T., Jr., and Rich, A. (1974). *Proc. Natl. Acad. Sci. U.S.A.* **71**, 3731–3735.

Kemper, B., Habener, J. F., Rich, A., and Potts, J. T., Jr. (1975). *Endocrinology* **96**, 903–912.

Kemper, B., Habener, J. F., Ernst, M., Potts, J. T., Jr., and Rich, A. (1976). *Biochemistry* **15**, 20–25.

Kemper, B., Habener, J. F., Rich, A., and Potts, J. T., Jr. (1977). *Science* **184**, 167–169.

Kinne, R., Shlatz, L. J., Kinne-Saffran, E., and Schwartz, I. L. (1975). *J. Membrane Biol.* **24**, 145–159.

Klahr, S., and Peck, W. A. (1980). *Adv. Cyclic Nucleotide Res.* **13**, 133–180.

Klein, D. C., and Raisz, L. G. (1970). *Endocrinology* **86**, 1436–1440.

Konijn, T. M., van de Meene, J. G. C., Chang, Y. Y., Barkley, D. S., and Bonner, J. T. (1969). *J. Bacteriol.* **99**, 510–512.

Kukreja, S. C., Hargis, G. K., Bowser, E. N., Henderson, W. J., Fisherman, E. W., and Williams, G. A. (1975). *J. Clin. Endocrinol. Metab.* **40**, 478–481.

Kukreja, S. C., Banerjee, P., Ayala, G., Bowser, E. N., Hargis, G. K., Henderson, W. J., and Williams, G. A. (1976). *Clin. Res.* **24**, 363 (abstr.).

Lacy, P. E., Howell, S. L., Young, D. A., and Fink, C. J. (1968). *Nature (London)* **219**, 1177–1179.

Lands, A. M., Arnold, A., McAuliff, J. P., Luduena, F. P., and Brown, T. G. (1967). *Nature (London)* **214**, 597–598.

Levine, M. A., Downs, R. W., Jr., Singer, M., Marx, S. J., Aurbach, G. D., and Spiegel, A. M. (1980). *Biochem. Biophys. Res. Commun.* **94**, 1319–1324.

Limbird, L. E., Gill, D. N., and Lefkowitz, R. J. (1980). *Proc. Natl. Acad. Sci. U.S.A.* **77**, 775–779.

Loreau, N., Lajotte, C., Wahbe, F., and Ardaillou, R. (1978). *J. Endocrinol.* **76**, 533–545.

Luben, R. A., Wong, G. L., and Cohn, D. V. (1976). *Endocrinology* **99**, 526–534.

MacGregor, R. R., Hamilton, J. W., and Cohn, D. V. (1975). *Endocrinology* **97**, 178–188.

MacGregor, R. R., Chu, L. L. H., and Cohn, D. V. (1976). *J. Biol. Chem.* **251**, 6711–6716.

McPartlin, J., Skrabanek, P., and Powell, D. (1978). *Endocrinology* **103**, 1573–1578.

Majeska, R. J., Rodan, S. B., and Rodan, G. A. (1978). *Exp. Cell Res.* **111**, 456–468.

Malbon, C. C., and Zull, J. E. (1974). *Biochem. Biophys. Res. Commun.* **56**, 952–958.

Malkinson, A. M., Krueger, B. K., Rudolph, S. A., Casnelli, J. E., Haley, B. E., and Greengard, P. (1975). *Metabolism* **24**, 331–341.

Marcus, R. (1975). *Endocrinology* **96**, 400–408.

Marcus, R., Wilber, J. F., and Aurbach, G. D. (1971). *J. Clin. Endocrinol. Metab.* **33**, 537–541.

Marcus, R., Arvesen, G., and Orner, F. B. (1979). *Endocrinology* **104**, 744–750.

Marks, S. C., Jr. (1973). *Am. J. Anat.* **138**, 165–189.

Martin, T. J., Ingleton, P. M., Underwood, J. C. E., Michelangeli, V. P., Hunt, N. H., and Melick, R. A. (1976). *Nature (London)* **260**, 436–438.

Marx, S. J., and Aurbach, G. D. (1975). *In* "Calcium Regulating Hormones" (R. V. Talmage, M. Owen, and J. A. Parsons, eds.), pp. 163–171. Excerpta Medica, Amsterdam.

Marx, S. J., and Aurbach, G. D. (1978). *In* "Endocrinology of Calcium Metabolism" (D. H. Copp and R. V. Talmage, eds.). Excerpta Medica, Amsterdam.

Marx, S. J., Hershman, J. M., and Aurbach, G. D. (1971). *J. Clin. Endocrinol. Metab.* **33**, 822–828.

Marx, S. J., Fedak, S. A., and Aurbach, G. D. (1972). *J. Biol. Chem.* **247**, 6913–6918.

Marx, S. J., Woodard, C., Aurbach, G. D., Glossmann, H., and Kentmann, H. T. (1973). *J. Biol. Chem.* **248**, 4797–4802.

Marx, S. J., Aurbach, G. D., Gavin, J. R., and Buell, D. W. (1974). *J. Biol. Chem.* **249**, 6812–6816.

Matsuzaki, S., and Dumont, J. E. (1972). *Biochim. Biophys. Acta* **284**, 227–234.

Mayer, G. P., Habener, J. F., and Potts, J. T., Jr. (1976). *J. Clin. Invest.* **57**, 678–683, 1976.

Mayer, G. P., Hurst, J. G., Barto, J. A., Keaton, J. A., and Moore, M. P. (1979a). *Endocrinology* **104**, 1181–1187.

Mayer, G. P., Keaton, J. A., Hurst, J. C., and Habener, J. F. (1979b). *Endocrinology* **104**, 1778–1784.

Melson, G. L., Chase, L. R., and Aurbach, G. D. (1970). *Endocrinology* **86**, 511–518.

Michelakis, A. M. (1970). *Proc. Soc. Exp. Biol. Med.* **135**, 13–16.

Milhaud, G., Rankin, J. C., Bolis, L., and Benson, A. A. (1977). *Proc. Natl. Acad. Sci. U.S.A.* **74**, 4693–4696.

Milhaud, G., Labat, M. L., Graf, B., and Thillard, M. J. (1978). *In* "Endocrinology of Metabolism" (D. H. Copp and R. V. Talmage, eds.), pp. 143–153. Excerpta med. Found., Amsterdam.

Minkin, C., Blackman, L., Newbrey, J., Pokress, S., Posek, R., and Walling, M. (1977). *Biochem. Biophys. Res. Commun.* **76**, 875–881.

Moran, J., Hunziker, W., and Fischer, J. A. (1978). *Proc. Natl. Acad. Sci. U.S.A.* **75**, 3984–3988.

Morrissey, J. J., and Cohn, D. V. (1978). *Endocrinology* **103**, 2081–2090.

Morrissey, J. J., and Cohn, D. V. (1979a). *J. Cell Biol.* **82**, 93–102.

Morrissey, J. J., and Cohn, D. V. (1979b). *J. Cell Biol.* **83**, 512-528.

Nagata, N., and Rasmussen, H. (1968). *Biochemistry* **7**, 3728-3733.

Nagata, N., and Rasmussen, H. (1970). *Biochim. Biophys. Acta* **215**, 1-16.

Nagata, N., Araki-Shimada, N., Ono, Y., and Kimura, N. (1978). *Acta Endocrinol.* **89**, 404-416.

Nakajima, S., Hirschowitz, B. I., and Sachs, G. (1971). *Arch. Biochem. Biophys.* **143**, 123-126.

Ng, B., Hekkelman, J. W., and Heersche, J. N. (1979). *Endocrinology* **104**, 1130-1135.

Nickols, G. A., Carnes, D. L., Anast, C. S., and Forte, L. R. (1979). *Am. J. Physiol.* **236**, 401-409.

Nielson, S. T., Buchanon-Lee, B., Matthews, E. W., Moseley, J. M., and Williams, C. C. (1971). *J. Endocrinol.* **51**, 455-464.

Nissenson, R. A. (1979). *J. Biol. Chem.* **254**, 1469-1475.

Nissenson, R. A., and Arnaud, C. D. (1979). *J. Biol. Chem.* **254**, 1469-1475.

Norberg, K.-A., Persson, B., and Granberg, P.-O. (1975). *Acta Clin. Scand.* **141**, 319-322.

Okano, K., Nakai, R., Fujita, T., and Hoshikawa, M. (1976). *Program Int. Cong. Endocrinol. 6th, 1976* Abstract 711.

Oldham, S. B., Fischer, J. A., Shen, L. H., and Arnaud, C. D. (1974). *Biochemistry* **13**, 4790-4796.

Oldham, S. B., Smith, R., Hartenbower, D. L., and Henry, H. L. (1979). *Adv. Exp. Med. Biol.* **103**, 509-516.

Ole-Moiyoi, O., Pinkus, G. S., Spragg, J., and Austen, K. F. (1979). *New Engl. J. Med.* **300**, 1289-1294.

Peck, W. A., and Burks, J. K. (1977). *In* "Mechanisms of Localized Bone Loss" (J. E. Horton, ed.), pp. 3-12. Information Retrieval, Washington, D.C.

Peck, W. A., and Klahr, S. (1979). *Adv. Cyclic Nucleotide Res.* **11**, 89-130.

Peck, W. A., Carpenter, J., and Messinger, K. (1974). *Endocrinology* **94**, 148-154.

Peck, W. A., Burks, J. K., Wilkins, J. Rodan, S. B., and Rodan, G. A. (1977). *Endocrinology* **100**, 1357-1364.

Pfeuffer, T. (1977). *J. Biol. Chem.* **252**, 7224-7234.

Pires, E. M. V., and Perry, S. V. (1977). *Biochem. J.* **167**, 137-146.

Pollard, H. B., Pazoles, C. J., Creutz, C. E., Ramu, A., Strott, C. A., Ray, P., Brown, E. M., Tack-Goldman, K. M., and Shulman, N. R. (1977). *J. Supramol. Struct.* **7**, 277-285.

Puschett. (1978). *In* "Endocrinology of Calcium Metabolism" (D. H. Copp and R. V. Talmage, eds.), pp. 226-229. Excerpta Medica, Amsterdam.

Raisz, L. G., Brand, J. S., Klein, D. C., and Au, W. Y. W. (1968). *In* "Progress in Endocrinology" (C. Gual, ed.), pp. 696-703. Excerpta Medica, Amsterdam.

Raisz, L. G., Wener, J. A., Trummel, C. L., Feinblatt, J. D., and Au, W. Y. W. (1971). *In* "Calcium, Parathyroid Hormone and the Calcitonins" (R. V. Talmage and P. L. Munson, eds.), pp. 446-453. Excerpta Medica, Amsterdam.

Raisz, L. G., Holtrop, J. J., and Simmons, H. A. (1973). *Endocrinology* **92**, 556-562.

Ramp, W. K., Cooper, C. W., Ross, A. J., III, and Wells, S. A., Jr. (1979). *Mol. Cell. Endocrinol.* **14**, 205-215.

Rao, L. G., Ng, B., Brunette, D. M., and Heersche, J. N. M. (1977). *Endocrinology* **100**, 1233-1241.

Rao, L. G., Moe, H. K., and Heersche, J. N. (1978). *Arch. Oral Biol.* **23**, 957-964.

Rasmussen, H., Goodman, D. B., Friedmann, N., Allen, J. E., and Kurokawa, K. (1976). *In* "Parathyroid Gland" (G. D. Aurbach, ed.), ["Handbook of Physiology" (R. O. Greep and E. B. Astwood, eds.), Vol. VII], pp. 225-264. Am. Physiol. Soc., Washington, D.C.

Ravazzola, M., Orci, L., Habener, J. F., and Potts, J. T., Jr. (1978). *Lancet* **1**, 371-372.

Reaven, E. P., and Reaven, G. M. (1975). *J. Clin. Invest.* **56**, 49-55.

Robinson, C. J., Martin, T. J., and MacIntyre, I. (1966). *Lancet* **2**, 83-84.

Rodan, G. A., Rodan, S. B., and Marks, S. C., Jr. (1978). *Endocrinology* **102**, 1501-1505.

Rodan, S. B., and Rodan, G. A. (1974). *J. Biol. Chem.* **249**, 3068-3074.

Rodbell, M., Birnbaumer, L., and Pohl, S. J. (1970). *J. Biol. Chem.* **245**, 718-722.

Rodbell, M., Birnbaumer, L., Pohl, S. J., and Krans, H. M. J. (1971). *J. Biol. Chem.* **246**, 1877-1882.

Rodriquez, H. J., Morrison, A., Slatapolsky, E., and Klahr, S. (1978). *J. Clin. Endocrinol. Metab.* **47**, 319-325.

Roos, B. A. (1977). *Endocrinology* **100**, 1679-1683.

Roos, B. A., and Deftos, L. J. (1976). *Endocrinology* **98**, 1284-1288.

Roos, B. A., Bundy, L. L., Baily, R., and Deftos, L. J. (1974). *Endocrinology* **95**, 1142-1149.

Rosenblatt, M., Callahan, E. N., Mahaffey, J. E., Pont, A., and Potts, J. T., Jr. (1977). *J. Biol. Chem.* **252**, 5847-5851.

Rosenblatt, M., Segre, G. V., Tyler, G. A., Shepard, G. L., Nussbaum, S. R., and Potts, J. T., Jr. (1980). *Endocrinology* **107**, 545-550.

Ross, E. M., Howlett, A. C., Ferguson, K. M., and Gilman, A. G. (1978). *J. Biol. Chem.* **253**, 6401-6412.

Roth, S. I., and Raisz, L. G. (1966). *Lab. Invest.* **15**, 1187-1211.

Roth, S. I., and Schiller, A. L. (1976). *In* "Parathyroid Gland" (G. D. Aurbach, ed.) [Handbook of Physiology, Endocrinology Section (R. O. Greep and E. B. Astwood, eds.), Vol. VII, Section 7], pp. 281-312. Am. Physiol. Soc. Washington, D.C.

Rubin, R. P. (1970). *Pharmacol. Rev.* **22**, 389-428.

Scarpa, A., Brinkley, F. J., and Dubyak, G. (1978). *Biochemistry* **17**, 1378-1386.

Segre, G. V., Rosenblatt, M., Reiner, B. L., Mahaffey, J. E., and Potts, J. T., Jr. (1979). *J. Biol. Chem.* **254**, 6980-6986.

Shah, J. H., Motto, G. S., Kukreja, S. C., Hargis, G. K., and Williams, G. A. (1975). *J. Clin. Endocrinol. Metab.* **41**, 692-696.

Sheppard, J. R. (1977). *Proc. Natl. Acad. Sci. U.S.A.* **74**, 1091-1094.

Sherwood, L. M., Potts, J. T., Jr., Care, A. D., Mayer, G. P., and Aurbach, G. D. (1966). *Nature (London)* **209**, 52-55.

Sherwood, L. M., Mayer, G. P., Ramberg, C. F., Jr., Kronberg, D. S., Aurbach, G. D., and Potts, J. T., Jr. (1968). *Endocrinology* **83**, 1043-1051.

Sherwood, L. M., Herrman, I., and Basset, C. A. (1970). *Nature (London)* **225** 1056-1058.

Shlatz, L. J., Schwartz, I. L., Kinne-Saffran, E., and Kinne, R. (1975). *J. Membr. Biol.* **24**, 131-144.

Simon, B., and Kather, H. (1977). *Digestion* **16**, 175-179.

Sloboda, R. D., Rudolph, S. A., Rosenbaum, J. L., and Greengard, P. (1975). *Proc. Natl. Acad. Sci. U.S.A.* **72**, 177-181

Smith, D. M., and Johnson, C. C., Jr. (1974). *Endocrinology* **95**, 130-139.

Smith, D. M., and Johnson, C. C., Jr. (1975). *Endocrinology* **96**, 1261-1269.

Sorensen, O. H., Hindberg, I., and Friis, T. (1972). *Acta Med. Scand.* **191**, 103-106.

Spiegel, A. M., Downs, R. W., Jr., and Aurbach, G. D. (1979). *J. Cyclic Nucleotide Res.* **5**, 3-17.

Sraer, J., Ardaillou, R., and Couette, S. (1974). *Endocrinology* **95**, 632-637.

Sraer, J., Sraer, J. D., Chansel, D., Jueppner, H., Hesch, R. D., and Ardaillou, R. (1978). *Am. J. Physiol.* **235**, F96-103.

Steiner, A. L., Pagliara, A. S., Chase, L. R., and Kipnis, D. M. (1972). *J. Biol. Chem.* **247,** 1114-1120.

Strewler, G. J., and Orloff, J. (1977). *Adv. Cyclic Nucleotide Res.* **8,** 311-361.

Sutcliffe, H. S., Martin, T. J., Eisman, J. A., and Pilczyk, R. (1973). *Biochem. J.* **134,** 913-921.

Tanaka, Y., DeLuca, H. F., Ghazarian, J. G., Hargis, G. K., and Williams, G. A. (1979). *Mineral Electrolyte Metab.* **2,** 20-25.

Targovnik, J. H., Rodman, J. S., and Sherwood, L. M. (1971). *Endocrinology* **88,** 1477-1482.

Tashjian, A. H., Jr., Wright, D. R., Ivey, J. L., and Pont, A. (1978). *Recent Prog. Hormone Res.* **34,** 285-334.

Teo, T. S., and Wang, J. H. (1973). *J. Biol. Chem.* **248,** 5950-5955.

Terasaki, W. L., and Brooker, G. (1977). *J. Biol. Chem.* **252,** 1041-1050.

Thomas, J.-P., Dorflinger, L. J., and Behrman, H. A. (1978). *Proc. Natl. Acad. Sci. U.S.A.* **75,** 1344-1348.

Tomlinson, S., Barling, P. M., Albano, J. D. M., Brown, B. L., and O'Riordan, J. L. (1974). *Clin. Sci. Mol. Med.* **47,** 481-492.

Torres, V. E., Hui, Y. S., Shah, S. V., Northrup, T. E., and Dousa, T. P. (1978). *Kidney Intl.* **14,** 444-451.

Vaes, G. (1968). *Nature (London)* **219,** 939-940.

Vesely, D. L., Lehotay, D. C., and Levey, G. S. (1978). *J. Studies Alcohol* **38,** 842-847.

Walker, D. G. (1977). *In* "Mechanisms of Localized Bone Loss" (J. E. Horton, ed), pp. 383-387. Information Retrieval, Washington, D.C.

Walker, D. G. (1978). *In* "Endocrinology of Calcium Metabolism" (D. H. Copp and R. V. Talmage, eds.), pp. 105-110. Excerpta Med. Found., Amsterdam.

Wilfong, R. F., and Neville, D. M., Jr. (1970). *J. Biol. Chem.* **245,** 6106-6112.

Williams, G. A., Hargis, G. K., Bowser, E. N., Henderson, W. J., and Martinez, N. J. (1973). *Endocrinology* **92,** 687-691.

Williams, G. A., Bowser, E. N., Hargis, G. K., Kukreja, S. C., Shah, J. H., Vora, N. M., and Henderson, W. J. (1978). *Proc. Soc. Exp. Biol. Med.* **159,** 187-191.

Williams, L. T., Gore, T. B., and Lefkowitz, R. J. (1977). *J. Clin. Invest.* **59,** 319-324.

Windeck, R., Brown, E. M., Gardner, D. G., and Aurbach, G. D. (1978). *Endocrinology* **103,** 2020-2025.

Wolff, D. J., and Brostrom, C. O. (1979). *Cyclic Nucleotide Res.* **11,** 27-88.

Wolff, J., and Williams, J. A. (1973). *Recent Prog. Horm. Res.* **29,** 229-285.

Wolfsdorf, J. I., Rosenfield, R. L., Fang, V. S., Kobayashi, R., Razdan, A. K., and Kim, M. H. (1978). *Acta Endocrinol. (Copenhagen)* **88,** 321-328.

Wong, G. L. (1979a). *J. Biol. Chem.* **254,** 34-37.

Wong, G. L. (1979b). *J. Biol. Chem.* **254,** 6337-6340.

Wong, G. L., and Cohn, D. V. (1974). *Nature (London)* **252,** 713-715.

Wrenn, R. W., and Biddulph, D. M. (1979). *J. Cyclic Nucleotide Res.* **5,** 239-250.

Yagi, K., Yazawa, M., Kakiuchi, S., Ohshima, M., and Uenishi, K. (1978). *J. Biol. Chem.* **253,** 1338-1340.

Zull, J. E., Malbon, C. C., and Chuang, J. (1977). *J. Biol. Chem.* **252,** 1071-1078.

VITAMINS AND HORMONES, VOL. 38

Recent Approaches to Fertility Control Based on Derivatives of LH-RH*

ANDREW V. SCHALLY, AKIRA ARIMURA, AND DAVID H. COY

The Veterans Administration Medical Center, Department of Medicine, School of Medicine, Tulane University, New Orleans, Louisiana

*This chapter is dedicated to the memory of Emanuel (Manny) M. Bogdanove, Professor of Physiology, Medical College of Virginia, colleague, collaborator, and friend, who contributed much to the concepts of regulation of pituitary gonadotropin secretion and whose untimely passing is a great loss to all endocrinologists.

257

I. General Introduction

Complicated political, economic, and social problems caused by uncontrolled population growth in many parts of the world have created widespread concern. Because of the size of our planet and its resources, infinite population expansion is impossible and eventual limitation to "zero growth" is inevitable. The need for regulation of our fertility to slow down the frightening rate of human population increase has been recognized for decades by various sociologists and to a lesser degree by political leaders, governments, and international agencies. The responsibility of scientists and physicians may go much further, since the achievement of better control of human fertility will require the development and testing of new methods of birth control that will be effective and at the same time safer and more convenient than the methods now available. Because of the inadequacies of present contraceptive methods, millions of pregnancies worldwide are unplanned and unwanted. Ironically, undeveloped, poorer nations have a faster population increase and are unable to effect significant control. Even in the United States, where effective contraceptives are available, about one-third of total pregnancies are unwanted (Connell, 1978; Mastroianni, 1978). The basis for success in the development of new and better contraceptive methods would appear to lie in a more complete understanding of all the complicated processes involved in human reproduction and in increased contraceptive research.

Among several contraceptive approaches presently being considered and developed is one based on analogs and derivatives of the hypothalamic hormone that controls the secretion of both luteinizing hormone (LH) and follicle-stimulating hormone (FSH) from the pituitary (Schally *et al.*, 1971a–d).

This hypothalamic hormone (Fig. 1) is called the LH- and FSH-releasing hormone, abbreviated as LH-RH/FSH-RH or simply gonadotropin-releasing hormone (Gn-RH) (Schally *et al.*, 1973a, 1978). However, while keeping in mind that LH-RH is generally accepted as the main or even the only FSH-releasing hormone, for the sake of convenience and in the interest of historical continuity we shall use the abbreviation LH-RH for naming its analogs. The IUPAC–IUB approved trivial name for this hormone has been rejected by most endocrinologists, by the Endocrine Society and its journals, and by most other scientists engaged in the study of reproduction (Schally *et al.*, 1978).

Approaches based on LH-RH may possibly lead in the forseeable future to the development of an easily applicable birth control method free of undesirable side effects. In this article we have attempted to

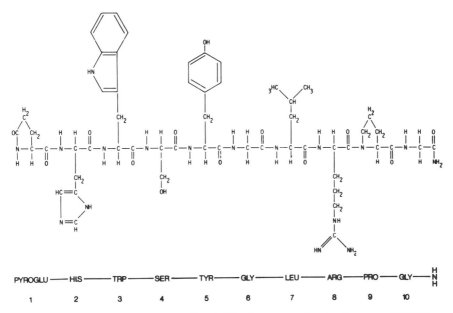

FIG. 1. The molecular structure of luteinizing hormone-releasing hormone (LH-RH).

compile and review significant information accumulated so far on LH-RH antisera and inhibitory analogs. The paradoxical antifertility effects that have been discovered to occur when relatively large doses of the superactive stimulatory analogs are used will also be discussed in detail. However, it is beyond the scope of this article to review the very extensive physiological and clinical studies carried out with LH-RH and its stimulatory analogs. As suggested by the editors, we shall emphasize our special interests and present the development of our ideas and hypotheses about the possible use of various derivatives of LH-RH for fertility control. We will also attempt to evaluate the medical significance of these findings.

It is our hope that the material covered will be a source for learning and a stimulus for further research. We would feel richly rewarded if our work could even in a small measure contribute to the regulation of human fertility.

II. Antisera to LH-RH

A. Introduction

After synthetic LH-RH became available in sufficient amounts, several groups of investigators succeeded in generating antisera to this hormone, developing radioimmunoassays (RIA), and using the antisera for immunocytochemistry as well as for other studies. Information obtained from these studies has expanded our knowledge of the hormone, including cellular and subcellular distribution, biosynthesis, release, metabolism, and elucidation of its physiological role.

Since LH-RH is a small peptide that is rapidly disintegrated *in vivo*, it rarely becomes immunogenic. Therefore, the incidence of antibody formation during or after a prolonged treatment of patients with LH-RH is extremely low. It is customary to couple or adsorb the LH-RH molecule to large carrier substances to increase immunogenicity when an attempt to generate the antiserum is made. In this section, we discuss methods for preparing immunogen for generating LH-RH antibody, characterization of antiserum generated, and change in reproductive functions that can be induced by passive and active immunization with LH-RH. We do not touch upon LH-RH radioimmunoassay or immunocytochemistry, for which several excellent reviews are available elsewhere (Hökfelt *et al.*, 1978; Nett and Niswender, 1979; Sétáló *et al.*, 1978; Zimmerman, 1976).

B. PRODUCTION OF ANTISERA

1. *Preparation of LH-RH Immunogen*

Synthetic LH-RH decapeptide can be chemically coupled to or simply adsorbed to large molecules, such as proteins or other high molecular weight substances. Thus the peptide may be prevented from being quickly metabolized *in vivo* and rapidly excreted in urine (Jeffcoate *et al.*, 1974; Redding *et al.*, 1973).

We prepared the LH-RH immunogen in a manner similar to that used for angiotensin (Worobec *et al.*, 1972). Synthetic LH-RH was dissolved in 0.9% NaCl to a concentration of 20 mg/ml. One milliliter of the LH-RH solution was mixed with 4 ml of 50% polyvinylpyrrolidone (PVP, 40,000 molecular weight, Mann Research Laboratory, New York) in 0.9% NaCl. After 2 hours, the mixture was emulsified with 5 ml of Freund's complete adjuvant (Difco Laboratories, Detroit, Michigan) by treatment in a Sorvall Omni-Mixer for 5 or 15 minutes. Five milligrams of LH-RH were injected into each animal in multiple sites for the primary immunization, followed by 1.3 or 1.6 mg for the booster injections at 1-month intervals (Arimura *et al.*, 1973). Julisz and Kerdelhué (1973) adsorbed LH-RH to Al_2O_3 for preparing the immunogen.

The LH-RH decapeptide can be chemically coupled with a protein molecule through its N or C terminus or through the phenol ring of tyrosine or histidine in position 5 or 2, respectively. Since both of the N and C termini of LH-RH decapeptide are blocked, it is necessary to prepare LH-RH analogs with free N or C termini that can be linked to protein by condensation with the carbodiimide reagent or by the mixed anhydride reaction. Synthetic Gly^{10}-LH-RH was conjugated with bovine serum albumin (BSA), emulsified with complete Freund's adjuvant, and administered to rabbits. The antibody thus generated showed an excellent standard curve in an RIA for LH-RH, but cross-reacted considerably with Gly^{10}-LH-RH. The binding site of our antiserum to Gly^{10}-LH-RH-BSA conjugate seemed to reside in the LH-RH hexapeptide fragment corresponding to positions 2 to 7. Synthetic Glu^{1}-LH-RH conjugated with a carrier protein such as human serum albumin (HSA) was also used as an immunogen preparation. The antiserum thus generated was found to be suitable for the LH-RH RIA, but also cross-reacted with the C-terminal tetrapeptide amide fragment for LH-RH. In other words, the N-terminal part of the LH-RH molecule was not needed for binding with this antibody (Arimura et al., 1975).

In an attempt to generate a highly specific antibody to LH-RH by using LH-RH-protein conjugate, LH-RH was also linked to protein through tyrosine or histidine by means of the bifunctional reagent (Nett et al., 1973), bisdiazotized benzidine, as in the case of TRH (Bassiri and Utiger, 1972). However, when a symmetrical bifunctional reagent is used in a one-step reaction, dimerization and oligomerization of LH-RH can occur. To avoid this, an asymmetric bifunctional reagent was used in a two-step coupling procedure in which p-diazonium-phenylacetic acid was attached to LH-RH and the resulting azo derivative was coupled to BSA with a carbodiimide reagent (Koch et al., 1973a). The antiserum thus generated showed very little cross-reaction with Gly^{10}-LH-RH but still exhibited 20% cross-reaction with des-pGlu^{1}-LH-RH.

Teuwissen et al. (1976) described a method for introducing one carboxyl group into the LH-RH molecule by carboxyl methylation of its histidine residue. The monocarboxymethylated LH-RH as a derivative for conjugation provides two advantages. First, it contains the intact glycine amide and pyroglutamyl terminal group. Second, the new compound may provide a well defined antigen that can react through its unique carboxyl with the amino group of the carrier molecule, forming a stable amide bond. The compound was conjugated by the classical carbodiimide method (Goodfriend et al., 1964) with poly-DL-alanyl chains (spacer group) polymerized on human lactoferrin. The conjugate was then emulsified in complete Freund's adjuvant and injected into the animals. An excellent standard curve for LH-RH RIA was established with the antiserum generated, but no information on the antigenic determinant at the antibody site was provided.

2. Characterization of Antiserum

The influence of the site of conjugation of hapten to protein on the specificity of the resulting antisera was reported for steroids (Niswender and Midgley, 1970). A similar study was made of antisera against LH-RH (Arimura et al., 1975). The specificity of several antisera as indicated by their crossactivity with synthetic peptides corresponding to fragments of LH-RH decapeptide or its analogs is shown in Table I. Antiserum 419 and 422 were generated in rabbits using PVP-adsorbed LH-RH as the immunogen. Antiserum 710 was generated against Gly[10]-LH-RH conjugated with BSA at the C terminus, as described by Goodfriend et al. (1964). Antisera 743, 744, and 745 were generated against Glu[1]-LH-RH coupled with human serum albumin (HSA) through the N terminus. Antisera 940, 942, and 944 were coupled with HSA or bovine serum albumin (BSA) using bisdiazotized benzidine (BDB) (Nett et al., 1973).

All antisera exhibited an ordinary inhibition curve in the RIA for LH-RH, except for antiserum 419, which showed a paradoxical or "hock type" standard curve in the low range of dose (Arimura et al., 1973). The extent of cross-reactivity (C) was expressed as follows:

$$C = \frac{L_{50}}{U_{50}} \times 100\%$$

where L_{50} = dose of LH-RH that shows 50% abscissa intercept and U_{50} = dose of peptide that shows 50% abscissa intercept. With antiserum 419, the peptides Nos. 1 to 6 did not show any cross-reactivity. Peptide No. 7, the C-terminal tetrapeptide itself, did not bind with the antiserum. Peptides Nos. 8 and 9, both lacking Trp[3], exhibited a slight but significant inhibition, but the slopes of the inhibition lines for these compounds were different from that of LH-RH.

The peptides Nos. 10–16, all containing Trp, showed cross-reactivity in various degrees in an RIA system using antiserum 419, and their slopes were parallel to that for LH-RH, although a larger mass was required for comparable inhibition. This suggests that pyroglutamic acid in position 1, histidine in position 2, and the C-terminal amide are not necessary for binding to antiserum 419. On the other hand, tryptophan in position 3 may be important for the antigen–antibody interaction, since the cross-reactivity of peptide No. 8 is considerably less than that of No. 15, and the inhibition slope for No. 8 is not parallel to

TABLE I

Cross-Reactivity[a] of Different Anti-LH-RH Sera with LH-RH Fragments and Analogs

Peptide No.	pyroGlu-His-Trp-Ser-Tyr-Gly-Leu-Arg-Pro-Gly-NH$_2$	Anti-LH-RH sera								
		419	422	710	743	744	745	940	942	944
LH-RH	Gly-NH$_2$									
1	pyroGlu————Leu-OH	0	0	+[b]	0	0	0	0	0	0
2	pyroGlu————Gly-OH	0	0	0	0	0	0	0	0	0
3	pyroGlu————T·p-OH	0	0	0	0	0	0	0	0	0
4	His————Leu-OH	0	0	+	0	0	0	0	0	0
5	Trp————Leu-OH	0	0	0	0	0	0	0	0	0
6	Ser————Leu-OH	0	0	0	0	0	0	0	0	0
7	————Leu-OH Gly-NH$_2$	0	0	0	0	0	0	0.02	1.0	0.04
8	Ser Gly-NH$_2$	0.5	0	0	0	32.1	0.98	0.66	6.6	4.5
9	pyroGlu( )————Gly-NH$_2$	0.5	0	0	0	56.3	22.7	4.1	6.6	8.6
10	pyroGlu( )————Gly-NH$_2$	10.4	0	15	11.4	90.0	45.5	6.6	3.1	8.6
11	His.————Gly-NH$_2$	16.8	0	>100	25.0	45.0	45.5	10.6	16.7	27.1
12	pyroGlu————Gly-OH	60.0	0	0	55.6	>100	100	35.4	0	0
13	Trp————Pro-OH	0.8	0	0	2.1	0	1.0	0	0	0
14	Trp————Pro-NH$_2$	13.0	0	0	25.0	0	0.4	0	0.1	0
15	Trp————Gly-NH$_2$	73.0	0	0	25.0	>100	>100	35.4	37.0	34.2
16	Trp————Arg-NH$_2$	+	0	0	0	0	0	0	0	0
17	pyroGlu————Pro-NH$_2$	73.0	0	100	>100.0	0	2.4	0	0.6	0.04
18	Glu————Gly-NH$_2$	—	1.2	23.8	33.3	>100	100.0	17.7	10.4	21.7

[a] The extent of cross-reactivity was expressed by the percentage ratio of the amounts of the analog and of LH-RH for B/B$_0$ = 50%, where B and B$_0$ represent the bound radioactivity with and without cold LH-RH, respectively, in the radioimmunoassay system for LH-RH. The inhibition curve is not parallel to that for LH-RH.

[b] + indicates that the peptide cross-reacts with the antiserum, but the inhibition curve is not parallel to that for LH-RH.

that for LH-RH. The NH$_2$ group at the C terminus enhances binding. These results suggest that the immunological binding site for antiserum 419 resides in the amino acid sequence from Trp at positions 3 to Pro at 9. A shorter peptide, No. 16, also showed a significant inhibition, but the slope was not parallel to that for LH-RH.

Antiserum 422 appears to be quite specific, reacting only with Glu[1]-LH-RH by 1.2%. Although this suggests that antiserum 422 requires both the N and C terminus of LH-RH for binding, these two ends could be in close proximity in the three-dimensional conformation of LH-RH (personal communication of Dr. R. P. Millar; Momany, 1978; Seprodi et al., 1978b).

For antiserum 710, peptides Nos. 12 and 16 showed complete cross-reaction. The N-terminal pyroglutamic acid may be moderately important but is not essential for binding, since the binding decreased in its absence. Peptide No. 10, which differs from LH-RH only by the absence of histidine, had no affinity. None of the peptides lacking histidine showed cross-reaction with this antiserum. This indicated that histidine plays a crucial role in the antigen–antibody binding. It was assumed that the amino acid sequence from positions 2 to 8 or 9 is the determinant of immunological binding for antiserum 710. The hexapeptide His-Trp-Ser-Tyr-Gly-Leu also showed a cross-reaction, although the inhibition slope was different from that for LH-RH.

With antiserum 743, directed toward the sequence from Trp[3] to Pro[9], the C-terminal amide enhanced binding. Antisera 744 and 745, both of which were generated against the same immunogen as that for antiserum 743, showed different antigenic determinants. Both of them directed toward C-terminal amino acid sequences, Leu[7] to Gly[10]-NH$_2$ for antiserum 744, and probably Ser[4] to Gly[10]-NH$_2$ for antiserum 745.

Antisera 940, 942, and 944 possessed similar antigenic determinants, directing toward the sequence from Ser[4] to Gly[10]-NH$_2$. The C-terminal amide was essential for binding.

The results indicate that the antigenic determinant of the antibody generally differs depending on the different type of conjugates and that the same immunogen preparation does not always generate antisera with identical binding sites.

It is important to obtain accurate information on the antigenic determinants of the antiserum to be used for an experiment whether it is RIA, immunocytochemistry, or another study. Otherwise, one must be extremely cautious in making interpretations of the results obtained. It is interesting that LH-RH-like activity in the pineal body was detected only by RIA using antiserum 710 (unpublished observation).

C. Physiological Events Induced by LH-RH That Were Revealed by Passive or Active Immunization with Synthetic LH-RH

1. Spermatogenesis and Follicular Maturation

It is generally accepted that FSH maintains the germinal epithelium, whereas LH facilitates the completion of spermatogenesis, stimulating the Leydig cells to produce testosterone (Gemzell and Roos, 1966). The administration of FSH to immature or mature hypophysectomized rats markedly increases the size of the testes but does not accelerate the appearance of mature sperm or increase the secretory activity of the Leydig cells. For completion of spermatogenesis, an androgenic influence is needed. It can be provided indirectly by the administration of LH or directly by the administration of testosterone (Means, 1975).

Suppression of the release or blockade of the action of LH-RH may eventually result in testicular atrophy and the arrest of spermatogenesis, because both LH and FSH secretions are probably regulated by hypothalamic LH-RH. After active immunization and the production of antibodies against LH-RH, testicular weight in one male rabbit decreased to 6% of that of the untreated control rabbit. Interstitial cells and seminiferous tubules were markedly atrophied, and the latter were devoid of germ cells. Pituitary LH content was markedly reduced in this rabbit (Arimura et al., 1973).

Immunization of adult rats with LH-RH–BSA conjugate resulted in atrophy of the testes and secondary sex organs. There was a considerable reduction in tubule diameter and the tubules were lined with Sertoli cells and spermatogonia, there being a total arrest of spermatogenesis (Fraser et al., 1974).

Immunization of marmoset monkeys caused a marked reduction of plasma testosterone in those monkeys that developed a high titer of antibody to LH-RH (Hodges and Hearn, 1977). Their testes became softer and smaller.

Immunization of a ewe with LH-RH-BSA conjugate resulted in disappearance of luteal tissue in most of the animals that produced antibody. Numerous follicles were found in all sheep. The number of antral follicles also decreased in the immunized ewes as compared to the control animals (Clarke et al., 1978).

Arrest of follicular maturation was also observed after passive immunization of cycling hamsters. In the ovaries of hamsters injected with the antiserum to LH-RH on diestrus day 1, only preantral follicles developed on the prospective proestrus. Unlike the intact hamsters, these animals did not show a gradual rise in circulating estrogens as they approached proestrus and did not ovulate spontaneously or even after the injection of LH-RH (de la Cruz *et al.*, 1976a).

Immunization of castrated rats with HSA–Glu¹-LH-RH conjugate resulted in a decrease in both LH and FSH levels associated with a rise of serum antibody titer against LH-RH (Arimura *et al.*, 1976a; Fraser *et al.*, 1975). On the other hand, both LH and FSH levels in HSA immunized rats or nonimmunized rats remained unsuppressed, and typical castration cells containing large vacuoles were found in the pituitary. Although there were castration cells in the pituitary of rats that produced antibody to LH-RH, these cells were markedly degranulated and secretory granules were scarce in the cytoplasm (Arimura *et al.*, 1976b).

Repeated administration of LH-RH antisera to the castrated rats, starting 1 day after castration, decreased both serum LH and FSH concentration to control levels. Castration cells were completely absent from the pituitaries, suggesting that castration cells are formed as a result of increased secretion of LH-RH. Antibody to the LH-RH decapeptide drastically affected both LH and FSH cells, additional evidence for the concept that LH-RH represents the physiological LH-RH and FSH-RH (Arimura *et al.*, 1976b).

2. *Estrous Cycle and Ovulation*

Neuroendocrine interplay in the hypothalamic–pituitary–gonadal axis that regulates estrous or menstrual cycles culminates at ovulation. It is generally accepted that LH-RH secretion is increased at proestrus in animals and at midcycle in primates and humans, thereby inducing the preovulatory surge of LH and FSH secretion. An increase of biologically active or immunoreactive LH-RH in the peripheral blood at proestrus in animals (Fraser *et al.*, 1973) and at midcycle in women (Arimura *et al.*, 1974b; Malacara *et al.*, 1972) was reported, but specificity of RIA for LH-RH in the peripheral plasma has been questioned. In monkeys anesthetized with phenylcyclidine hydrochloride, blood collected from the sectioned pituitary stalk contained immunoreactive LH-RH in levels ranging from a low of 20–75 pg/ml to a high of 800 pg/ml at midcycle. There was also a pulsatile increase of LH-RH release (Camel *et al.*, 1976). Immunoreactive LH-RH concentration in blood from the rat pituitary stalk rose in the afternoon of proestrus when alfaxalone (Althesin) was used as the anesthetic (Sarkar *et al.*, 1976). An injection of the LH-RH antiserum to LH-RH into cycling rats in the morning of proestrus completely suppressed the preovulatory surge of both LH and FSH and prevented ovulation (Koch *et al.*, 1973b; Arimura *et al.*, 1974a; Kerdelhué *et al.*, 1976).

Serum prolactin levels remained unaltered (Koch *et al.*, 1973b). Immunization of female rats with LH-RH resulted in abolition of regular cyclic patterns of vaginal smears, the absence of luteal tissue, and blockade of ovulation. Follicular growth varied among rats and appeared to be dependent on whether the inhibition of LH-RH had been sufficient to affect the secretion of basal levels of gonadotropins. Low levels of gonadotropins were associated with poor follicular development, uterine atrophy, and leukocyte vaginal smears, whereas levels of gonadotropins, comparable to those in diestrous control rats, led to adequate follicular growth in the absence of ovulation, the production of cystic follicles, uterine stimulation, and persistent vaginal estrus (Fraser and Baker, 1977; Takahashi *et al.*, 1978).

A single injection of a small amount of anti-LH-RH serum into normal cycling rats provoked a long-term alteration in the hypothalamic–gonadal axis that included a transient diestrous period followed by persistent estrus with large cystic follicles. Marked hyperprolactinemia occurred after transient hypoprolactinemia (Kerdelhué *et al.*, 1976). Ewes immunized with LH-RH failed to show estrus or ovulate when the antibody titer to LH-RH increased. Plasma LH significantly decreased with elevated levels of prolactin and unaltered FSH levels (Clarke *et al.*, 1978).

Injections of 0.5 ml of our sheep anti-LH-RH serum completely blocked ovulation when administered i.v. or s.c. at any stage of the estrous cycle in hamsters. This antiovulatory activity lasted 12–13 days. Injections of LH-RH on the afternoon of proestrus induced ovulation in the antiserum-treated hamsters when the antiserum was injected in proestrus, but not when injected in diestrus 1 or diestrus 2. This suggests that the anti-LH-RH serum acts differently in blocking ovulation during diestrus and proestrus by suppressing follicular development and inhibiting the preovulatory surge of gonadotropins, respectively. Serum estradiol levels were significantly reduced, but not completely suppressed, after injection of 0.5 ml of antiserum. 17-β-Estradiol administered 22 hours before the presumptive preovulatory LH surge improved significantly the LH response to LH-RH in the antiserum-blocked hamsters. This indicates a direct modulation of pituitary LH responsiveness by estradiol in the absence of endogenous LH-RH activity (de la Cruz *et al.*, 1976a). McCormack *et al.* (1977) reported that single i.v. injections of a rabbit antiserum against synthetic LH-RH promptly suppressed LH and FSH concentrations in ovariectomized rhesus monkeys. Gonadotropin levels remained depressed for 10–21 days, the approximate duration of enhanced LH-RH binding activity in the circulation. Doses of LH-RH antiserum sufficient to reduce tonic gonadotropin secretion did not modify the time course or magnitude of estrogen-induced gonadotropin surges. It is possible that the circulating levels of antibody may not have been high enough to intercept a functionally significant proportion of a presumptive bolus of LH-RH during its brief sojourn in the hypophysial portal circulation.

3. *Implantation of Ova and Gestation*

Although the importance of pituitary LH in the implantation of fertilized ova and the maintenance of fetuses during early pregnancy in animals has been well documented, the extent of dependence of LH secretion on hypothalamic LH-RH during pregnancy has remained unclarified. Our group demonstrated the importance of endogenous LH-RH in both implantation and the maintenance of fetuses during early pregnancy (Arimura *et al.*, 1976a; Nishi *et al.*, 1976a). In the first experiment, a proestrous rat was caged with two male rats that had been proved to be fertile. If vaginal lavage on the following morning contained spermatozoa, that day was designated as pregnancy day 1. Anti-LH-RH sheep γ-globulin (anti-LH-RHG) was administered i.v. to the rats once daily from day 1 through day 7 or from day 3 to day 5 of the pregnancy. Viable sites in the uterus were hardly distinguishable on day 8 in the anti-LH-RHG-treated rats when an exploratory laparotomy was performed; however, they became distinguishable on day 14 in some of these animals. On the other hand, administration of normal sheep γ-globulin (NSG) did not interfere with normal implantation. Inhibition of implantation was observed even when a single injection of anti-LH-RHG was administered to the rat on day 4, but not on days 3 or 5. The suppressive effect of anti-LH-RHG was completely prevented by a simultaneous injection of two doses of 1 μg of LH-RH in 16% gelatin/0.9% saline and was nearly completely reversed by a single dose of 1 μg of estradiol (Arimura *et al.*, 1976a).

The effect of anti-LH-RHG on gestation after implantation was also examined. After pregnancy was confirmed by a laparotomy on day 7, the rats were given anti-LH-RGH or NSG daily from days 7 to 11. In all the anti-LH–RHG-treated rats resorption of fetuses occurred, as indicated by a second exploratory laparotomy on day 14. Yet, no vaginal bleeding accompanied this resorption. Gestation was not disturbed in the NSG-treated animals. It was found that a single injection of anti-LH-RHG on day 9 or 10 caused complete resorption of fetuses in all the treated rats. Injection on day 8, 11, or 12 was only partially effective. These results indicate that the critical days are 9 and 10, when LH-RH is essential for the maintenance of viable fetuses (Nishi *et al.*, 1976a).

Administration of LH-RH twice daily from days 9 to 12 of pregnancy completely overcame the effect of anti-LH-RH. Treatment with 4 mg of progesterone daily from days 7 to 12 of gestation also prevented the resorption of fetuses by anti-LH-RHG. Serum progesterone levels were elevated on day 7 of gestation and reached a peak on days 13 to 14 in the control animals. Injection of anti-LH-RHG on day 9 or 10 drastically reduced plasma progesterone levels on day 11 and thereafter. The suppression of progesterone was slight or absent when the anti-LH-RHG was injected on day 12 (Nishi *et al.*, 1976a). Therefore there is a good correlation between the termination of gestation and the decrease in serum progesterone. Because, in the control animals, circulating LH levels during days 9 and 10 of pregnancy declined to the point of being barely detectable by our radioimmunoassay, the possible reduction of LH levels by anti-LH-RGH could not be confirmed. However, the results of these studies indicate that the hypothalamic LH-RH plays an important role in the early pregnancy of rats. On day 4, LH-RH, probably through LH, stimulates estrogen secretion, which is essential for implantation of fertilized ova, and on days 9 and 10 LH-RH stimulates progesterone secretion, which is essential for the maintenance of viable fetuses (Nishi *et al.*, 1976a).

The reproductive capacity of rats immunized with LH-RH was tested by caging them with normal male rats from 3 weeks after immunization. Although mating occurred in 3 out of 8 immunized rats during the first month, none of them produced offspring. After subsequent exposure to the male rats, there were no signs of mating (Fraser and Baker, 1977).

Generation of high titer of antibody against LH-RH by active immunization in a pregnant marmoset monkey resulted in abortion that was associated with a drop of plasma progesterone levels (Hodges and Hearn, 1977). These results demonstrate that immunization against LH-RH is also an effective way of suppressing gonadal activity in the primate.

D. CONCLUSION

Although LH RH has little immunogenicity, chemical or physical coupling of the peptide with large molecules enhances the antigenicity. Binding sites of the antibody generated against LH-RH conjugate vary, depending on the method of conjugation. However, even the same immunogen preparation does not necessarily induce antibodies with identical binding sites. Different antigenic determinants at the antibody site as well as different affinities affect the results of RIA and immunocytochemical studies. On the other hand, physiological events regulated by blood-borne endogenous LH-RH were suppressed or inhibited by passive or active immunization of LH-RH, regardless of the different LH-RH conjugates for immunization that were used.

Administration of LH-RH antiserum or generation of LH-RH antibody by active immunization uniformly results in a decrease in circulating LH and FSH levels, abolishment of estrous or menstrual cycle, blockage of ovulation, gonadal atrophy, suppression of secretion of gonadal steroids, delayed implantation, and blockage of gestation in rats, hamsters, ewe, and marmoset and rhesus monkeys. The extent of the effect of LH-RH antibody on the gonadal functions varies, depending on the titer of antibody generated or administerd. Although the necessity for Freund's adjuvant for active immunization and the rather drastic effect of complete suppression of gonadal function that was often observed in the animal experiments preclude its adaptability as a method of human fertility control at present, it may still be possible to develop a new approach to contraception by suppression of action of LH-RH either immunologically or by the use of competitive LH-RH antagonists. In any case, the findings described in this section will provide fundamental information on the effect of nullification of the actions of endogenous LH-RH.

III. Stimulatory Analogs of LH-RH

A. Introduction

In the 8 years since the isolation of LH-RH (Schally *et al.*, 1971a,c,d) and the determination of its structure and synthesis (Matsuo *et al.*, 1971a,b; Baba *et al.*, 1971) (Fig. 1), an estimated 1000 analogs of LH-RH have been synthesized. The enormous amount of information gathered from the biological testing of these compounds has let to clarification of the role of individual amino acid residues, to the discovery of many agonistic analogs of greater therapeutic usefulness than the parent hormone, and to the continued development of inhibitory antagonistic analogs.

There is little doubt that, in addition to basic scientific reasons for determining structure-function relationships for this hormone, a strong interest in possible veterinary and medical applications of LH-RH derivatives stimulated this synthetic undertaking. As early as 1971 we postulated that agonistic LH-RH analogs and derivatives might be useful not only for the stimulation of fertility in domestic animals and human beings (including cryptorchidism, delayed puberty, and hypogonadotropic hypogonadism), but also for the control of fertility by the disruption of the menstrual cycle, prevention of the ovulatory LH-surge, functional luteolysis, and standardization of the rhythm method as well (Schally and Kastin, 1971). The correctness of these predictions has been well proved, although the exact clinical regimens are still lacking. We also envisioned that inhibitory analogs of LH-RH could be used for the development of a new birth control method. The feasibility of this approach was also clearly confirmed, and, although we still do not have inhibitory analogs powerful enough to be practical, we are rapidly approaching this goal. Some of the key available information that has been accumulated on these topics is reviewed below.

B. METHODS OF DETERMINATION OF ACTIVITY OF STIMULATORY AND INHIBITORY LH-RH ANALOGS

1. *In Vitro Assays*

a. *Release of LH and FSH from Rat Pituitary Halves or Quarters in Vitro.* Fragments of rat pituitaries are incubated in 1 ml Krebs-Ringer bicarbonate buffer containing glucose and bovine serum albumin according to the *in vitro* method used for CRF assay by Saffran and Schally (1955), with some modification as described previously for LH-RH (Schally *et al.*, 1972b, 1973c; Arimura and Schally, 1980).

b. *Release of LH and FSH from Monolayer Cultures of Rat Pituitary Cells*

i. *Stimulatory Activity.* LH-RH and its analogs stimulate the release of LH and FSH from cultured pituitary cells in a dose-related manner (Vale *et al.*, 1972a, 1977). *In vitro* activities of some LH-RH analogs as measured by this method are sometimes different from *in vivo* potencies (Labrie *et al.*, 1976b).

ii. *Inhibitory Activity.* Suppression of response to LH-RH by inhibitory analogs can be measured in the same system. After 4 or 5 days in culture, the cells were washed and incubated for 5 hours at 37°C in Dulbecco-modified Eagle's medium in the presence or the absence of 3 × 10^{-9} M LH-RH. Inhibitory LH-RH analogs are added 10 minutes prior to LH-RH (Labrie *et al.*, 1976b; Coy *et al.*, 1975d).

2. *In Vivo Assays*

a. *LH Release in Ovariectomized, Estrogen- and Progesterone-Treated Rats (Ramirez and McCann, 1963).* This animal preparation is most sensitive to LH-RH. Elevation of serum LH after injection of test materials is used as the response parameter. In our hands, the minimum detectable dose of LH-RH is 0.2 ng/rat. Serum LH is assayed by RIA. This preparation is however, insensitive to FSH-RH activity. This assay can be used for inhibitory analogs, which are injected or infused for 2 hours prior to administration of LH-RH (2.5 ng) (Vilchez-Martinez et al., 1974b, 1975a).

b. *LH and FSH Release in Immature Male Rats*

i. *Stimulatory Analogs.* Prolonged infusion of LH-RH analogs into immature rats can increase serum LH and FSH in a dose-related manner (Arimura et al., 1972; Vilchez-Martinez et al., 1975a). Serum LH and FSH are determined by RIA.

ii. *Inhibitory Analogs—Blockade of LH and FSH Release.* Anti-LH/FSH releasing activities of analogs can be screened over a 4-hour period of time with the immature male rat assay (Vilchez-Martinez et al., 1975a,b, 1976a). Animals were injected s.c. with analogs or with vehicle alone. Two hundred nanograms of synthetic LH-RH or saline solution were injected s.c. at the same time or at different times thereafter. Blood was collected 30 minutes after LH-RH or saline administration. In order to diminish the aleatory errors between different experimental assays, the anti-LH/FSH-RH were calculated as a percentage of inhibition (% inhib.) of gonadotropin release using the following mathematical approach:

$$\% \text{ inhib.} = \frac{100\ [(E{-}C)(E{-}Ea) + (Ea{-}C)(Ca{-}C)]}{(E{-}C)^2}$$

Each letter represents the plasma value of gonadotropins of different experimental groups: E = LH-RH + vehicle; Ea = analog + LH-RH; Ca = analog + saline; and C = vehicle + saline. Moreover, intrinsic LH/FSH-RH activity (IA) of the inhibitory analogs was determined by the following method: IA = $100\ (Ca{-}C)/(E{-}C)$.

c. *Inhibition of LH and FSH Response to LH-RH in Chimpanzees.* This inhibition can be measured in a similar fashion (Gosselin et al., 1979). LH-RH antagonists greatly inhibit the LH-RH-induced LH response in chimpanzees.

d. *Induction of Ovulation by Stimulatory Analogs*

i. *In Proestrus Rats Blocked with Pentobarbital.* Vaginal smears were checked every morning as described by Everett (1974), and only rats exhibiting at least two consecutive 4-day estrous cycles were selected. On the day of proestrus, the rats were anesthetized with an i.p. injection of 3.5 mg of pentobarbital (Nembutal)/100 gm body weight at 12:30 PM and analogs were injected s.c. at 2 PM. Animals were killed the next morning and the oviducts were examined for the presence of ova. Rats treated with phenobarbital or fluophenazine can also be used for this test (Banik and Givner, 1977).

ii. *In Diestrus Rats (Vilchez-Martinez et al., 1974b; Rippel et al., 1975).* Four-day cycling rats were used, and the analog was injected i.v. or s.c. at 2 PM on the second day of diestrus. On the following day, the oviduct was inspected. Androgen-sterilized diestrus rats can also be used (Dutta *et al.*, 1978).

iii. *Golden Hamsters Blocked with Phenobarbital.* The animals are examined every morning for a vaginal discharge, and only animals exhibiting at least two consecutive 4-day estrous cycles are used. At 12:30–1 PM on the day of proestrus, the hamsters were injected s.c. with 13 mg of phenobarbital/100 gm body weight to block the spontaneous ovulation. Analogs are administered s.c. This preparation is very sensitive, 75 ng LH-RH being the minimal effective dose for inducing full ovulation. The animals were killed the next morning, and their oviducts were inspected for the presence of ova (Arimura *et al.*, 1971).

e. *Blockade of Ovulation by Inhibitory Analogs*

i. *In Proestrous Rats.* Antiovulatory tests can be performed with adult female Charles River CD rats that weigh approximately 200 gm. They are kept under controlled temperature and light conditions. Daily vaginal smears are taken starting 14 days after arrival, and only rats that show at least two successive regular 4-day cycles are used. Analogs dissolved in propylene glycol/saline solution or corn oil are injected s.c. usually at 12 noon on the proestrus day. Control groups are injected with vehicle alone. On the following morning, the oviducts of the animals are inspected for ova under a dissecting microscope (de la Cruz *et al.*, 1976b; Vilchez-Martinez *et al.*, 1976a; Corbin and Beattie, 1975a,b). The results obtained from antiovulatory tests can be expressed by binomial data, using 1 for ovulation and 0 for no ovulation; they can be subjected to analysis of variance and then compared by Duncan's new multiple range test. However, the most convenient way to express their potency is to compare the percentage of blockade of ovulation in response to a certain dose of inhibitory analog. We have observed a good correlation between the activity of LH-RH analogs in inhibiting the gonadotropin release induced by LH-RH in immature male rats and their ability to block ovulation (Pedroza *et al.*, 1978).

ii. *In Golden Hamsters.* Only the animals exhibiting at least two consecutive 4-day estrous cycles are used (see Section B,2,d,iii). At 12:30 PM on the day of proestrus, hamsters are injected s.c. with phenobarbital. LH-RH analogs are injected s.c. at various times before s.c. injection of 75 ng of LH-RH (Nishi *et al.*, 1976b). However, this method is less convenient than the blockade of ovulation in rats, since the hamsters are more difficult to block with inhibitory analogs (de la Cruz *et al.*, 1976a).

iii. *Inhibition of Ovulation Caused by Mating or Induced by LH-RH in Rabbits.* Mature female rabbits are used. Inhibitory analogs can be injected 3–5 times at half-hour intervals beginning 30 minutes prior to mating or administration of 500 ng/kg of synthetic LH-RH. Reduction in plasma LH levels and blockade of ovulation are measured (Phelps *et al.*, 1977).

3. *Binding Affinity—Receptor Assay for LH-RH and Analogs*

Binding affinity to pituitary receptor sites for most analogs seems to be closely related to their ability to trigger gonadotropin release. Since the mechanism of action of LH-RH involves interaction with pituitary plasma membrane receptors, an *in vitro* assay, in which highly purified pituitary cell membrane preparations are used, was also developed in our laboratory (Pedroza *et al.*, 1977a,b). We have determined that the number of binding sites for LH-RH is approximately 2.36 pmol per milligram of protein with a high affinity constant of 7.1 $\times$ 10^9 M^{-1}.

4. *Radioimmunoassay for LH-RH*

A considerable number of RIA for LH-RH have been reported (Arimura *et al.*, 1973; Nett *et al.*, 1973; Koch *et al.*, 1973a; Jonas *et al.*, 1975). Details of the methods are described elsewhere (Arimura *et al.*, 1973; Nett *et al.*, 1973; Arimura and Schally, 1980).

Although the RIA methods are specific, they detect various analogs to different degrees depending on the antibody used. The recognition sites vary from one antibody to another.

C. Relationship between Structure and Biological Activity of LH-RH

It is beyond the scope of this article to review in detail the role of the amino acids residues in the LH-RH molecule and all the studies which have contributed to the present state of knowledge of the relationship between structure and biological activity of LH-RH. This topic was the subject of several of our previous reviews (Coy and Schally, 1978; Coy *et al.*, 1979; Schally and Coy, 1977; Schally *et al.*, 1976, 1978). It may suffice to reemphasize the amino-terminal tripeptide and tetrapeptide fragments of LH-RH as well as the carboxyl-terminal nonapeptide and octapeptide of LH-RH have very little or no LH-RH activity (Schally *et al.*, 1972a). This indicates that very active small fragments cannot be obtained from LH-RH. In contrast to early reports, the tetrapeptide pyroGlu-Tyr-Arg-Trp-NH$_2$, which is not part of the LH-RH sequence, has only one part in 12,000 of the activity of the LH-RH decapeptide and an equivalent FSH-RH activity. No dissociation of LH-RH activity from that of FSH-RH has been found for any LH-RH analog.

Certain amino acids can be replaced in the LH-RH molecule without a major loss of activity. For instance, tyrosine in position 5 can be replaced by phenylalanine or by closely related amino acids with aromatic side chains (Coy *et al.*, 1973a,b). Leucine in position 7 may be substituted by valine, isoleucine, or norleucine (Fujino *et al.*, 1972a). Replacement of serine in the 4 position by threonine or by alanine results in molecules with 20% and 5% of LH-RH activity, respectively (Coy *et al.*, 1973b; Geiger *et al.*, 1972). Analogs with lysine, ornithine, or homoarginine in position 8 in place of arginine possess 7.6%, 5.5%, and 21.7% of LH-RH activity, respectively (Geiger *et al.*, 1974). Few analogs have been synthesized in which proline in position 9 was replaced, but the low activity of Ala^9-LH-RH (Coy *et al.*, 1973b) indicates that proline exerts important conformational effects on that part of the peptide chain (Coy *et al.*, 1975a).

Many modifications including substitutions of proline, leucine, glycine, or orotic acid (Yanaihara *et al.*, 1973a) for the pyroglutamic acid residue result in almost complete loss of activity. The fact that Glu^1-LH-RH has 6% activity can be explained by partial cyclization to pyroglutamic acid under physiological conditions (Yanaihara *et al.*, 1973a); D-pyroGlu^1-LH-RH has 8% LH-RH activity (Hirotsu *et al.*, 1974). Some acylated glycine analogs have higher activity. Formyl-sarcosine^1-LH-RH has 64% activity, and acetyl-sarcosine^1-LH-RH has 72% activity. Incorporation of 2-pyrrolidone-4-carboxylic acid, which is an isomer of pyroGlu, or its N-methyl analog into LH-RH in place of pyroglutamic acid gives rise to compounds with 19% and 58% LH-RH activity, respectively (Nikolics *et al.*, 1977).

These extensive structure–activity studies (Nikolics *et al.*, 1977) on pyroglutamic acid in position 1 led us to suggest that the maintenance of biological activity was dependent on hydrogen bonding between the pyrrolidone carboxyl group and the glycine amide NH$_2$ group at position 10. The close proximity of the N and C termini of LH-RH appears to be confirmed by the significant activities (0.5–1.5%) of ring analogs such as cyclic-[β-Ala^1,D-Ala^6, Gly^{10}]-LH-RH that have been made from inactive linear precursors (Seprodi *et al.*, 1978a). In addition, although D-Ala^{10}-LH-RH has less than 0.01% of gonadotropin-releasing activity of LH-RH, the D-Ala^{10}-analogs of several typical LH-RH antagonists have essentially unchanged inhibitory effects. This again suggests a complex conformational interaction between the ends of the peptide chain.

In conclusion, amino acids in positions 1 and 4 to 10 may be involved only in binding to the receptors and/or in exerting conformational effects. However, histidine and tryptophan could exert a functional effect in addition to providing receptor-binding capacity, since simple substitutions or deletions in positions 2 or 3 greatly decrease or abolish LH-RH activity and yet still maintain binding affinity in some antagonist compounds. Indeed, the His-Trp sequence may constitute an "active center" in LH-RH. Thus, the imidazole group of histidine in position 2 possesses features, such as aromaticity, acid-base character, and hydrogen bonding capacity, that render it necessary for expression of activity; and replacement or deletion of histidine virtually eliminates agonist activity. The low potencies (0.01–0.03%) of Ser^2-, Arg^2-, Leu^2-, and Gln^2-LH-RH (Arnold et $al.$, 1974; Yanaihara et $al.$, 1973a,b) as compared to 2–40%, respectively, of Phe^2-LH-RH and Trp^2-LH-RH indicated the need for aromaticity in position 2. Some structures related to L-histidine that possess acid-base properties and hydrogen donor and acceptor capability have considerable LH-RH activity. Among them are 1-N-imidazolemethyl-His^2-LH-RH (6% activity) (Rivier et $al.$, 1972), (β-pyrazolyl-3-Ala)^2-LH-RH (19% activity) (Coy et $al.$, 1974a) and (β-pyrazolyl-l-Ala)^2-LH-RH (1% activity) (Coy et $al.$, 1975c).

Similarly, the deletion or replacement of tryptophan in position 3 by nonaromatic amino acids also results in nearly complete loss of activity. This crucial role of Trp may be linked in some way to the electron-donating capacity of the indole nucleus of tryptophan. Thus, Leu^3-LH-RH and Ala^3-LH-RH are virtually inactive (Yanaihara et $al.$, 1973b), but Tyr^3-LH-RH and Phe^3-LH-RH (Coy et $al.$, 1973b; Yanaihara et $al.$, 1973b) have a low but definite potency (0.1% to 0.4%). Also, pentamethylphenylalanine^3-LH-RH possesses high LH-RH activity, probably because of its electron-transfer capability (Coy et $al.$, 1974c). D-Trp^3-LH-RH has only 0.1% activity (Hirotsu et $al.$, 1974), indicating that the conformation in position 3 is important. The replacement of the hydrogen atom in position 5 of the tryptophan ring, as in 5-fluoro-Trp^3-LH-RH, lowers the LH-RH activity to 6% (Coy et $al.$, 1974c), possibly because of a reduction in the electron density of the aromatic ring. Thus, most alterations in the 2 and/or 3 position(s) of LH-RH destroy the gonadotropin-releasing mechanism, while preserving or increasing the binding affinity of the molecule. The functional character of histidine and tryptophan in positions 2 and 3 of LH-RH was further inferred by synthesis of many inhibitors of LH-RH with changes in these positions (see Section IV).

D. SUPERACTIVE ANALOGS OF LH-RH

The C-terminal residue of LH-RH can be altered in various ways without too much loss of activity (Fujino et al., 1973b). For instance, Ala^{10}-LH-RH and the $desGly^{10}$-analog of LH-RH have about 10% LH-RH activity (Fujino et al., 1972a). Fujino et al. (1972a, 1973b) were the first to report that replacement of glycinamide by ethylamide or propylamide groups produces analogs more active than LH-RH. Thus, $desGly^{10}$-LH-RH ethylamide is 3–5 times more potent than LH-RH, and its activity is also prolonged (Arimura et al., 1974d; Fujino et al., 1972b). Analogs with glycinamide groups substituted by other alkylamides also have considerable LH-RH activities. Among these analogs are the methylamide (100% activity), ethanolamide (150% activity), pyrrolidinamide (80% activity) (Fujino et al., 1972b), allylamide (170% activity), and propargylamide (47% activity) (Coy et al., 1975b), and isopropylamide (100% to 283% activity) (Fujino et al., 1973a). $DesGly^{10}$-LH-RH 2-chloroethylamide is equipotent with LH-RH, and $desGly^{10}$-LH-RH 2,2,2-trifluoroethylamide is 5–9 times as active as LH-RH (Coy et al., 1975e). The increased activity of these analogs could be due to better binding conformation at the C terminus and/or to a decreased rate of enzymic breakdown.

Replacement of glycine in the 6 position of LH-RH can also lead to an increase in biological activity. Monahan et al. (1973) were the first to report that $D-Ala^6$-LH-RH was much more active than LH-RH. The potency of this analog was estimated to be 6–7 times greater than that of LH-RH (Coy et al., 1974b; Monahan et al., 1973), a phenomenon attributed to better binding conformation than in LH-RH. We synthesized $D-Leu^6$-LH-RH, which was 5–9 times more active than LH-RH (Vilchez-Martinez et al., 1974a), and later other analogs with D-amino acid substitutions in position 6. The activities of the D-6-amino acid analogs appear to increase with the size of the side chain. The most active were $D-Phe^6$-LH-RH and $D-Trp^6$-LH-RH, which were 10 and 13 times more potent in vivo, respectively, than LH-RH, and which showed prolonged activity (Coy et al., 1976c). In vitro, in monolayer cultures of rat pituitary cells, these two analogs were 90 and 100 times more potent than LH-RH, respectively (Coy et al., 1975d, 1976c). The latest clinical results also indicate that the potency of $D-Trp^6$-LH-RH in humans is 50–100 times greater than that of LH-RH.

The incorporation of both changes, i.e., ethylamide (EA) in the 10 position and a D-amino acid in the 6 position, produces analogs 30–100 times more potent than LH-RH, and they cause prolonged release of LH and FSH (Arimura et al., 1974c; Coy et al., 1974d; Fujino et al., 1974a,b; Vilchez-Martinez et al., 1974a). D-Ala⁶, desGly¹⁰-LH-RH EA (Fig. 2), and D-Leu⁶, desGly¹⁰-LH-RH EA (Fig. 3) released 50–60 times as much LH and 15 times as much FSH as did similar doses of LH-RH when administerd to immature male rats. The integrated levels of gonadotropins over a 6-hour period were used for the comparisons (Arimura et al., 1974c; Vilchez-Martinez et al., 1974a). The ovulatory activity of these compounds in rats is also 50–80 times greater than that of LH-RH (Fujino et al., 1974a,b). D-Ala⁶,-desGly¹⁰-LH-RH EA also caused prolonged release of LH and FSH (6–10 hours) in rats when administered orally and intravaginally (de la Cruz et al., 1975c). How ever, the doses needed for oral administration were about 1000 times, and for the intravaginal 100 times, larger than those causing comparable elevation by the subcutaneous route. Rectal absorption is about 0.25%; and intranasal, approximately 1% in rats. In vitro, LH- and FSH-releasing activities of D-Leu⁶, desGly¹⁰-LH-RH EA determined using anterior pituitary cells in monolayer cultures were both 30 times higher than those of LH-RH.

D-Ser-(Buᵗ)⁶-LH-RH EA (H766) (Fig. 4) was reported (König et al., 1975; Sandow et al., 1978b) also to be 50–100 times more potent than LH-RH. Fragments containing residues 3–9, 4–9, or even 5–9 of this analog were recently reported to retain a small degree of ovulatory activity (Sandow and König, 1979). This is in contrast to His- or Trp-lacking C-terminal fragments of LH-RH, which are devoid of activity (Schally et al., 1972a).

In conclusion, the changes in the 6 and 10 positions reinforce each other and produce superactive, long-acting analogs. These superactive analogs of LH-RH are active when administered i.v., s.c., i.m., orally, intravaginally, intranasally, or rectally in rats (de la Cruz et al., 1975c; Sandow et al., 1978b; Schally et al., 1976).

Antisera against LH-RH do not cross-react with the potent, long-acting analogs of LH-RH. In rats immunized against LH-RH, gonadotropin levels decreased and gonadal atrophy ensued (Sandow et al., 1978b). However, the injection of D-Ser-(Buᵗ)⁶-LH-RH EA returned

$$\text{pGlu-His-Trp-Ser-Tyr-D-Ala-Leu-Arg-Pro-NH-CH}_2\text{-CH}_3$$

FIG. 2. The molecular structure of D-Ala⁶-LH-RH ethylamide.

pGlu-His-Trp-Ser-Tyr-D-Leu-Leu-Arg-Pro-NH-CH$_2$-CH$_3$

FIG. 3. The molecular structure of D-Leu⁶-LH-RH ethylamide.

plasma gonadotropins to normal levels and reversed gonadal atrophy. This indicated another therapeutic potential of these analogs in the case of antibody formation after prolonged treatment with LH-RH (Sandow *et al.*, 1978b).

Contrary to initial predictions, the ethylamide analogs of D-Phe⁶- and [D-Trp⁶]-LH-RH, which are more active than D-Ala⁶- and D-Leu⁶-LH-RH, have only about the same activity as the parent peptides *in vivo*. This also strongly indicates that the position 6 and 10 modifications are contributing in varying degrees to similar favorable conformational changes in the decapeptide. Unfortunately, it seems that once the ideal situation has been achieved, no further improvement is possible utilizing these types of changes. Thus, as another example, the trifluoroethylamide analog of D-Leu⁶-LH-RH has identical *in vivo* gonadotropin-releasing activity (Coy *et al.*, 1975e) as the ethylamide analog, despite desGly-NH$_2$¹⁰-LH-RH trifluoroethylamide being at least twice as active as desGly-NH$_2$¹⁰-LH-RH ethylamide. The increase in biological activity of the superactive LH-RH analogs with substitutions in positions 6 and 10 can probably be attributed to better and more prolonged binding to the pituitary receptors, a slower inactivation (Benuck and Marks, 1976; Koch *et al.*, 1977; Marks and Stern, 1974), or a combination of both factors (Monahan *et al.*, 1973; Schally *et al.*, 1976; Vale *et al.*, 1977). It was reported that analogs substituted in position 6 and 10 are less readily broken by peptidases in rat serum and pituitary or hypothalamic homogenates (Benuck and Marks, 1976; Koch *et al.*, 1977; Marks and Stern, 1974). However, the finding that the magnitude and time of binding of monoiodinated D-Ala⁶- and D-Leu⁶, desGly¹⁰-LH-RH EA, and other analogs to the pituitary tissue are much greater than for LH-RH may explain the prolonged activity of these analogs better than decreased inactivation (Reeves *et al.*, 1977). We have also observed (Pedroza *et al.*, 1977a) that the agonist

(Bu^t)
|
PYRO - GLU - HIS - TRP - SER - TYR - D-SER - LEU - ARG - PRO - NH-CH$_2$-CH$_3$

   1   2   3   4   5   6   7   8   9

FIG. 4. The molecular structure of D-Ser (Bu^t)⁶-LH-RH EA (HOE 766).

D-Trp[6]-LH-RH, competes with LH-RH for its pituitary plasma membrane receptors, displacing the ^{125}I-labeled LH-RH more strongly than its parent hormone. Therefore, both stimulatory analogs of LH-RH apparently exert their action through the same pituitary plasma membrane receptors as those of LH-RH.

E. CLINICAL STUDIES WITH LH-RH AND ITS AGONISTIC SUPERACTIVE LONG-ACTING ANALOGS AIMED AT FERTILITY STIMULATION

Because this article is devoted to contraception rather than stimulation of fertility, a detailed description of the clinical studies with LH-RH and its analogs aimed at treatment of infertility in men and women would be beyond its scope. However, a brief synopsis of these studies is given below in view of a subsequent section on clinical studies utilizing paradoxical antifertility effects of LH-RH and its stimulatory LH-RH analogs for the development of new contraceptive approaches.

LH-RH has been used therapeutically, particularly for inducing ovulation in women (Nillius and Wide, 1975; Potashnik *et al.*, 1978; Zañartu *et al.*, 1974; Zarate *et al.*, 1974), for treating hypogonadism and oligospermia in men (Aparicio *et al.*, 1976; Mortimer *et al.*, 1974; Schwarzstein *et al.*, 1975) and cryptorchidism in boys (Happ *et al.*, 1978a; Illig *et al.*, 1977).

Long-acting superactive analogs of LH-RII, particularly D-Phe[6]-LH-RH and D-Trp[6]-LH-RH, D-Ala[6]-LH-RH ethylamide (EA), D-Leu[6]-LH-RH EA, and D-Ser(Bu[t])[6]-LH-RH EA, which are 50–100 times more potent than LH-RH and other analogs, were also used in clinical studies. It was shown that D-Ala[6]-LH-RH EA and D-Leu[6]-LH-RH EA given systemically raise LH and FSH levels in the blood in men and women for as long as 24 hours (de Medeiros-Comaru *et al.*, 1976; Soria *et al.*, 1975; Wass *et al.*, 1979).

Normal men respond even to oral administration to 10 mg of D-Leu[6]-LH-RH EA with an elevation of plasma LH and FSH levels (Gonzalez-Barcena *et al.*, 1975). However, the doses required for oral administration are more than 1000 times larger than those that are active i.v. This analog also was tested in normal men by intranasal application and proved to be active (Gonzalez-Barcena *et al.*, 1976; Happ *et al.*, 1978c). Intranasal therapy of cryptorchidism with D-Leu[6]-LH-RH EA in prepubertal cryptorchid boys for 5–12 weeks caused a complete testicular descent in 4 of the 11 boys (Happ *et al.*, 1978b).

In normal women, D-Leu[6]-LH-RH EA was also very effective when given intravaginally in doses of 2 mg in the form of Carbowax suppositories, as well as when given rectally (Saito *et al.*, 1977). After intravaginal administration of D-Leu[6]-LH-RH EA, plasma estrogen remained elevated at both 24 and 48 hours. Repeated administration of large doses of D-Ala[6]-LH-RH EA reestablished normal menstrual cycles in three out of seven women with secondary amenorrhea, and the cycles still continue more than 3 years after the treatment (de Medeiros-Comaru *et al.*, 1976).

Attempts have been made by Zañartu *et al.* (1975) to program ovulation in normal women by treatment with estrogen and D-Leu[6]-LH-RH EA. When a single injection of 0.5–0.8 mg of this analog was administered on day 13 of the cycle to normal women pretreated with 50 μg of ethynylestradiol, signs of recent ovulation were observed on day 15 or 16 in 22 out of 24 treated subjects (91%). In the control group only 55% of the women ovulated on day 15 or 16. This regimen may possibly be useful for obtaining pregnancy in ovulatory women in whom artificial insemination by donor is indicated.

For the past 3 years we have been studying the clinical effect of D-Trp[6]-LH-RH in men and women. Given i.v., s.c., or i.m. in England, Mexico, Spain, and Brazil, it raised serum LH, FSH, testosterone, and 17β-estradiol levels for a period of at least 6 hours (Jaramillo-Jaramillo *et al.*, 1977, 1978a; Wass *et al.*, 1979). When administered intranasally in doses of 500 μg, it elevated plasma LH and FSH levels for up to 24 hours, but the 500 μg doses of LH-RH were not effective (Wass *et al.*, 1979). The intranasal activity of LH-RH analogs increased the probability of their therapeutic usefulness.

Treatment with D-Trp[6]-LH-RH was reported to induce a relatively high percentage of ovulations and pregnancies in women previously treated unsuccessfully with human menopausal gonadotropin (HMG) or clomiphene (Jaramillo-Jaramillo *et al.*, 1978b). In other recent studies by Zañartu *et al.* (1979) in women with hypothalamic–pituitary dysfunction, 70% ovulated after combined treatment with D-Trp[6]-LH-RH and α-bromoergocryptine (C.B. 154) and about 40% became pregnant.

Treatment of men with hypogonadotropic hypogonadism with 10 μg of D-Trp[6]-LH-RH per day for 90 days resulted in great improvements in their condition (Jaramillo-Jaramillo *et al.*, 1978c). Preliminary results also indicate that administration of small doses (2–5 μg) of D-Trp[6]-LH-RH every day or every other day can lead to increases in sperm counts in oligospermics (Guitelman *et al.*, 1980), by analogy to similar studies carried out previously with LH-RH (Aparicio *et al.*, 1976; Schwarzstein *et al.*, 1975).

D-Ser(Bu^t)^6-LH-RH EA (H766) also was found to be a potent stimulant of the release of LH and FSH in men (Happ *et al.*, 1978c; Wiegelmann *et al.*, 1976), normally cycling women (Dericks-Tan *et al.*, 1977; Friedrich *et al.*, 1978), and in amenorrheic women (Hanker *et al.*, 1978; Nillius and Wide, 1977). This analog can be administered in the form of a nasal spray and has been used for treatment of women with secondary amenorrhea and for induction of ovulation (Katzorke *et al.*, 1980). Thus, it was reported recently that prolonged intranasal treatment of amenorrheic women with D-Ser(Bu^t)^6-LH-RH EA in doses of 87–174 µg/day reestablished normal cycles in 7 out of 10 women (Katzorke *et al.*, 1980). Increases in secretion of sex steroids also were reported in both women and men in response to D-Ser(Bu^t)^6-LH-RH EA.

The finding that a single administration of superative analogs causes prolonged elevation of serum LH and FSH in humans should permit the design of suitable regimens for induction of ovulation in amenorrheic women and more convenient treatment of male infertility. Moreover, except for one report of secondary drug failure because of antibody formation in one hypogonadal patient treated for more than 1 year with LH-RH (Brown *et al.*, 1977; Van Loon and Brown, 1975), no side effects of treatment with LH-RH or analogs have been detected.

However, in spite of some positive results (Jaramillo-Jaramillo *et al.*, 1978c; Zañartu *et al.*, 1979), the overall degree of success in clinical therapy with the long-acting analogs in other studies was low (Canales *et al.*, 1980a; Forsbach *et al.*, 1976), perhaps because of the largely empirical regimens and also because our current knowledge of how to use these hormones in therapy of infertility is inadequate. Suitable regimens that can consistently give a high percentage of clinical response have not yet been devised. A successful long-term therapy in humans will require standardization of optimal doses and time of administration.

In view of paradoxical antifertility effects of relatively large pharmacological doses of LH-RH and its long-acting superactive analogs, the doses of analogs administered parenterally should be limited to 2–40 µg/day. Development of suitable clinical regimens for parenteral and intranasal administration may lead to increasingly successful use of long-acting superactive analogs for induction of follicular maturation and ovulation, for treatment of hypogonadotropic hypogonadism and oligospermia, and in pediatric endocrinology.

F. Paradoxical Antifertility Effects of Large Doses of LH-RH and Its Long-Acting Superactive Analogs in Animals

1. *Introduction*

A delicate qualitative and quantitative interplay between hypothalamus, pituitary, and ovary, LH, FSH, ovarian steroids, and in some species prolactin, is essential for follicular maturation, ovulation, implantation, nidation, and maintenance of gestation. Many agents, including the hormones themselves, if administered at an inappropriate time, could interfere with these mechanisms and would thus be expected to produce antifertility effects. Thus, exogenous LH or hCG were found to induce regression of corpora lutea in rabbits (Keyes and Nalbandov, 1968; Spies *et al.*, 1966). A similar luteolytic effect of exogenous LH in pseudopregnant rats was reported by Rothchild and Schwartz (1965) and MacDonald *et al.* (1970). Interference with pregnancy in rats and hamsters by administration of PMS or hCG was reported by Yang and Chang (1968) and by Banik (1975). Banik (1974) further claimed that hCG and PMS could be used for inducing menses or early abortion in monkeys and human beings if administered between 14 and 35 days of gestation. These antifertility effects were ascribed to alterations in production of ovarian steroids.

Later, Hsueh *et al.* (1976, 1977) reported marked loss of LH receptors and steroidogenic response to gonadotropins in the rat after daily injections of LH or hCG. This ability of gonadotropins to induce loss of their own receptors appears to be analogous to the effect of insulin, TRH, GH, and other hormones on the levels of their own receptors in the respective target tissues.

A variety of recent studies demonstrated antifertility effects of large pharmacological doses of LH-RH and some long-acting, superactive stimulatory analogs of LH-RH. Prolonged treatment with these compounds causes impairment of reproductive functions. These effects initially have been termed paradoxical, because LH-RH and its analogs were considered strictly to be profertility hormones. However, these properties may be more correctly defined as contraceptive or antifertility effects, and they encompass a variety of actions, which are described below.

2. *Effects in Female Animals*

a. Precoital Contraceptive and Other Effects. Banik and Givner (1975) were the first to report that advancement of ovulation in diestrous rats by administration of 10–80 ng D-Ala^6-LH-RH EA interfered with the mating behavior and pregnancy during the treatment cycle. The antifertility effect disappeared during the following cycle.

In a subsequent study, Banik and Givner (1976) showed that rhythmic administration of 20–120 ng doses of D-Ala[6]-LH-RH EA every third day starting in the afternoon of diestrus to 4-day cyclic rats will interfere with mating and fertility for a period of approximately four cycles, when the females were allowed constant cohabitation with fertile males, except for 24 hours after treatment. It was presumed that the antifertility effect of this analog was achieved through its capacity to induce ovulation at a physiologically "wrong time" (i.e., 1 day before the expected day of proestrus). They suggested that analogs of LH-RH could be potentially useful for a more reliable rhythm method of birth control in humans, by timing ovulation and narrowing the fertile period of the cycle.

Recently, Banik and Givner (1980) also have shown that the synthetic LH-RH, D-Ala[6]-LH-RH EA, and D-Trp[6]-LH-RH are effective in enhancing ovulation, mating behavior, and pregnancy in rats and mice if administered i.m. at a "*physiologically right time*," i.e., when the follicles are nearly or fully mature. On the basis of their experimental evidence, they suggested that these preparations could be useful either for enhancing or controlling fertility in animals and humans by timely inducing ovulation and allowing or precluding insemination.

Parallel or subsequent studies with other analogs or LH-RH itself extended these findings. Johnson *et al.* (1976) reported that in mature rats given 1–10 μg/day of D-Leu[6]-LH-RH EA twice daily for 32–77 days there was a reduction of ovarian and uterine weight and cessation of cycling. Termination of treatment was followed by prompt restoration of normal ovarian weight and function. Prolonged treatment (30 days) of female rats with 50 ng/day of D-Ser(Bu[t])[6]-LH-RH EA caused a reduction of uterine weight and an increase in progesterone, but there was a decrease in estrogen production (Sandow *et al.*, 1978b).

When a series of LH-RH analogs containing an AzGly[10] modification (e.g., D-Ser(Bu[t])[6]-AzGly[10]-LH-RH or D-Phe[6], AzGly[10]-LH-RH) and having potent agonist properties were given in high concentration, 0.5 and 5.0 μg/rat twice daily to intact female rats, plasma LH and FSH were raised to extremely high levels after administration of the compounds for 14 days, but plasma estradiol concentrations were reduced to those in ovariectomized rats. The weights of the ovary and uterus were also markedly reduced (Maynard and Nicholson, 1979).

LH-RH itself, administered precoitally to "Nembutalized" rats (anesthetized with pentobarbital), but not to unblocked rats, in a dose of 10 μg, produced a 50% reduction in the pregnancy rate and a 38%

decrease in the number of viable pups delivered (Corbin *et al.*, 1978a). Chronic precoital injections of LH-RH (100 μg) for 7 days also caused a contraceptive effect and inhibited pregnancy (Beattie and Corbin, 1977).

The mechanism of this action was studied by various investigators. The possibility of a direct effect of LH-RH on the ovary was first suggested by Neves-e-Castro *et al.* (1974) and Neves-e-Castro and Reis-Valle (1975). Rippel and Johnson (1976b) were the first to observe that hypophysectomy did not alter the inhibitory effect of LH-RH on the ovarian weight gain caused by hCG (see also next section). Concomitant treatment of hypophysectomized female rats with FSH and D-Leu[6], (N^{α}-Me)Leu[7]-LH-RH or D-Trp[6]-LH-RH EA suppressed the FSH-induced increase in ovarian weight and in ovarian aromatase. Granulosa cells havested from hypophysectomized rats treated with LH-RH analogs produced a significantly smaller amount of estrogen than did the cells from rats treated with FSH alone (Hsueh and Erickson, 1979a). Ying and Guillemin (1979) reported that treatment with D-Trp[6]-LH-RH EA inhibited follicular development induced by PMS in hypophysectomized rats.

Kledzik *et al.* (1978b) demonstrated that, in cycling female rats, administration of D-Ala[6]-LH-RH EA on diestrus day 1, in doses as low as 8 ng, caused a marked reduction in ovarian LH-hCG receptors lasting for 3 days in the case of a 25-μg dose. This was not related to the occupancy of binding sites by LH, since LH levels returned to normal in 12 hours. FSH receptors, uterine weight, and plasma progesterone were also reduced. These results are in agreement with our own studies, which showed that treatment with D-Trp[6]-LH-RH also decreased LH/hCG binding sites in ovaries of normal as well as hypophysectomized female rats (Arimura *et al.*, 1979a, 1980). Immature female rats were primed with PMS, followed by hCG. Half of the animals were hypophysectomized on the next day of hCG injection. Saline or 0.2-μg doses of D-Trp[6]-LH-RH were injected s.c. to these rats daily for 7 days starting on the day of hypophysectomy. All rats were sacrificed by decapitation 24 hours after the last injection. Ovaries were excised, and their LH/hCG receptors were measured by incubating ovarian tissue and ^{125}I-hCG for 16–20 hours at room temperature. Daily injection of 2 μg of D-Trp[6]-LH-RH caused a significant reduction of ovarian LH/hCG receptors in both intact and hypophysectomized rats. Greater depletion was seen with 2 μg than with 0.2 μg of the analog. Serum LH and FSH levels in hypophysectomized rats were barely detectable and were not altered by injection of the LH-RH agonist. The extent of reduction of ovarian LH/hCG receptors by D-

Trp⁶-LH-RH in hypophysectomized rats was comparable to that observed in normal rats. These results suggest that the reduction of ovarian LH/hCG receptors can be accounted for by some other mechanism than "down regulation" and are in agreement with the data of Hsueh and Erickson (1979a) and other investigators, suggesting some direct effect of superactive LH-RH directly on the ovary.

b. *Studies in Immature and Pubertal Rats.* Johnson *et al.* (1976) reported that inhibition of ovarian and uterine weight increases in immature rats within 3 days when doses of 0.5 to 3 μg/day of D-Leu⁶-LH-RH EA were given for 55 days starting on day 22 of age. Chronic administration of this analog also caused delay of vaginal opening and absence of normal cyclicity. LH and FSH responses of immature rats to this analog decreased after day 1, but gonadotropin levels still remained elevated throughout treatment with the analog as compared with controls. Cessation of treatment led to restoration of normal ovarian function.

D-Ala⁶-LH-RH also delayed puberty (i.e., vaginal canalization) and retarded the growth of the ovaries, uteri, and anterior pituitary glands (Corbin *et al.*, 1978a). This delay of puberty in immature rats was in agreement with antifertility effects seen in adult animals.

Various other studies have explored these effects in greater detail. D-Leu⁶-LH-RH EA given in doses of 0.2–5 μg for 3 days also inhibited the ovarian and uterine weight augmentation in immature intact or hypophysectomized rats induced by 50–500 U of human chorionic gonadotropin (hCG) (Rippel and Johnson, 1976b). Clear dose-response inhibition of hCG was obtained. Other LH-RH analogs also had inhibitory effects in proportion to their LH- and FSH-releasing activity. The data were said to constitute the first evidence for direct inhibitory effects of superactive analogs of LH-RH on the ovary and uterus. Subsequent investigations provided data in support of this hypothesis. Mayer *et al.* (1979) reported inhibition of the uterine or ovarian growth of intact or hypophysectomized rats by treatment with D-Leu⁶-LH-RH EA (5 μg/day for 3 days) alone or in combination with hCG. The uptake of ¹³¹I-labeled D-Leu⁶-LH-RH EA observed in the pituitary gland and ovary was inhibited by the treatment with unlabeled analog. This study also indicates that the superactive analogs may act directly on the ovary.

Our own studies with D-Trp⁶-LH-RH (Vilchez-Martinez *et al.*, 1979) extended these findings. Treatment of immature female rats 30 days old with 1 μg/day of D-Trp⁶-LH-RH for 10 days decreased the uterine weight, elevated serum gonadotropins, and lowered pituitary LH as well as the responsiveness to LH-RH. The body weight and the pituitary weight were not changed, but ovarian weight was increased. A delay of vaginal opening was also observed. A dose of 50 ng/day produced few changes. A decrease in the specific uptake of [^{125}I]LH-RH indicated that D-Trp^6-LH-RH competes with LH-RH for binding to the pituitary receptor sites for LH-RH. Serum estradiol was not modified, suggesting that the effect in uterine weight was extrapituitary. D-Trp^6-LH-RH at a dose of 1 μg also decreased the uterine binding sites for estradiol on days 38 and 42 of age. Since a similar effect was also observed in hypophysectomized, oophorectomized animals treated with D-Trp^6-LH-RH, this offers the proof for a direct effect of D-Trp^6-LH-RH on the uterus (Vilchez-Martinez and Pedroza, 1978).

c. Postcoital Contraceptive and Other Effects. Corbin and his collaborators (Corbin and Beattie, 1975b; Corbin *et al.*, 1976, 1977; Beattie *et al.*, 1977; Beattie and Corbin, 1977) were the first to report that LH-RH and its analogs interfered with pregnancy. A dose of 1000 μg given on days 1 to 7 or 7 to 12 terminated 100% of the pregnancies in rats. A dose of 1000 μg/kg in rabbits also terminated 80% of the pregnancies. Even smaller doses of LH-RH (200 μg) given daily over days 1 to 7 were sufficient to inhibit pregnancy. A 48-hour delay in the preimplantation rise in E$_2$ and a fall in progesterone on days 3 to 7 were also noted during this treatment. They suggested that LH-RH induced the rise in serum LH that is luteolytic during early pregnancy and delayed the serum estradiol surge necessary for normal implantation. Corbin *et al.* (1976) extended these investigations to D-Ala^6-LH-RH EA and found that it also had postcoital contraceptive effects in rats and rabbits. It could terminate pregnancy in rats when injected s.c. in doses of 1–100 μg daily on days 1 to 3, 1 to 7, or 7 to 12 of pregnancy. This analog was also effective in blocking uterine implantation sites of mated rats when given by a minipump in doses of ca 6 μg/day for 4 days (Bowers and Folkers, 1976). Other analogs of the D-Ala^6 or D-Trp^6 series with or without the 9-ethylamide group also displayed a powerful postcoital contraceptive effect (Corbin *et al.*, 1978a, 1979).

The effects of LH-RH and its analogs in pregnant rats were investigated by Humphrey *et al.* (1976, 1977, 1978). They determined that pregnancy could be terminated in rats by injection of 500 μg of LH-RH twice daily on days 9, 10, or 11. This was reversed by administration of progesterone. They concluded that the postnidatory effect of LH-RH was mediated by functional luteolysis. During the prenidatory period, pregnancy was terminated in rats by doses of 150 μg twice daily from day 1 to day 7. Since estrogen normalized the effect of LH-RH treatment, the delay in nidation could be due to ovarian estrogen failure.

LH-RH EA produced similar effects and was even more potent than LH-RH in terminating pregnancy when injected in 30-μg doses over days 1 to 7 or 7 to 12 (Humphrey *et al.*, 1976).

The actual luteolytic effect of superactive analogs was first demonstrated by Rippel and Johnson (1976a), who showed that D-Leu^6-LH-RH EA in a dose of 50 μg caused regression of corpora lutea in pseudopregnant or pregnant rabbits and a fall in progesterone levels. Yoshinaga (1979) reported that the interruption of pregnancy by LH-RH and its agonists was not reproduced by continuous infusion of large doses of LH in pregnant rats. Kledzik *et al.* (1978a) demonstrated that the postcoital contraceptive activity of 25 μg of D-Ala^6-LH-RH EA was associated with an inhibition of ovarian hCG/LH and FSH receptor levels. Rivier *et al.* (1978) investigated LH-RH and one of its highly potent analogs, D-Trp^6-LH-RH EA, for their effects on pregnancy. Daily doses of the analog prevented implantation and/or caused resorption of implanted blastocysts in mated female rats. This effect was dose-related and was most evident when given in regimens including days 5 to 7 or days 9 to 10 of pregnancy. LH-RH also has antigonadal effects, but at much higher doses than the analog. Rivier *et al.* suggested that termination of pregnancy in analog- or LH-RH-treated rats is most probably due to the markedly diminished progesterone levels, which could result from secretion of biologically inactive gonadotropins, reduced pituitary responsiveness to endogenous LH-RH, or down-regulation of gonadal receptors for LH.

Our own studies with D-Trp^6-LH-RH indicate that this analog administered in doses of 6 μg/day during early pregnancy (days 1 to 5) completely prevented implantation of ova and was associated with a dramatic reduction of progesterone secretion and some reduction in estradiol. These effects were different from those of large doses of hCG, which did not affect steroid levels though they eventually terminated pregnancy (Arimura *et al.*, 1978).

3. Effects in Male Animals

Large doses of LH-RH or its analogs can also cause gonadal inhibition in male rats, golden hamsters, and dogs (Sandow *et al.*, 1978b). In male hamsters with gonadal atrophy induced by blinding, spermatogenesis was resumed after administration of 50–100 ng LH-RH daily for 4 weeks, whereas doses of 500–1000 ng severely impaired the spermatogenesis. Similar suppressive effects were observed with D-Ser(Bu^t)^6-LH-RH EA (HOE 766) (Sandow, 1976). Administration of 50–200 μg/kg of body weight of D-Ser(Bu^t)^6-LH-RH EA for 3–4 weeks to rats and dogs reduced the testosterone content of testes and caused atrophy of the testes, seminal vesicles, and prostate gland. A negative nitrogen balance also was caused by this treatment, reduction in hypothalamic LH-RH content also was seen in rats after 10 days of treatment with this analog.

In immature male rats, treatment with 50 ng/day s.c. of D-Ser(Bu^t)^6-LH-RH EA for 4 weeks decreased the weight of androgen-dependent organs (ventral prostate, seminal vesicles, and levator ani muscle), but not testicular weight. Serum and pituitary LH also were decreased and testicular testosterone content was lowered to less than 10% of the control after 4 weeks of treatment. A more physiological dose of analog, such as 5 ng/day s.c., initially increased the testosterone content, which was followed by a slight reduction after 3 weeks. Changes in testicular morphology and inhibition of spermatogenesis were observed only with 50 ng/day. This inhibition of testicular function was reversible 6 weeks after cessation of treatment. In castrated male rats treated with 50 ng/day of D-Ser(Bu^t)^6-LH-RH EA s.c. for 4 weeks plasma LH levels were reduced from days 14 to 28 and plasma FSH levels from days 21 to 28 of treatment. Pituitary LH and FSH concentrations were also decreased. The plasma prolactin levels were low on day 14 of treatment. These findings indicate a direct inhibitory effect of the analog on gonadotropin secretion in the absence of gonads (Sandow *et al.*, 1978a).

Other superactive analogs of LH-RH have similar effects. Treatment of adult male rats with 0.6–75 μg of D-Leu^6-LH-RH EA or 50 IU of human chorionic gonadotropin three times a day for 1 week caused a marked decline in LH receptors in testicular tissue (Auclair *et al.*, 1977b). Testicular weight also was significantly decreased by these treatments, whereas plasma testosterone levels were decreased by administration of the analog and increased after hCG. A single injection of 125 μg of this analog or hCG also induced a long-lasting loss of testis LH/hCG binding sites with receptor levels returning to control values at 8 days (Auclair *et al.*, 1977b). Since the amount used was thought to be high, the effect of lower doses was also studied (Auclair *et al.*, 1977a). Daily administration of as little as 8 ng of D-Leu^6-LH-RH EA three times a day for 1 week to male rats resulted in a 30% reduction of testicular LH/hCG and prolactin receptors with a maximal reduction of 80% at 40 ng. FSH receptor levels were not affected, but testosterone levels were reduced.

D-Ala^6-LH-RH EA was also studied in male rats. Pelletier *et al.* (1978) evaluated the effect of treatment with this analog injected at a dose of 100 ng, twice a week, on testicular morphology and on spermatogenesis in the rat. Significant degenerative changes of seminiferous tubules could be observed after 2 weeks of treatment. These changes were progressive and led to a marked inhibition of spermatogenesis after 4–8 weeks of treatment. Testis weight was decreased to approximately 50% of control after 8 weeks of treatment. Bex and Corbin (1978) and Corbin and Bex (1979) reported that chronic administration of D-Ala[6]-LH-RH EA to mature male rats reduced the weights of the testes, seminal vesicles, and ventral prostate, inhibited spermatogenesis, lowered testosterone levels and testicular binding of LH, and decreased mating performance and fertility. Administration of this analog to immature males produced only a depression of gonadal weight; these effects were reversible. Chronic treatment of hypophysectomized immature males let to a reduction in testes weight, suggesting a direct (extrapituitary) gonadal effect.

Rivier *et al.* (1980) reported that daily administrations of D-Trp[6]-LH-RH EA to male rats caused a reduction in the diameter of testicular tubules, loss of LH receptor sites in the testes, and decreased plasma testosterone and prolactin levels, but increased plasma progesterone. The mitotic activity of the testes was restored 4 weeks after cessation of treatment. Some of the effects on the testes were deemed to be direct.

In our own studies in male rats we have used D-Trp[6]-LH-RH. Male rats were hypophysectomized and treated with 2 μg of D-Trp[6]-LH-RH daily for 7 days with or without 1 IU of hCG every 2 days. Testicular LH/hCG binding sites in agonist-treated rats were 40 ± 7 (SE)% of those in control hypophysectomized rats. The testis weight of hCG-treated rats was higher than that of the control, but binding sites were 63 ± 10% of the control. Binding sites of rats treated with both hCG and agonist were only 17 ± 8% of the control. In another experiment, uptake by rat testis of radioactivity 30 min after injection of ^{125}I-labeled-D-Trp[6]-LH-RH was decreased to 62% of the control by pretreatment with 2.5 μg of cold D-Trp[6]-LH-RH, implying that the testis possesses a specific receptor for the LH-RH agonist. Together, these results suggest that the paradoxical effect of LH-RH agonist on the gonad results at least in part from a direct action that leads to the reduction of LH/hCG receptors (Arimura *et al.*, 1979a).

Similarly, treatment with D-Trp[6]-LH-RH decreased testicular LH/hCG binding sites in hypophysectomized immature rats whether pretreated with PMS or not. Injection of 50 IU of PMS 67 hours before hypophysectomy caused an increase in the testicular weight as well as an increase in LH/hCG binding sites. However, PMS did not affect the LH/hCG receptor-reducing effect of D-Trp[6]-LH-RH (Arimura *et al.*, 1979a, 1980). Reduction of testicular LH/hCG receptor by D-Leu[6], (N^α-Me)Leu[7]-LH-RH or D-Leu[6], (N^α-Me)Leu[7]-LH-RH EA in hypophysectomized rats was also reported by Hseuh and Erickson (1979b). Testes from the agonist-treated, hypophysectomized rats released considerably smaller amounts of testosterone (Hsueh and Erickson, 1979b). Heber *et al.* (1978) reported the presence of specific high-capacity, low-affinity LH-RH binding sites in the testes. It is possible that LH-RH agonists exert their inhibitory effect by direct action on the testes through the reduction of gonadal receptors.

G. ANTIFERTILITY EFFECTS OF SUPERACTIVE LH-RH ANALOGS IN HUMANS

Tamada and Matsumoto (1969) showed that ovulation can be suppressed in women with previously normal ovulatory cycles by administration of 1000–2000 i.v. hCG daily for 6–16 days. Recent clinical studies indicate that superactive LH-RH analogs can also exert antifertility effects in humans when used in relatively large doses or given by repeated administration. Tharandt *et al.* (1977) reported that, in patients with idiopathic isolated gonadotropin deficiency, s.c. administration of 100 μg of D-Leu[6]-LH-RH EA induced LH and FSH increases for more than 12 hours after the very first application. However, long-term therapy with the analog (100 μg s.c./day) did not improve hypogonadism. Paradoxically, in 8 patients on daily treatment with D-Leu[6]-LH-RH EA the FSH serum levels fell after 1 week and the LH levels after 8 weeks.

Happ *et al.* (1978d) studied the effect of the same analog when administered for prolonged periods of time to eugonadotropic males and postmenopausal females. In six eugonadotropic males, a significant decrease in responsiveness of LH and FSH to a standard dose of LH-RH and a fall in basal testosterone secretion were observed after 2 and 4 weeks of s.c. administration of 5 μg of D-Leu[6]-LH-RH EA twice daily. However, in two eugonadotropic males, these effects could not be observed after intranasal administration of 50 μg of this analog for 4 weeks. In two postmenopausal women, long-term s.c. administration of 5 μg of this analog produced a marked decrease of basal serum levels and decreased LH and FSII responses within 2 weeks of application. These changes were reversible 3 months after termination of treatment.

Chronic stimulation with D-Ser(Bu^t)[6]-LH-RH EA can also lead to a decreased responsiveness of the pituitary gland. Dericks-Tan *et al.* (1977) showed that D-Ser(Bu^t)[6]-LH-RH greatly stimulated LH and FSH release in normally cyclic women, maximal serum gonadotropin levels being found 4 hours after the injection. However, when 5 μg was injected every 8 hours for 3 days, the initially high release of LH and FSH declined progressively to almost nil. Similar effects were obtained in normal males (Wiegelmann et al., 1977) and in amenorrheic women (Hanker et al., 1978). When six women with long-standing functional amenorrhea were treated with 5 μg of D-Ser(Bu^t)^6-LH-RH EA twice daily for 14 days, LH and FSH responses to 25 μg of LH-RH varied widely before the treatment was started, whereas at the end of it they were uniformly low. In all patients, D-Ser(Bu^t)^6-LH-RH EA induced gonadotropin release, the peak values occurring between day 1 and day 3 of therapy. Despite further injections, mean gonadotropin levels declined rapidly thereafter and remained in the basal range for the rest of the study.

Baumann et al. (1978) also reported that daily i.m. administration of 10 μg of D-Ser(Bu^t)^6-LH-RH EA could cause a shift in ovulation and prolongation of cycle. Katzorke et al. (1978) administered this analog in doses of 87 μg/day in the form of nasal spray. Administration on days 12, 13, and 14 caused a delay or inhibition of ovulation, and only 27% of the women ovulated on day 13, 14, or 15. However, when it was given on day 13 only, it triggerred ovulation in 80% of the women on day 15 or 16. They suggested the potential usefulness of treatment with the analog for timing of ovulation for purposes of artificial insemination.

The actual contraceptive potential of superactive LH-RH analogs was revealed from studies on inhibition of ovulation or luteolysis in women when relatively large doses or repeated administration was used. Nillius et al. (1978) administered D-Ser(Bu^t)^6-EA^{10}-LH-RH s.c. once daily in a dose of 5 μg to four regularly menstruating women. Treatment was instituted within the first 3 days of the menstrual bleeding and continued for 22–30 days. The maximum FSH and LH responses to the LH-RH analog were obtained during the first few days of treatment. The gonadotropin responses then gradually decreased. This change in the pituitary responsiveness probably prevented the release of a normal preovulatory LH surge, and ovulation was inhibited in all the women during the treatment cycle. After the treatment, all the women resumed normal ovulatory menstrual cycles. Later, they reported that chronic intranasal administration of 400–600 μg daily of D-Ser(Bu^t)^6-LH-RH EA in the form of spray to 27 regularly menstruating women could also inhibit ovulation. There were no serious side effects (Bergquist et al., 1979; Nillius et al., 1980).

LH-RH itself and various superactive analogs of LH-RH have also been used for induction of luteolysis. Lemay et al. (1978) reported that s.c. administration of LH-RH in doses of 250 μg at 4-hour intervals for 6 days, between day 2 and day 7 after ovulation, caused a fall in serum progesterone and early onset of menstruation (2–3 days earlier) in four normal women. Later, the same group (Lemay et al., 1979) extended these findings by demonstrating that similar effects could be obtained when such a regimen was administered for 1–2 days only. Thus, five subcutaneous injections of 250 μg of LH-RH at 4-hour intervals, on 1 or 2 consecutive days between days 1 and 9 following the LH surge in normal women, shortened the luteal phase from 1 to 4 days in 16 of 17 treatment cycles. Treatment was more effective when LH-RH was administered on days 6 to 9 after the LH surge, the luteal phase being shortened by 3.3 ± 0.2 days. The serum progesterone level decreased to $44\% \pm 6\%$ of control levels when LH-RH was injected late in the luteal phase. These data demonstrated a luteolytic effect of LH-RH when given repeatedly in the luteal phase to normal women. Similar luteolytic effects could also be obtained with other superactive analogs of LH-RH (Lemay et al., 1980). Koyama et al. (1978) used LH-RH EA (desGly-$NH_2{}^{10}$, Pro-ethylamide^9-LH-RH) and administered it s.c. in a dose of 100 μg once daily for 5 days during the postovulatory period in six women with regular menstrual cycles. They found a suppression of plasma progesterone during the treated luteal phase as compared with that of the control luteal phase. Casper and Yen (1979) reported that s.c. injection of 50 μg of D-Trp^6-LH-RH EA on each of two successive days during midluteal phase in normally cycling women induced a short luteal phase and premature menstruation. These events were associated with luteolysis, as evidenced by premature decline of progesterone and estradiol levels compared with control cycles. These findings (Casper and Yen, 1979; Koyama et al., 1978; Lemay et al., 1979) suggest that repetitive, massive, administration of LH-RH or its analogs during the luteal phase of the cycle may induce functional luteolysis. This approach may prove to be useful in the prevention or interception of implantation.

The paradoxical antifertility effects of superactive LH-RH analogs could perhaps be used for the development of a male contraceptive that would inhibit spermatogenesis and thus decrease male fertility without decreasing libido, or a female contraceptive based on ovulation inhibition or luteolysis. However, the failure rate of any of these presumptive contraceptive methods based on superactive analogs of LH-RH has not yet been established, and it cannot be excluded that it could be relatively high. Work on these approaches or evaluation of such methods is actively proceeding in several centers in the United

States and other countries. Among the questions that have to be answered are the effectiveness, safety, side effects, and acceptance rate of these methods.

IV. Inhibitory Analogs of LH-RH

A. Theoretical Considerations for Antagonists of LH-RH

The design of modified structures that might compete with a biologically active compound for the same receptor sites and yet exhibit little intrinsic activity is an old concept that has been used to develop a number of drugs. For example, many microorganisms require p-aminobenzoic acid to form the vitamin folic acid, and sulfanilamide, a structural analog of p-aminobenzoate, can block folic acid synthesis. Other classical examples could include 5-fluorouracil, which is a pyrimidine antagonist and antimetabolite used for treatment of tumors.

Classical competitive inhibition occurs at the substrate binding (catalytic) site or receptor site, the receptor being defined as that membrane component of the cell that binds the hormone in a reversible interaction. The chemical structure and stereochemistry of an inhibitory analog must resemble that of the substrate or the hormone.

However, this approach has only recently met with any degree of success in the peptide field, and at the time we proposed development of inhibitory analogs of LH-RH (Schally and Kastin, 1971), the concept of a peptide endowed with anti-LH-RH activity was based purely on theoretical considerations. Knowledge of the essential structural features (active site) in a peptide is the primary step for the synthetic development of specific antagonists. We correctly forecast that replacement or deletion of one or more amino acids in LH-RH might result in analogs that possess features requisite for effective binding but lack those that might be necessary for a functional effect, i.e., the stimulation of LH and FSH release (Schally and Kastin, 1971). Such analogs would be competitive inhibitors of LH-RH; that is, they would be devoid of LH-RH activity but, by competing for attachment to the receptor site with endogenous LH-RH, would lead to a decrease of LH and FSH secretion (Schally and Coy, 1977). Another type of possible effective antagonist could be noncompetitive and be based on the introduction of a group that would react covalently with a site on the receptor and bind irreversibly. However, not enough is known about the structure of the receptor to design such inhibitors at this time.

It must be emphasized that such LH-RH antagonists are intended primarily for female contraception. They would not need to abolish the basal secretion of LH and FSH. Indeed, a complete inhibition of LH and FSH release would be undesirable, since it would interfere with the ovarian steroidogenesis, which might have undesirable effects on women. The role of the antagonists of LH-RH would be to decrease or block the midcycle surge of LH and FSH that is necessary for ovulation. To be practical, a contraceptive polypeptide might have to be given by a route of administration other than parenteral. Judging from clinical experiences with LH-RH or its stimulatory analogs, intranasal administration appears to be the most likely practical method at this time. However, such an inhibitor could also possibly be administered with depot carriers or implanted after coupling to a suitable polymer that would allow its slow release. LH-RH appeared to be an ideal candidate for the development of a new contraceptive method based on its antagonists, since they could disrupt the reproductive cycle relatively safely.

B. DEVELOPMENT OF INHIBITORY ANALOGS OF LH-RH

The enormous structural complexity of a decapeptide and the short physiological half-lives of most peptides make the task of finding an inhibitor of greater binding affinity and duration of action than the endogenous hormone very laborious. With studies of this type, it is first necessary to find some modification to the molecule that will destroy biological activity without completely destroying binding affinity. Hence, this usually requires the alteration of some active center and the synthesis and examination of many analogs. The information gained from studies on various stimulatory analogs of LH-RH has been used to guide attempts to create synthetic inhibitors of LH-RH.

One of the analogs, desHis^2-LH-RH, was reported to antagonize competitively LH-RH in monolayer cultures of rat anterior pituitary cells when present in dosages 10,000 times greater than LH-RH (Vale et al., 1972b). However, in our hands, desHis^2-LH-RH did not show significant anti-LH-RH activity in vivo when given to ovariectomized, estrogen- and progesterone-treated rats in doses 4000 times greater than LH-RH prior to administration of LH-RH (Schally et al., 1973b). Similarly, desHis^2-LH-RH added in vitro to pre- and incubation medium containing rat pituitaries in doses of 10 μg/ml or 2500 times greater than LH-RH (4 ng/ml) did not inhibit the response to LH-RH over a 6-hour incubation period. Moreover, 2.5 mg of desHis^2-LH-RH given i.v. 3 minutes before LH-RH did not inhibit the ovulation caused by 1 μg of LH-RH in three estrous rabbits (Schally et al., 1973b).

It was attempted, nevertheless, to increase the weak antagonist activities of the parent peptide by introducing some of the superactive modifications already discussed, since these appear to operate by increasing binding affinity. We synthesized the corresponding peptide containing the C terminus modified with ethylamide (EA) in the hope that it would improve the inhibitory activity of the parent peptide (Coy et al., 1973c, 1974b). In vivo assays for inhibitory activity of desHis^2, desGly^{10}-LH-RH EA in ovariectomized, steroid-treated rats, revealed that the significant release of LH provoked by a standard dose of LH-RH was abolished by prior treatment with 100 μg of this peptide antagonist. Later experiments demonstrated that the peptide, infused into the carotid artery of the ovariectomized, steroid-treated rats, inhibited LH-RH-induced LH release. Doses of 0.001, 0.01, 0.1, and 1.0 μg of the inhibitor gave a characteristic competitive binding curve, and significant lowering of LH levels were obtained down to 10 ng. This was the first peptide that significantly reduced LH secretion in response to LH-RH in vivo (Vilchez-Martinez et al., 1974b). DesHis^2, desGly^{10}-LH-RH EA has also proved to be capable under some conditions of inhibiting spontaneous or LH-RH-induced ovulation in rats.

Tryptophan in position 3 could also be replaced to give peptides with some inhibitory activity, such as Leu^3-LH-RH (Vilchez-Martinez et al., 1975a). However, this peptide and desTrp^3, desGly^{10}-LH-RH EA inhibited LH-RH less effectively than desHis^2, desGly^{10}-LH-RH EA, but desHis^2-, D-Ala^6-LH-RH was found to be even more potent (Monahan et al., 1973).

A whole series of potential antagonists were synthesized and assayed in immature male rats. This assay permitted us to compare accurately the effectiveness of LH-RH antagonists by measuring the inhibition of the response to LH-RH in their presence. Thus, the administration of desHis^2, desGly^{10}-LH-RH EA; desHis^2, Leu^3, desGly^{10}-LH-RH EA; desHis^2, D-Ala^6, desGly^{10}-LH-RH EA; and desHis^2, D-Ala^6-LH-RH in doses of 200 μg/rat, and desHis^2, Leu^3, D-Ala^6, desGly^{10}-LH-RH EA in doses ranging from 100 to 400 μg/rat caused a significant inhibition of LH-RH-induced release of LH and FSH. On the other hand, desHis^2, desGly^{10}-LH-RH propylamide, and Leu^2, Leu^3, D-Ala^6, desGly^{10}-LH-RH EA failed to block the response to LH-RH. Among these peptides, desHis^2, D-Ala^6, desGly^{10}-LH-RH EA and Leu^2, Leu^3, D-Ala^6, desGly^{10}-LH-RH EA in doses of 200 μg, and desHis^2, Leu^3, D-Ala^6, desGly^{10}-LH-RH EA in a dose of 400 μg/rat, showed some intrinsic LH- and FSH-releasing activities (Vilchez-Martinez et al., 1975b). Leu^3, desGly^{10}-LH-RH EA, Gly^2, Leu^3, desGly^{10}-LH-RH EA, Leu^2, desGly^{10}-LH-RH EA, desHis^2, D-Leu^6-LH-RH, and D-pyroGlu^1, desHis^2, desGly^{10}-LH-RH EA also showed anti-LH-releasing activity, but no significant differences were found between these analogs tested and desHis², desGly¹⁰-LH-RH EA (Vilchez-Martinez *et al.*, 1975a). It appeared that, for a given antagonist, inhibition was improved by incorporating either the D-amino acid in the 6 position, or a C-terminal ethylamide group. However, if both these modifications were incorporated within the same analog, increased inhibition was often marked by an increase in inherent agonist activity. Other conclusions that could be deduced were that, although tryptophan in position 3 could be replaced by simple amino acids with some retention of competitive binding, no spectacular advantages resulted. The results *in vitro* indicated a similar degree of inhibition to that obtained *in vivo* for these analogs.

As in the case of the corresponding agonist peptides, the substitution of D-alanine, D-leucine, D-phenylalanine, or D-tryptophan in position 6 of a particular inhibitor increased antagonist activity, in that order, *in vitro* (Coy *et al.*, 1976b) and *in vivo* (Coy *et al.*, 1976a). However, the greatest amount of work was carried out on desHis², D-Ala⁶, D-Leu⁶, and D-Phe⁶ analogs because of poorer yields obtained when synthesizing peptides with more than one residue of Trp. For instance, when assayed in immature male rats, desHis², D-Phe⁶-LH-RH caused maximal inhibition of LH-RH, when it was injected simultaneously with the analog. At 240 minutes, the inhibitory ability of the peptide disappeared and at no time was there significant release of LH by the analog alone. The pattern of inhibition of FSH release was similar (Coy *et al.*, 1976a).

Another important discovery was that D-Phe²-LH-RH (Rees *et al.*, 1974) was far more effective than desHis²-LH-RH *in vivo* and *in vitro*. Inhibition of LH release produced by desHis², D-Leu⁶-LH-RH, D-Phe², D-Leu⁶-LH-RH, and D-Phe², D-Phe⁶-LH-RH in immature male rats was 61–79% when these peptides were injected s.c. in doses of 200 μg simultaneously with 200 ng of LH-RH. However, the inhibition by D-Phe², D-Phe⁶-LH-RH increased to 91% when it was injected 30 minutes before LH-RH. FSH release was also inhibited to a similar extent (Coy *et al.*, 1976a). When the inhibitory effects of these peptides were tested over a prolonged period of time in immature male rats in doses of 500 μg/rat, D-Phe², D-Leu⁶-LH-RH and D-Phe², D-Phe⁶-LH-RH were found to be considerably more potent than desHis², D-Leu⁶-LH-RH and desHis², D-Phe⁶-LH-RH, respectively. The maximum inhibition of LH release for both peptides occurred at 30–60 minutes, D-Phe², D-Leu⁶-LH-RH causing 81% and D-Phe², D-Phe⁶-LH-RH, 88% inhibition, respectively. The inhibitory effect lasted for at least 4 hours (Coy *et al.*, 1976a).

When tested in pituitary cells in culture, desHis²-LH-RH, desHis²,

D-Leu[6]-LH-RH,   desHis[2],   D-Phe[6]-LH-RH,   D-Phe[2]-LH-RH,   D-Phe[2],
D-Leu[6]-LH-RH, and D-Phe[2], D-Phe[6]-LH-RH inhibited 50% of LH release
induced by LH-RH at molar ratios (MR$_{50}$'s) of 3000, 500, 60, 1000, 150,
and 25, respectively. These *in vitro* experiments indicated, in agreement with *in vivo* results, that substitution of D-phenylalanine for
histidine at position 2 of LH-RH leads to compounds more potent than
the corresponding desHis[2]-analogs (Ferland *et al.*, 1976). In general,
the D-Phe[2]-analogs were about three times more active than the corresponding desHis[2] -analogs *in vitro* (Coy *et al.*, 1976b), and both were
more potent and longer-acting *in vivo* (Coy *et al.*, 1976a).

Direct comparisons were also made between the inhibitory activities
of D-Phe[2]-peptides with D-Ala, D-Leu, or D-Phe in position 6, and it was
found that their effectiveness increased progressively in that order.
The most potent of the three peptides, D-Phe[2], D-Phe[6]-LH-RH, produced
significant inhibition of LH for 6 hours and of FSH for 8 hours after
injection into immature male rats, which is 2-3 hours longer than with
the D-Ala[6]- and D-Leu[6]-analogs (Vilchez-Martinez *et al.*, 1976a,b).

Thus, several of the D-Phe[2] peptides that were developed appeared to
be suitable for attempts to block ovulation in rats, hamsters, and rabbits. Initial experiments were carried out with D-Phe[2], D-Leu[6]-LH-RH
in naturally cycling hamsters; after some exploratory work, 750 μg
doses of the analog injected subcutaneously at 3, 4, 5, and 6 o'clock on
the afternoon of proestrus led to an 83% lowering of the LH surge (de la
Cruz *et al.*, 1975b). This was accompanied by only 30% suppression of
ovulation when animals were examined the following morning. The
reason for this was discovered later when it was shown that hamsters
were able to ovulate fully with approximately only 10% of the gonadotropins normally released during proestrus (de la Cruz *et al.*, 1976a).

Subsequent experiments in 4-day cycling rats showed a much higher
blockade of ovulation. This assay has become the most rapid and convenient method for testing the new generation of relatively potent
antagonists. The best results with these inhibitory analogs were obtained when multiple doses of large amounts were given, since their
length of action was not sufficient to produce complete inhibition of the
LH surge that takes place over an 8-hour period in the rat. Analogs
such as D-Phe[2], D-Ala[6]- and D-Phe[2], D-Leu[6]-LH-RH were able to block
ovulation (Beattie *et al.*, 1976; Corbin and Beattie, 1975a; Yardley *et
al.*, 1975) and the preovulatory gonadotropin surge in cycling rats
when multiple doses in the region of 12 mg/kg of body weight were
given during the afternoon of proestrus. In 4 day cycling rats, D-Phe[2],
D-Leu[6]-LH-RH caused 82% blockade of ovulation after three injections
of 2 mg on the proestrous day (de la Cruz *et al.*, 1976b) (Table II). When

TABLE II

Comparison of LH-RH Antagonists Modified in Positions 2 and 6; 2, 3, and 6; 2, 3, 6, and 1; and 2, 3, 6, and 10

LH-RH analog	Dose (mg)	Blockade of ovulation (%)
D-Phe^2,D-Trp^6	6 ?	89
D-Phe^2,D-Leu^6	2 (×3)	82
D-Phe^2,D-Phe^3,D-Phe^6	1 (×3)	100
D-Phe^2,D-Phe^3,D-Phe^6	1.5	100
D-Phe^2,D-Phe^3,D-Phe^6	1.0	33
D-Phe^2,D-Trp^3,D-Phe^6	1.0	90
	0.5	0
D-pyroGlu^1,D-Phe^2,D-Trp^3,D-Phe^6	1.0	100
	0.5	80
D-Phe^2,D-Trp^3,D-Lys^6	1.5	0
D-pyroGlu^1,D-Phe^2,D-Trp^3,D-Lys^6	1.5	80
D-Phe^2,D-Trp^3,D-Phe^6,D-Ala^{10}	1.5	80
D-Phe^2,D-Trp^3,D-Phe^6,D-Phe^{10}	1.5	0

D-Phe^2, D-Leu^6-LH-RH and D-Phe^2, D-Ala^6-LH-RH were administered in equal doses on the afternoon of the day of proestrus in 4-day cycling rats, D-Phe^2, D-Leu^6-LH-RH more completely inhibited the ovulation occurring on the following morning than did D-Phe^2, D-Ala^6-LH-RH (Vilchez-Martinez et al., 1976a), the inhibition of ovulation after a single injection of 5 mg of peptide being 30% for the former and 11% for the latter compound. Analogs such as D-Phe^2, D-Phe^6-LH-RH and D-Phe^2, D-Trp^6-LH-RH were effective in single doses of about 6 mg/kg in the rat (Coy et al., 1977).

The 2 position in LH-RH has been the subject of extensive efforts to discover modifications that are even better than the D-phenylalanine replacement. Other naturally occurring D-amino acids substituted at this position were all found to be less effective (Rees et al., 1974). D-p-flouro-Phe^2-LH-RH was reported (Beattie et al., 1975) to be more active than the D-Phe^2-analog; however, D-p-nitro-Phe^2- and D-p-amino-Phe^2-analogs were only equally as effective as the corresponding D-Phe^2-peptides. Interestingly, the D-p-amino-Phe^2-analog had good solubility in water, whereas the D-Phe^2-inhibitory peptides are very insoluble and must be administered in propylene glycol solutions or as suspensions in oil. D-Pentafluoro-Phe^2, D-Trp^3, D-Phe^6-LH-RH was less active than the corresponding D-Phe^2-peptide, so that increased lipophilicity in this position is presumably not advantageous. Likewise, diphenyl-Gly^2, Phe^3, D-Phe^6-LH-RH was less active than the D-Phe^2-

analog, which could be due to the presence of symmetry or the two bulky phenyl side chains at position 2 in this analog. Other modified analogs of D-Phe², D-Phe⁶-LH-RH were also synthesized. Dutta *et al.* (1978) reported that D-Phe², D-Phe⁶, AzGly¹⁰-LH-RH in a dose of 15 μg/rat completely blocked the ovulation induced by 0.5 μg of LH-RH in adrogen-sterilized constant estrus rats. In contrast to the results with the D-Phe²-analogs, L-Phe²-peptides have very poor inhibitory properties.

Attempts were then made to synthesize peptides with lower LH-RH activity that retained the desirable properties of D-Phe², D-Phe⁶-LH-RH. Position 3 was thus extensively investigated. D-Phe², Phe³, D-Phe⁶-LH-RH, was essentially equivalent as an inhibitor to D-Phe², D-Phe⁶-LH-RH; this is good evidence for an active role for tryptophan in the mechanism of gonadotropin secretion, since Phe³-LH-RH had LH-releasing activities of 0.1% of LH-RH itself. Five hundred micrograms of D-Phe², Phe³, D-Phe⁶-LH-RH suppressed LH and FSH release in male rats in response to LH-RH (200 ng) for at least 4 hours (de la Cruz *et al.*, 1976b). A single s.c. injection of 1.5 mg of D-Phe², Phe³, D-Phe⁶-LH-RH given at noon on the proestrous day resulted in 95% reduction of preovulatory LH surge and 84% reduction of the FSH surge (de la Cruz *et al.*, 1976b). Three s.c. injections of 1 mg each of D-Phe², Phe³, D-Phe⁶LH-RH into proestrous rats at noon, 2:30 PM, and 5 PM completely suppressed spontaneous ovulation. Later it was determined repeatedly that a single injection of 1.5 mg of this peptide at noon was sufficient to block spontaneous ovulation completely, in contrast to the first experiment in which this treatment suppressed ovulation by 86.4%. Four injections of 3 mg of desHis², D-Phe⁶-LH-RH blocked only 11% of spontaneous ovulations in proestrous rats (de la Cruz *et al.*, 1976b) (Table II).

Since Phe⁵-LH-RH has only 50% of LH-RH activity, attempts were also made to lower the inherent LH-RH activity of D-Phe², D-Phe⁶-LH-RH by incorporating this modification. D-Phe², Phe⁵, Phe⁶-LH-RH behaved quite similarly to the D-Phe², Phe³, D-Phe⁶-LH-RH (Ferland *et al.*, 1976). In female rats anesthetized with thiamylal (Surital), D-Phe², Phe⁵, D-Phe⁶-LH-RH given at about 1:00 PM on proestrous day at a 500 molar ratio inhibited the plasma LH rise induced by 200 ng of LH-RH by 75% up to 5 hours after its injection. When administered at 12:00 noon at the dose of 2 mg, this analog inhibited the spontaneous proestrous LH surge and ovulation by 85% and 75%, respectively (Ferland *et al.*, 1976). D-Phe², D-Phe⁶, D-Phe⁷-LH-RH, D-Phe², Phe³, D-Phe⁶-LH-RH, and D-Phe², Phe⁵, D-Phe⁶-LH-RH also inhibited 50% of LH release *in vitro* in monolayer cultures of rat pituitary cells at MR_{50} values of 400, 100, and 75, respectively (Coy *et al.*, 1976b; Ferland *et al.*, 1976).

Attempts to increase inhibitory activity by the substitution of D-Trp in position 2 were unsuccessful. For instance, D-Trp^2, Phe^3, D-Phe^6-LH-RH did not block ovulation at 3-mg doses (Coy *et al.*, 1977). D-Leu in position 7 gave a peptide with no observable inhibitory properties. Antagonists with D-Trp in position 6 had properties almost indistinguishable from those of corresponding D-Phe^6-peptides.

However, the replacement of Trp by D-Trp in position 3 appears to increase the potency of inhibitory peptides significantly (Coy *et al.*, 1977). D-Phe^2, D-Trp^3, D-Phe^6-LH-RH (Fig. 5) is both longer acting (nearly 10 hours in the rat) and a more potent inhibitory peptide than D-Phe^2, Phe^3, D-Phe^6-LH-RH. In tests for inhibition of ovulation, D-Phe^2, D-Trp^3, D-Phe^6-LH-RH was approximately twice as effective as D-Phe^2, D-Phe^3, D-Phe^6-LH-RH (Coy *et al.*, 1977; Pedroza *et al.*, 1978) (Table II). These data would suggest that D-Trp^3-LH-RH, which has very low LH-releasing activity (Hirotsu *et al.*, 1974), might still bind quite well to the pituitary receptors (Coy *et al.*, 1977). In fact we have actually observed (Pedroza *et al.*, 1977a) that D-Phe^2, D-Trp^3, D-Phe^6-LH-RH competes with LH-RH for its pituitary plasma membrane receptors, displacing [^{125}I]LH-RH more strongly than its parent hormone (see Section IV, E). Therefore, the inhibitory analogs of LH-RH probably exert their action on the same pituitary receptors as those for LH-RH.

Other replacements of position 3 and 6 residues of the LH-RH sequence also produced quite potent inhibitory analogs, for instance, D-Phe^2, Pro^3, D-Trp^6-LH-RH and D-Phe^2, Leu^3, D-Trp^6-LH-RH (Humphries *et al.*, 1976). When the D-Phe^2, Pro^3, D-Trp^6-LH-RH was infused by a minipump at the rate of 375 μg/day for 4 days to cycling rats, ovulation was inhibited; when administered to castrated male rats, serum LH levels were decreased. D-Phe^2, Leu^3, D-Trp^6-LH-RH was less effective in inhibiting ovulation but also lowered the serum LH levels of castrated rats (Bowers and Folkers, 1976). D-Phe^2, Pro^3, D-Phe^6-LH-RH was also claimed (Humphries *et al.*, 1976) to be a more

p-GLU-D-PHE-D-TRP-SER-TYR-D-PHE-LEU-ARG-PRO-GLY-NH$_2$

1   2   3   4   5   6   7   8   9   10

D-PHE^2,D-TRP^3,D-PHE^6-LH-RH

FIG. 5. The molecular structure of D-Phe^2, D-Trp^3, D-Phe^6-LH-RH.

potent inhibitor than either the corresponding L-Trp³- or L-Phe³-peptides. However, D-Phe², Pro³, D-Trp⁶-LH-RH was said to be about three times weaker *in vitro* than D-Phe², D-Trp³, D-Trp⁶-LH-RH and of about the same potency as D-Phe², D-Trp³, D-Phe⁶ (Vale *et al.*, 1977). Our own assays indicate that D-Phe²-Pro³-D-Phe⁶-LH-RH is about half as active as D-Phe², D-Trp³, D-Phe⁶-LH-RH in the tests for blockade of ovulation.

Another major development in antagonistic activity resulted from the replacement of L-pyroGlu by the D-pyroGlu group in the inhibitor molecule (Rivier and Vale, 1978). Although D-pyroGlu¹-LH-RH (Coy *et al.*, 1975a) has only 10% LH releasing activity, antagonists containing D-pyroGlu are more active than the corresponding L-pyroGlu-peptides in the standard blockade of the ovulation assay in the rat (Table II). Similarly, D-Ala¹⁰-LH-RH has very low LH-releasing activity, whereas D-Phe², D-Trp³, D-Ala¹⁰-LH-RH retains essentially full inhibitory activity.

Another important approach that we have used for increasing the inhibitory activity of competitive antagonists has been the substitution of D-Lys for Gly in position 6 and the use of its ε-amino as (*a*) a peptide branching and (*b*) a dimerization point (Coy *et al.*, 1979; Seprodi *et al.*, 1978a). In this way, analogs with much increased antiovulatory activity have been obtained that appear to be more effective as a result of their ability to bind to two receptor sites simultaneously. Thus, the introduction of large aromatic groups (e.g., benzoyl, indomethacinyl, acetylsalicylyl) onto the ε-amino group of the D-Lys residue resulted in no increase in antiovulatory activity (Table III). However, the branched-chain (Y) peptide [D-Phe², D-Trp³, *N*-(pyroGlu-

TABLE III

BLOCKADE OF OVULATION BY BRANCHED-CHAIN COMPOUNDS

$$\overset{\text{X}}{\underset{\mid}{}}$$

pyroGlu-D-Phe-D-Trp-Ser-Tyr-D-Lys-Leu-Arg-Pro-Gly-NH₂ or,

Peptide, X=	Dose[a] (mg)	Blockade of ovulation (%)
Control	—	0
H	1.5	0
Benzoyl	1	10
Indomethacinyl	1	0
Acetylsalicylyl	1	10
pyroGlu-D-Phe-D-Trp-Ser-Tyr	1	73

[a] All were injected at noon of day of proestrus.

D-Phe-D-Trp-Ser-Tyr)-D-Lys⁶]-LH-RH had far greater inhibitory activity than D-Phe², D-Trp³, D-Lys⁶-LH-RH on a weight basis, despite its higher molecular weight (Table III). It is possible to attribute this increased activity to the presence of two N termini in one molecule that could interact with and block two receptor sites simultaneously. However, this effect is peculiar to the N terminus, since branched-chain peptides with an extra C-terminal portion as expected did not have increased inhibitory activity. A peptide with three N-termini also had much decreased activity, presumably owing to steric problems between chains.

We extend this approach to full dimers and trimers of D-Phe², D-Trp³, D-Lys⁶-LH-RH and were able to derive some even more potent inhibitors. The best of the series (Table IV) were the isophthaloyl followed by the succinoyl dimers of the D-Lys⁶-peptide. Trimeric molecules were inactive again, most probably because of steric problems. One of the most active compounds in this series was the isophthaloyl dimer of D-Phe², D-Trp³, D-Lys⁶-LH-RH (Fig. 6 and Table IV), which gave significant blockade of ovulation in the rat at a single dose of 0.5 mg, an improvement over the best monomeric analogs of that time, such as

TABLE IV

BLOCKADE OF OVULATION IN THE RAT BY MONOMERIC AND BY DIMERIC ANALOGS OF LH-RH

Peptide	Dose (mg)	Blockade of ovulation (%)
Isophthaloyl dimer of D-Phe², D-Trp³, D-Lys⁶-LH-RH	1	89
	0.5	60
Succinoyl dimer of D-Phe², D-Trp³, D-Lys⁶-LH-RH	1	80
	0.5	40
D-Phe², D-Trp³, N-Ala-D-p-NH₂-Phe⁶-LH-RH (a) (L-pyroGlu)	1	20
D-Pyro-Glu¹, D-Phe², D-Trp³, N-Ala-D-p-NH₂-Phe⁶-LH-RH (b)	0.5	30
Isophthaloyl dimer of (a) (L-pyroGlu)	0.25	40
	0.125	0
Isophthaloyl dimer of (b) (D-pyroGlu)	0.25	80
	0.125	33
D-pyroGlu¹, D-Phe², D-Trp³, D-Lys⁶-LH-RH (c)	1.5	100
	0.5	25
Isophthaloyl dimer of (c)	0.25	100
	0.125	30
D-pyroGlu¹, D-p-Cl-Phe², D-Trp³, D-Lys⁶-LH-RH (d)	1	60
Isophthaloyl dimer of (d)	0.25	100
	0.125	53
D-pyroGlu¹, D-p-Cl-Phe², D-Trp³, D-Trp⁶-LH-RH	0.25	30

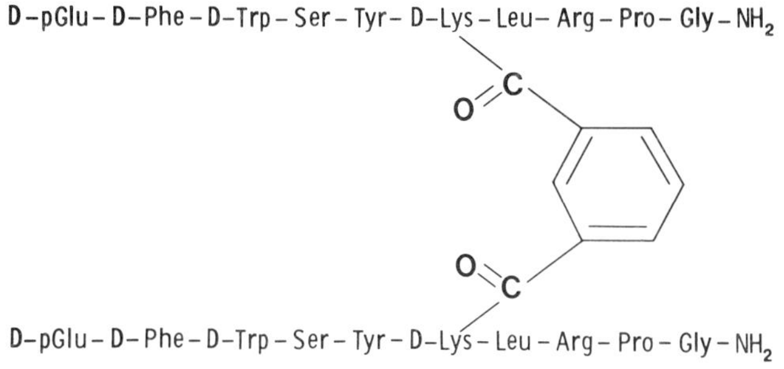

D –pGlu– D–Phe – D–Trp – Ser – Tyr– D–Lys– Leu– Arg – Pro– Gly – NH$_2$

D–pGlu– D–Phe – D–Trp – Ser – Tyr– D–Lys – Leu – Arg – Pro– Gly – NH$_2$

FIG. 6. The molecular structure of N^ϵ,N^ϵ-isophthaloyl-bis(D-pyro-Glu^1, D-Phe^2, D-Trp^3, D-Lys^6-LH-RH).

D-Phe^2, D-Trp^3, D-Phe^6-LH-RH, which were fully active in the 1.5 mg range.

Several ways were tried for improving activity still further, including the replacement of D-Lys by N^ϕ-Ala, D-p-NH$_2$-Phe since aromatic D-amino acids in position 6 are more effective than those with alkyl side chains for improving binding affinity (Coy and Schally, 1978). The inhibitory activities (Table IV) of these isophthaloyl dimers of N^ϕ-Ala-D-p-NH$_2$-Phe were approximately twice as high as the analogous D-Lys^6 dimers. However, in this series, the D-pyroGlu^1 modification had a far less beneficial effect than it did when incorporated in less active monomeric analogs.

In parallel with the studies on dimers, structure–activity work was continued on position 2, particularly the effects of various substituents on the benzene ring of the D-Phe residue. Beattie *et al.* (1975) reported a modest increase in inhibitory activity with D-p-F-Phe^2, D-Ala^6-LH-RH; however, this observation had not been extended to a new series of inhibitors. The effects of D-p-F-, D-p-Cl-, and D-p-Br-Phe in the second position of several antagonists were examined, and it was found that the p-Cl-peptides, both dimers and monomers, had slightly improved activities (Table IV).

In addition to the D-pyroGlu^1 modification, Channabasavaiah and Stewart (1979) reported that acylated D-amino acids, including D-Phe, in position 1 also give excellent results. D-Phe^1, D-Phe^2, D-Trp^3, D-Trp^6-LH-RH was prepared in our laboratory and, as expected for the nonacylated peptide, had no activity at a 1 mg dose. However, replacement of D-Phe by D-p-Cl-Phe in position 2 of this peptide greatly increased antiovulatory activity (Table V) so that 82% blockade of ovulation was obtained with a 0.25 mg dose (Coy *et al.*, 1980). Acetylation of the free amino terminus improves activity still further, so that N-Ac-D-Phe^1, D-p-Cl-Phe^2, D-Trp^3, D-Trp^6-LH-RH gave good blockade of

TABLE V

BLOCKADE OF OVULATION IN THE RAT BY ANTAGONISTS WITH D-PHE[1] MODIFICATIONS

Peptide		Dose (mg)	Blockade of ovulation (%)
D-Phe[1], D-Phe[2], D-Trp[3], D-Phe[6]-LH-RH		1	0
D-Phe[1], D-p-Cl-Phe[2], D-Trp[3], D-Phe[6]-LH-RH	[a]	0.25	82
Ac-D-Phe[1], D-p-Cl-Phe[2], D-Trp[3,6]-LH-RH	[a]	0.062	100
	[a]	0.031	64
	[b]	0.031	100
	[b]	0.016	20

[a] Propylene glycol–saline.
[b] Corn oil.

ovulation at an unprecedentedly low dose of 62 μg when injected in propylene glycol–saline solution (Table V). When administered as a suspension in corn oil, complete blockade was observed with 31 μg and partial blockade with 16 μg, possibly because of prolongation of release and activity in this carrier (Table V). Comparing the activity of the chloropeptide with N-Ac-D-Phe[1], D-Phe[2], D-Trp[3], D-Trp[6]-LH-RH, it is clear that the chloro modification increases inhibitory activity roughly 10-fold. Whether these improvements are due to steric or electronic considerations still remains to be clarified. Excellent possibilities exist for further increases in inhibitory activity (Coy *et al.*, 1980).

C. PHYSIOLOGICAL STUDIES WITH LH-RH ANTAGONISTS

1. Rats

a. Correlation between Inhibition of LH and FSH Release in Male Rats and Blockade of Ovulation. Most of the studies in rats are described in Section IV,B on the development of antagonists. Pedroza *et al.* (1978) found a good correlation between the inhibition of LH-RH-induced gonadotropin release in the immature male rat assay and the suppression of ovulation by the LH-RH analogs. In *in vivo* inhibition of the release of LH and FSH in response to LH-RH over a 4-hour period of time and the antiovulatory activity of these analogs were parallel to each other. D-Phe[2], D-Trp[3], D-Phe[6]-LH-RH was the most potent analog in the series available at that time and tested.

b. *Effects of Administration of Inhibitory Analogs on Stages of the Rat Estrous Cycle.* Corbin and Beattie (1975a) reported that injections of D-Phe², D-Ala⁶-LH-RH at "appropriate times" on any day prior to the gonadotropin surge result in high degrees of blockade of ovulation. However, no details were given concerning their experimental designs.

Vilchez-Martinez *et al.* (1978) studied D-Phe², Phe³, D-Phe⁶-LH-RH and injected it during the different stages of the estrous cycle in rats at a dose of 1.5 mg/rat. When it was administered at noon of day of proestrus, a 100% blockade was observed. This decreased to 33% and 17% when the analog was injected at 9 AM on proestrus and diestrus 2, respectively. No blockade of ovulation was observed after the injection of the analog on diestrus 1 or on the previous estrus. The sequential administration of the analog twice daily on the day of estrus, diestrus 1 and 2, brought about almost complete suppression of the LH surge on proestrus and an 86% blockade of ovulation without altering the cyclic vaginal smear pattern. Serum levels of estradiol were not modified, but progesterone levels were significantly lower on proestrus as compared to control rats.

c. *Intravaginal Administration of Analogs.* Intravaginal administration of D-Phe², Phe³, D-Phe⁶-LH-RH could also block spontaneous ovulation in proestrus rats (de la Cruz *et al.*, 1975a), but doses three times larger than when given s.c. were needed.

d. *Termination or Prevention of Pregnancy.* D-Phe², D-Ala⁶-LH-RH has been rigorously tested by Corbin and Beattie (1975a). They found that this peptide in addition to inhibiting ovulation could also prevent pregnancy when administered precoitally to rats on the day of proestrus (Beattie *et al.*, 1976). Our preliminary experiments in which D-Phe², Phe³, D-Phe⁶-LH-RH and D-Phe², D-Trp³, D-Phe⁶-LH-RH were administered to pregnant rats did not lead to termination of pregnancy.

e. *Effect of LH-RH Antagonists on the Reproductive Status of Immature Female Rats.* Corbin (1978) reported that administration of the LH-RH antagonist D-Phe², D-Ala⁶-LH-RH to immature female rats from day 25 to day 35 of age was without significant effect on the day of vaginal opening, on weights of the ovaries, uteri, and anterior pituitary, and on ovarian histology on autopsy day 39, which is at variance with previous results derived from studies employing mature female animals.

f. *Effect on Pituitary Levels of Gonadotropins.* Two weeks of treatment of immature male rats with D-Phe², D-Trp³, D-Phe⁶-LH-RH (1 mg or 0.5 mg × 2 injections per rat per day) caused a significant depletion of the pituitary gonadotropin content without significantly affecting the serum levels of gonadotropins (de la Cruz *et al.*, 1978).

g. Effect on Biosynthesis of LH in Vitro. When pituitary glands from ovariectomized rats were incubated with [³H]glucosamine in the presence of increasing doses of LH-RH, addition of the antagonist desHis², D-Ala⁶-LH-RH to the incubation system inhibited LH-RH-induced synthesis of [³H]LH and release of [³H]LH and immunoreactive LH (IR-LH). The dose required for half-maximal inhibition of LH-RH-induced release of either IR-LH or [³H]LH was 0.4 times that required for half-maximal inhibition of synthesis (Liu and Jackson, 1979).

These studies are in agreement with our own work (Chowdhury *et al.*, 1979), where addition of D-Phe², D-Trp³, D-Phe⁶-LH-RH into the incubation medium containing rat pituitaries or the pretreatment of rats *in vivo* with this antagonist resulted in significant inhibition of [³H]leucine incorporation into gonadotropins. This again suggests that antagonistic analogs of LH-RH can suppress *in vitro* synthesis of gonadotropins.

2. Golden Hamsters

As we have already mentioned, initial experiments with early analogs were carried out in normally cycling hamsters. D-Phe², D-Leu⁶-LH-RH injected s.c. in 750-μg doses at 3, 4, 5, and 6 PM on the afternoon of proestrus led to an 83% lowering of the LH surge (de la Cruz *et al.*, 1975b). However, this was accompanied by only 30% suppression of ovulation. The reason for this was discovered later (de la Cruz *et al.*, 1976a) when it was shown that hamsters were able to ovulate fully with approximately only 10% of the gonadotropins normally released during proestrus. Nishi *et al.* (1976b) also examined D-Phe², D-Phe⁶-LH-RH, D-Phe², D-Leu⁶-LH-RH, D-Phe², D-Ala⁶-LH-RH, DPhe², D-Phe³, D-Phe⁶-LH-RH, DesHis², D-Leu⁶-LH-RH, and desHis², D-Phe⁶-LH-RH for their ability to suppress LH-RH-induced ovulation in phenobarbital-blocked hamsters. In contrast to results in rats, only D-Phe²-D-Leu⁶-LH-RH caused a significant suppression of ovulation when injected 60 minutes before LH-RH. For reasons explained above, subsequent studies in hamsters were abandoned.

3. Rabbits

Plasma LH levels and ovulation were studied in female rabbits after administration of LH-RH inhibitors before and after mating with experienced males. A single s.c. injection of D-Phe², Phe³, D-Phe⁶-LH-RH (6 mg/kg) given 30 minutes before mating in four rabbits resulted in a 30- to 60-minutes delay in the coitus-induced release of LH, but all the does ovulated (Phelps *et al.*, 1977). When multiple dosages of 4 mg/kg body weight of D-Phe², Phe³, D-Phe⁶-LH-RH were administered 3–5 times at half-hour intervals beginning 30 minutes prior to mating, there was a considerable reduction in plasma LH elevations at 0.5, 1.0, 2.0, and 4.0 hours after mating, and three out of five treated rabbits showed partial or complete blockade of ovulation. Similar results were obtained with D-Phe^2, D-Trp^3, D-Phe^6-LH-RH.

LH-RH-induced ovulation could also be blocked in rabbits. An early sharp peak in the plasma LH level and full ovulation could be stimulated in six out of six does by a single i.v. injection of synthetic LH-RH (500 ng/kg), but three half-hourly s.c. injections (4 mg/kg) of D-Phe^2, Phr^3, D-Phe^6-LH-RH beginning 30 minutes before administering LH-RH greatly reduced the rise in plasma LH ($p < 0.01$) and completely blocked ovulation in all of the same six rabbits (Phelps et al., 1977). Corbin and Beattie (1975a) had reported previously that 25 mg of D-Phe^2, D-Ala^6-LH-RH blocked LH-RH-induced ovulation in rabbits.

4. Primates

a. Rhesus Monkeys (Macaca mulatta). Administration of nine injections of 16 mg each of D-Phe^2, Phe^3, D-Phe^6-LH-RH at 6-hour intervals tended to inhibit partially the estradiol-induced LH surge (Spies et al., 1980). In another experiment, D-Phe^2, Phe^3, D-Phe^6-LH-RH and D-Phe^2, D-Trp^3, D-Phe^6-LH-RH in doses of 40 mg suppressed LH release induced by electrical stimulation in some animals (Spies et al., 1980).

b. Baboons. In the baboon, administration of LH-RH causes a biphasic LH release. Administration of 40 mg of D-Phe^2, Phe^3, D-Phe^6-LH-RH i.m. 1 hour before 100 μg of synthetic LH-RH during the luteal phase partially suppressed the second LH peak (Hagino et al., 1977).

c. Marmosets. The work by Hearn et al. at the M.R.C. Reproductive Biology Unit in Edinburgh indicates that D-Phe^2, Phe^3, D-Phe^6-LH-RH administered i.m. in doses of 1 mg to male marmoset monkeys blocked the LH release induced by 0.5 μg of LH-RH. The best inhibition was obtained when this antagonist was given 60 minutes before LH-RH, but even administration 2 hours prior to LH-RH caused a significant suppression of LH release. This analog was also able to reduce basal levels of LH in marmoset monkeys (Hearn et al., 1980).

d. Chimpanzees (Pan troglodytes). Chimpanzees respond to single injections of LH-RH in a manner closely approximating the human response, whereas the response of other nonhuman primate species is sometimes inconsistent. D-Phe^2, D-Trp^3, D-Phe^6-LH-RH in doses of 35 mg inhibited the LH response of chimpanzees given 10 μg of LH-RH to 33% of the amount released by control animals without altering basal gonadotropin levels (Gosselin et al., 1979). These results indicate that LH-RH antagonists can diminish the response to exogenous LH-RH without acutely affecting basal gonadotropin secretion. They also suggest that a nonhuman primate model may be used to test the efficacy of these compounds as potential contraceptive agents.

e. Crab-Eating Macaque (Macaca fascicularis). D-Phe^2, D-Ala^6-LH-RH was also studied in the female crab-eating macaque. However, neither the length of the menstrual cycle nor the quality of the cervical mucus was dramatically altered during treatment with this analog. Of the nine macaques that were treated with 25 mg/kg body weight per day for 6 days, only two had anovulatory cycles associated with premature LH surges and one was devoid of an LH surge. Although this antagonist is relatively weak, the general lack of effect indicates that the macaque may be an inappropriate model for these studies (Corbin *et al.*, 1978b).

f. Fish. Addition of D-Phe^2, Phe^3, D-Phe^6-LH-RH to the incubation medium powerfully inhibited the *in vitro* release of gonadotropin from the pituitaries of rainbow trout in response to LH-RH, but the basal release of gonadotropin was not lowered (Crim *et al.*, 1981). This is in agreement with previous *in vivo* results in brown trout.

D. EFFECT OF INHIBITORY ANALOGS OF LH-RH ON CYCLIC AMP (cAMP)

It has been reported that seven antagonists of LH-RH, including D-Phe^2, D-Phe^6-LH-RH, inhibited the adenohypophysial accumulation of cyclic adenylate 3',5'-monophosphate (cAMP) *in vitro,* parallel to the suppression of LH-RH-induced LH and FSH release. This was in agreement with the suggestion that cAMP is a mediator in the action of LH-RH (Beaulieu *et al.*, 1975; Borgeat *et al.*, 1974; Labrie *et al.*, 1976a).

However, there is conflicting evidence about the role of cAMP in the LH-RH-induced release of LH. Conn *et al.* (1979) recently reexamined the actions of LH-RH on LH release and cAMP production in primary cultures of dispersed rat pituitary cells. Addition of 10^{-10} to 10^{-6} M LH-RH to cultured cells caused rapid release of LH into the incubation medium. In contrast, LH-RH caused no significant change in intracellular or extracellular cAMP. Neither dibutyryl cAMP nor methylisobutylxanthine stimulated LH production to the same level as LH-RH. These results demonstrate the independence of LH release from cAMP accumulation in cultured cells, suggesting that cAMP is not required for stimulation of LH release from these cells and that LH-RH acts on LH secretion by a different mechanism (Conn *et al.*, 1979).

This report is in agreement with other recent studies in which binding of LH-RH to purified pituitary plasma membranes was found to occur without activation of adenylate cyclase (Clayton *et al.*, 1978), and with an earlier report on the absence of adenylate cyclase stimulation by LH-RH (Theoleyre *et al.*, 1976). Other *in vitro* studies utilizing pituitaries from rats of both sexes and cultured pituitary cells of female rats (Naor *et al.*, 1978; Nakano *et al.*, 1978) have also suggested that cAMP may not have an intermediate role in LH-RH-induced gonadotropin release and/or that cGMP may be involved instead.

E. EFFECT OF INHIBITORY ANALOGS ON THE UPTAKE OF LABELED LH-RH BY PITUITARY MEMBRANE RECEPTORS IN RATS

The exact mechanism of action of antagonists of LH-RH has not been completely clarified, but some antagonists should inhibit the binding of LH-RH to pituitary receptors in a competitive fashion. Spona (1974) showed that the early antagonist desHis², desGly¹⁰-LH-RH EA competes with LH-RH for LH-RH binding sites on the pituitary plasma membrane. Since the investigation of binding of antagonists of LH-RH with adenohypophysial plasma membranes should help in designing better inhibitory analogs, we have studied the interaction of some of our most advanced inhibitory analogs with pituitary receptors for LH-RH. In our studies, rat pituitary homogenate was incubated with radioiodinated LH-RH ([¹²⁵I]LH-RH) (5 nM) in the presence of different concentrations of either cold LH-RH (5–80 nM) or D-Phe², D-Trp³, D-Phe⁶-LH-RH (10–1000 nM). LH-RH competed for the receptor sites with the tracer, but the analogs, at the same concentration as LH-RH, displaced the tracer from the receptor sites to a greater degree than did the parent hormone (Pedroza *et al.*, 1977b). Similarly, the displacement of [¹²⁵I]LH-RH by cold LH-RH in the adenohypophysial plasma membrane preparations was also smaller than that produced by D-Phe², D-Trp³, D-Phe⁶-LH-RH. The blockade of ovulation inhibitory analogs of LH-RH, such as D-Phe², D-Trp³, D-Phe⁶-LH-RH could be explained by the mechanism of binding to LH-RH pituitary receptors.

Heber and Odell (1978) found some correlation between *in vivo* LH and FSH releasing activity and high-affinity receptor-binding affinity of stimulatory analogs. However, in contrast to our results, they found that antagonistic analogs did not bind to the high-affinity receptor.

F. CLINICAL STUDIES WITH INHIBITORY ANALOGS OF LH-RH

In the course of development of antagonistic analogs of LH-RH, as the inhibitory activity improved, we felt that it would be of critical importance to show that these analogs were active in man. This task was made possible by the fact that inhibitory analogs of LH-RH showed a complete absence of toxicity in animals and had no visible side effects in humans.

The earliest clinical trial was carried out with desHis^2, desGly^{10}-LH-RH ethylamide, which was infused i.v. for 1–2 hours at doses of 1 mg and 2 mg. No inhibition of the gonadotropin response to 25 μg of LH-RH was seen after this analog. This is in agreement with its weaker inhibitory activities in the rat. Similarly, D-Phe^2, Phe^3, D-Phe^6-LH-RH in doses of 10 mg, 30 mg, and 60 mg i.m. did not block the LH and FSH responses to 25 μg LH-RH in normal men; no diminution of release was seen to the repeated injections of this small dose of LH-RH (Gonzalez-Barcena et al., 1977). The persistence of uniform responses of the gonadotropins to injections of 25 μg of LH-RH 1, 4, 8, and 24 hours after D-Phe^2, Phe^3, D-Phe^6-LH-RH served as a control for the first successful clinical study in which we were able to show that D-Phe^2, D-Trp^3, D-Phe^6-LH-RH is capable of blocking LH and FSH release in normal men after injection of LH-RH (Gonzalez-Barcena et al., 1977).

Five adult men without any known endocrine abnormalities volunteered for this study, which was carried out in Mexico. These volunteers were given 25 μg of synthetic LH-RH i.v. on the first day. On the second day, 90 mg of D-Phe^2, D-Trp^3, D-Phe^6-LH-RH were injected i.m., and 25 μg of LH-RH were injected i.v. as a bolus 1, 4, 8, and 24 hours later. Blood samples were collected before LH-RH injection and then every 15 minutes for 1 hour for plasma gonadotropin assay. In 4 out of 5 men, the single i.m. injection of this analog significantly suppressed the LH release at 1, 4, and 8 hours, and occasionally at 24 hours. FSH release showed a similar pattern of inhibition. Inhibition of gonadotropin increase, when expressed as maximal increase, was statistically significant at 1, 4, 8, and 24 hours after injection of the inhibitory analog. When expressed as an integrated amount released, it was also statistically significant for LH at 1, 4, 8, and 24 hours.

Basal levels of LH and FSH, 1, 4, 8, and 24 hours after administration of the inhibitory analog were not suppressed in the four subjects. This maintenance of basal gonadotropin levels was also observed in a fifth man, whose resting LH and FSH levels were unexpectedly found to be moderately elevated, even though his LH response to LH-RH decreased after the inhibitor. These results demonstrated for the first time that inhibitory analogs of LH-RH are active in man and validated our suggestion, made several years ago, that inhibitory analogs of

LH-RH would be effective in human beings (Schally and Kastin, 1971). The observations on the lack of alteration in basal levels of LH and FSH, while the gonadotropin response to exogenous or endogenous surge of LH-RH is suppressed, considerably enhanced the promise of inhibitory analogs of LH-RH for the development of new methods of birth control.

This study was extended in normal women. Intramuscular administration of 90 mg of D-Phe^2, D-Trp^3, D-Phe^6-LH-RH to eight normal women diminished the gonadotropin response to 50 μg of LH-RH given 3 and 6 hours later; however, the response to LH-RH was not blocked 24 hours after the injection of this inhibitory analog. The menstrual cycle was disrupted in all eight cases, and ovulation did not occur (Canales et al., 1980b).

The next step was to investigate the influence of this inhibitory analog alone on endogenous elevated gonadotropin levels in oophorectomized or postmenopausal patients. Our results show that the administration of 90 mg of D-Phe^2, D-Trp^3, D-Phe^6-LH-RH to a 45-year-old woman 12 years after oophorectomy decreased the LH values up to 8 hours after the injection. In another woman who had undergone oophorectomy, resting FSH levels also decreased up to 24 hours after injection in response to the inhibitor. A simultaneous suppression of LH and FSH serum levels occurred in a 35-year-old woman with ovarian amenorrhea. The results of Gonzalez-Barcena et al. (1978) and Canales et al. (1980b) confirmed and extended the conclusion of the first study and again showed that this inhibitory analog of LH-RH is active in humans (Schally et al., 1979a,b). The isophthaloyl dimer of D-Phe^2, D-Trp^3, D-Lys^6-LH-RH was active in women in doses of 50 mg (Gonzalez-Barcena et al., 1980). The inhibitory analogs are already of sufficient potency to enable extensive trials on blockade of ovulation in normal women to take place. In these trials, the analogs will be injected i.m. in oil, but eventually more convenient routes of administration, such as nasal spray, will be used.

In conclusion, we feel that the feasibility of creating, by synthetic approaches, peptides related to LH-RH that would inhibit LH and FSH release and ovulation has been clearly proved. Since still more potent LH-RH competitive inhibitors than those reported so far can be synthesized, this type of synthetic approach is reasonable and practical. Thus, it is possible that some of the inhibitors of LH-RH might eventually form the basis of new birth control methods. These methods would be based on the blockade of the ovulatory midcycle peak of LH-RH or on inhibition of implantation by antagonists of LH-RH. The inhibitory

LH-RH analogs could also be useful for treatment of precocious puberty, endometriosis, and postmenopausal symptoms.

Parallel to the synthesis of more potent inhibitors, work on the routes of administration of these compounds will also have to be carried out and suitable routes devised. Frequent parenteral administration would be inconvenient and, hence, impractical; and oral administration would probably have a very low degree of effectiveness on the order of about 1/1000, as compared with parenteral. Hence, the most practical route of administration appears to be intranasal, which was successful for LH-RH and its analogs, or that based on using suitable depot carriers for i.m. administration. A long-acting contraceptive peptide free of the side effects of existing antifertility steroids would be a welcome addition to the existing methods of control of human fertility.

V. Conclusions

We have reviewed the most recent advances on antisera to LH-RH and the agonistic and antagonistic analogs of this hormone. Work with antisera to LH-RH should be continued to investigate the possibilities of temporary active immunization against LH-RH.

The theoretical considerations (Schally and Kastin, 1971) about the validity of contraceptive methods based on analogs of LH-RH have been accepted by leading scientists in the field of physiology of reproduction (Short, 1974). The feasibility of use of inhibitory analogs of LH-RH for contraception was proved by our clinical work (Gonzalez-Barcena et al., 1977, 1978; Canales et al., 1980b). Continued research and testing along these lines may lead to the development of contraceptives based on inhibitory analogs of LH-RH that could be conveniently applied as a nasal spray and that would be free of undesirable side effects.

Basic and clinical research should also be continued on the phenomena of paradoxical fertility inhibition by large doses of superactive long-acting LH-RH analogs. We have to determine whether the demonstration of inhibition of ovulation (Bergquist et al., 1979; Nillius et al., 1978) and luteolysis (Casper and Yen, 1979; Lemay et al., 1978, 1979) by the appropriate administration of the superactive analogs could lead to their practical use as contraceptives. Moreover, if the research in primates in progress shows that the inhibition of spermatogenesis with analogs of LH-RH is reversible, such a method could be considered for male contraception. Further exploration of the fertility stimulating and inhibiting potential of superactive agonistic analogs and development of more potent inhibitory analogs should lead to new methods of birth control.

ACKNOWLEDGMENTS

We are grateful to Miss Cheryl A. Meyers and Miss Irene McFadries for their excellent help in the preparation of this manuscript. Some of the work described here was supported by NIH Contract NICHD HD-8-2819, NIH Research Grants AM-07467, AM-09094, and HD-06555, and the Veterans Administration.

REFERENCES

Aparicio, N. J., Schwarzstein, L., Turner, E. A., de Turner, D., Mancini, R., and Schally, A. V. (1976). *Fertil. Steril.* **27**, 549.

Arimura, A., and Schally, A. V. (1980). *In* "Hormones in Blood" (C. H. Gray and V. H. T. James, eds.), 3rd ed. p. 2. Academic Press, New York.

Arimura, A., Matsuo, H., Baba, Y., and Schally, A. V. (1971). *Science* **174**, 511.

Arimura, A., Debeljuk, L., and Schally, A. V. (1972). *Endocrinology* **91**, 529.

Arimura, A., Sato, H., Kumasaka, T., Worobec, R. B., Debeljuk, L., Dunn, J., and Schally, A. V. (1973). *Endocrinology* **93**, 1092.

Arimura, A., Debeljuk, L., and Schally, A. V. (1974a). *Endocrinology* **95**, 323.

Arimura, A., Kastin, A. J., Schally, A. V., Saito, M., Kumasaka, T., Yaoi, Y., Nishi, N., and Ohkura, K. (1974b). *J. Clin. Endocrinol. Metab.* **38**, 510.

Arimura, A., Vilchez-Martinez, J. A., Coy, D. H., Coy, E. J., Hirotsu, Y., and Schally, A. V. (1974c). *Endocrinology* **95**, 1174.

Arimura, A., Vilchez-Martinez, J. A., and Schally, A. V. (1974d). *Proc. Soc. Exp. Biol. Med.* **146**, 17.

Arimura, A., Sato, H., Coy, D. H., Worobec, R. B., Schally, A. V., Yanaihara, N., Hashimoto, T., Yanaihara, C., and Sukura, N. (1975). *Acta Endocrinol. (Copenhagen)* **78**, 222.

Arimura, A., Nishi, N., and Schally, A. V. (1976a). *Proc. Soc. Exp. Biol. Med.* **152**, 71.

Arimura, A., Shino, M., de la Cruz, K. G., Rennels, E. G., and Schally, A. V. (1976b). *Endocrinology* **99**, 291.

Arimura, A., Pedroza, E., Vilchez-Martinez, J. A., and Schally, A. V. (1978). *Endoc. Res. Commun.* **4**, 357.

Arimura, A., Serafini, P. C., and Sonntag, W. (1979a). *Program 61st Annu. Meet. Endocr. Soc.* Abstract No. 284, p. 144.

Arimura, A., Serafini, P., Talbot, S., and Schally, A. V. (1979b). *Biochem. Biophys. Res. Commun.* **90**, 687.

Arimura, A., Talbot, S., Serafini, P. C., and Schally, A. V. (1980). *Int. J. Fertil.* **25**, 151.

Arnold, W., Flouret, G., Morgan, R., Rippel, R., and White, W. (1974). *J. Med. Chem.* **17**, 314.

Auclair, C., Kelly, P. A., Coy, D. H., Schally, A. V., and Labrie, F. (1977a). *Endocrinology* **101**, 1890.

Auclair, C., Kelly, P. A., Labrie, F., Coy, D. H., and Schally, A. V. (1977b). *Biochem. Biophys. Res. Commun.* **76**, 855.

Baba, Y., Matsuo, H., and Schally, A. V. (1971). *Biochem. Biophys. Res. Commun.* **44**, 459.

Banik, U. K. (1974). U.S. Patent 3,816,617.

Banik, U. K. (1975). *J. Reprod. Fertil.* **42**, 67.

Banik, U. K., and Givner, M. L. (1975). *J. Reprod. Fertil.* **44**, 87.

Banik, U. K., and Givner, M. L. (1976). *Fertil. Steril.* **27**, 1078.

Banik, U. K., and Givner, M. L. (1977). *Fertil. Steril.* **28**, 1243.

Banik, U. K., and Givner, M. L. (1980). *In* "Reproductive Processes and Contraception" (K. W. McKerns, ed.), p. 143. Plenum, New York.

Bassiri, R. M., and Utiger, R. D. (1972). *Endocrinology* **90**, 722.

Baumann, R., Kuhl, H., Taubert, H. D., and Sandow, J. (1978). *42nd Meet. Ger. Soc. Gynecol. Obstet., 1978* Abstract No. 327.

Beattie, C. W., and Corbin, A. (1977). *Biol. Reprod.* **16**, 333.

Beattie, C. W., Corbin, A., Foell, T. J., Garsky, V., McKinley, W. A., Rees, R. W. A., Sarantakis, D., and Yardley, J. P. (1975). *J. Med. Chem.* **18**, 1247.

Beattie, C. W., Corbin, A., Foell, T. J., Garsky, V., Rees, R. W. A., and Yardley, J. (1976). *Contraception* **13**, 341.

Beattie, C., Corbin, A., Cole, G., Corry, S., Jones, R. C., Koch, K., and Tracy, J. (1977). *Biol. Reprod.* **16**, 322.

Beaulieu, M., Labrie, F., Coy, D. H., Coy, E. J., and Schally, A. V. (1975). *J. Cyclic Nucleotide Res.* **2**, 243.

Benuck, M., and Marks, N. (1976). *Life Sci.* **19**, 1271.

Bergquist, C., Nillius, S. J., and Wide, L. (1979). *Lancet* **2**, 215.

Bex. F. J., and Corbin, A. (1978). *Am. Soc. Androl., 1978* Abstract No. 6.

Borgeat, P., Labrie, F., Cote, J., Ruel, F., Schally, A. V., Coy, D. H., and Yanaihara, N. (1974). *Mol. Cell. Endocrinol* **1**, 7.

Bowers, C. Y., and Folkers, K. (1976). *Biochem. Biophys. Res. Commun.* **72**, 1003.

Brown, G. M., VanLoon, G. R., Hummel, B. C. W., Grota, L. J., Arimura, A., and Schally, A. V. (1977). *J. Clin. Endocrinol. Metab.* **44**, 784.

Camel, P. W., Araki, S., and Ferin, M. (1976). *Endocrinology* **99**, 243.

Canales, E. S., Montvelinsky, H., Fonseca, M. E., Zarate, A., Kastin, A. J., Coy, D. H., and Schally, A. V. (1980a). *Int. J. Fertil.* **25**, 193.

Canales, E. S., Montvelinsky, H., Zarate, A., Kastin, A. J., Coy, D. H., and Schally, A. V. (1980b). *Int. J. Fertil.* **25**, 190.

Casper, R. F., and Yen, S. S. C. (1979). *Science* **205**, 408.

Channabasavaiah, K., and Stewart, J. (1979). *Biochem. Biophys. Res. Commun.* **86**, 1266.

Chowdhury, M., de la Cruz, A., Coy, D. H., Schally, A. V., and Steinberger, E. (1979). *Biol. Reprod.* (submitted for publication).

Clarke, I. J., Fraser, H. M., and McNeilly, A. S. (1978). *J. Endocrinol.* **78**, 39.

Clayton, R., Shakespear, R., and Marshall, J. C. (1978). *Mol. Cell. Endocrinol.* **11**, 63.

Conn, P. M., Morrell, D. V., Dufau, M. L., and Catt, K. J. (1979). *Endocrinology* **104**, 448.

Connell, E. B. (1978). *Draper Fund Rep.* No. 6, Summer, p. 3.

Corbin, A. (1978). *Experientia* **34**, 813.

Corbin, A., and Beattie, C. W. (1975a). *Endocr. Res. Commun.* **2**, 1.

Corbin, A., and Beattie, C. W. (1975b). *Endocr. Res. Commun.* **2**, 445.

Corbin, A., and Bex, F. J. (1979). *Pan Am. Conf. Androl. 1st, 1979*, Abstract No. 251.

Corbin, A., Beattie, C. W., Yardley, J. and Foell, T. J. (1976). *Endocr. Res. Commun.* **3**, 359.

Corbin, A., Beattie, C. W., Rees, R., Yardley, J., Foell, T. J., Chai, S. Y., McGregor, H., Gorsky, V., Sarantakis, D., and McKinley, W. A. (1977). *Fertil. Steril.* **28**, 471.

Corbin, A., Beattie, C. W., Tracy, J., Jones, R. W., Foell, T. J., and Rees, R. W. A. (1978a). *Int. J. Fertil.* **23**, 81.

Corbin, A., Jaszczak, S., Peluso, J., Shandilya, N. L., and Hafez, E. S. E. (1978b). *Contraception* **18**, 105.

Corbin, A., Bex, F. J., Yardley, J. P., Rees, R. W., Foell, T. J., and Sarantakis, D. (1979). *Endocr. Res. Commun.* **6**, 1.

Coy, D. H., and Schally, A. V. (1978). *Ann. Clin. Res.* **10**, 139.

Coy, D. H., Coy, E. J., and Schally, A. V. (1973a). *J. Med. Chem.* **16**, 827.

Coy, D. H., Coy, E. J., and Schally, A. V. (1973b). *J. Med. Chem.* **16**, 1140.

Coy, D. H., Vilchez-Martinez, J. A., Coy, E. J., Arimura, A., and Schally, A. V. (1973c). *J. Clin. Endocrinol. Metab.* **37**, 331.

Coy, D. H., Coy, E. J., Hirotsu, Y., and Schally, A. V. (1974a). *J. Med. Chem.* **17**, 140.

Coy, D. H., Coy, E. J., Schally, A. V., Vilchez-Martinez, J. A., Debeljuk, L., Carter, W. H., and Arimura, A. (1974b). *Biochemistry* **13**, 323.

Coy, D. H., Coy, E. J., Hirotsu, Y., Vilchez-Martinez, J. A., Schally, A. V., van Nispen, J. W., and Tesser, G. I. (1974c). *Biochemistry* **13**, 3550.

Coy, D. H., Coy, E. J., Schally, A. V., Vilchez-Martinez, J. A., Hirotsu, Y., and Arimura, A. (1974d). *Biochem. Biophys. Res. Commun.* **57**, 335.

Coy, D. H., Coy, E. J., and Schally, A. V. (1975a). *Res. Methods Neurochem.* **3**, 393.

Coy, D. H., Coy, E. J., Schally, A. V., and Vilchez-Martinez, J. A. (1975b). *J. Med. Chem.* **18**, 275.

Coy, D. H., Hirotsu, Y., Redding, T. W., Coy, E. J., and Schally, A. V. (1975c). *J. Med. Chem.* **18**, 948.

Coy, D. H., Labrie, F., Savary, M., Coy, E. J., and Schally, A. V. (1975d). *Biochem. Biophys. Res. Commun.* **67**, 576.

Coy, D. H., Vilchez-Martinez, J. A., Coy, E. J., Nishi, N., Arimura, A., and Schally, A. V. (1975e). *Biochemistry* **14**, 1848.

Coy, D. H., Coy, E. J., Vilchez-Martinez, J. A., de la Cruz, A., Arimura, A., and Schally, A. V. (1976a). *In* "Hypothalamus and Endocrine Functions" (F. Labrie, J. Meites, and G. Pelletier, eds.), p. 339. Plenum, New York.

Coy, D. H., Labrie, F., Savary, M., Coy, E. J., and Schally, A. V. (1976b). *Mol. Cell. Endocrinol.* **5**, 201.

Coy, D. H., Vilchez-Martinez, J. A., Coy, E. J., and Schally, A. V. (1976c). *J. Med. Chem.* **19**, 423.

Coy, D. H., Vilchez-Martinez, J. A., and Schally, A. V. (1977). *Pept. 1976, Proc. Eur. Pept. Symp. 14th, 1976* p. 463.

Coy, D. H., Seprodi, J., Vilchez-Martinez, J. A., Pedroza, E., Gardner, J., and Schally, A. V. (1979). *In* "Central Nervous System Effects of Hypothalamic Hormones and Other Peptides" (R. Collu, ed.), p. 317. Raven, New York.

Coy, D. H., Mezo, I., Pedroza, E., Nekola, M. V., Vilchez-Martinez, J. A., Piyachurawatana, P., Schally, A. V., Seprodi, J., and Teplan, I. (1980). *Pro. Am. Pept. Sympt., 6th, 1979*, 775.

Crim, L., Evans, D. M., Coy, D. H., and Schally, A. V. (1980). *Life Sci.* **28**, 129.

de la Cruz, A., Coy, D. H., Coy, E. J., and Schally, A. V. (1975a). *Clin. Res.* **23**, 478A.

de la Cruz, A., Coy, D. H., Schally, A. V., Coy, E. J., de la Cruz, K. G., and Arimura, A. (1975b). *Proc. Soc. Exp. Biol. Med.* **149**, 576.

de la Cruz, A., de la Cruz, K. G., Arimura, A., Coy, D. H., Vilchez-Martinez, J. A., Coy, E. J., and Schally, A. V. (1975c). *Fertil. Steril.* **26**, 894.

de la Cruz, A., Arimura, A., de la Cruz, K. G., and Schally, A. V. (1976a). *Endocrinology* **98**, 490.

de la Cruz, A., Coy, D. H., Vilchez-Martinez, J. A., Arimura, A., and Schally, A. V. (1976b). *Science* **191**, 195.

de la Cruz, A., Chowdhury, M., Tcholakian, R. K., Coy, D. H., Schally, A. V., and Steinberger, A. (1978). *Biol. Reprod.* **19**, 364.

de Medeiros-Comaru, A. M., Rodrigues, J., Povoa, L. C., Franco, S., Dimetz, T., Coy, D. H., Kastin, A. J., and Schally, A. V. (1976). *Int. J. Fertil.* **21**, 239.

Dericks-Tan, J. S. E., Hammer, E., and Taubert, H. D. (1977). *J. Clin. Endocrinol. Metab.* **45**, 597.

Dutta, A. S., Furr, B. J. A., Giles, M. B., Valcaccia, I., and Walpole, A. L. (1978). *Biochem. Biophys. Res. Commun.* **81**, 382.

Everett, J. W. (1974). *In* "Major Problems in Neuroendocrinology" (D. Bajusz and G. Jasmin, eds.), p. 346, Karger, Basel.

Ferland, L., Labrie, F., Savary, M., Beaulieu, M., Coy, D. H., Coy, E. J., and Schally, A. V. (1976). *Clin. Endocrinol., Suppl.* **6**, 279S.

Forsbach, G., Ayala, A., Zarate, A., Canales, E. S., Soria, J., Schally, A. V., Kastin, A. J., Coy, D. H., and Coy, E. J. (1976). *Arch. Invest. Med.* **7**, 43.

Fraser, H. M., and Baker, T. G. (1977). *J. Endocrinol.* **77**, 85.

Fraser, H. M., Jeffcoate, S. L., Holland, D. T., and Gunn, A. (1973). *J. Endocrinol.* **59**, 735.

Fraser, H. M., Gunn, A., Jeffcoate, S. L., and Holland, D. T. (1974). *J. Endocrinol.* **63**, 399.

Fraser, H. M., Jeffcoate, S. L., Gunn, A., and Holland, D. T. (1975). *J. Endocrinol.* **64**, 191.

Friedrich, E., Etzrodt, A., Becker, H., Hanker, J., Keller, E., Kleisel, P., Pinto, V., Schindler, A. E., Schneider, H. P. G., Vanderbecke, A., Werder, H., and Wyss, H. I. (1978). *Acta Endocrinol. (Copenhagen)* **87**, 19.

Fujino, M., Kobayashi, S., Obayashi, M., Fukuda, T., Shinagawa, S., Yamazaki, I., Nakayama, R., White, W. F., and Rippel, R. H. (1972a). *Biochem. Biophys. Res. Commun.* **49**, 698.

Fujino, M., Kobayashi, S., Shinagawa, S., Obayashi, M., Fukuda, T., Kitada, C., Nakayama, R., Yamazaki, I., White, W. F., and Rippel, R. H. (1972b). *Biochem. Biophys. Commun.* **49**, 863.

Fujino, M., Shinagawa, S., Obayashi, M., Kobayashi, S., Fukuda, T., Yamazaki, I., and Nakayama, R. (1973a). *J. Med. Chem.* **16**, 1144.

Fujino, M., Shinagawa, S., Yamazaki, I., Kobayashi, S., Obayashi, M., Fukuda, T., Nakayama, R., White, W. F., and Rippel, R. H. (1973b). *Arch. Biochem. Biophys.* **154**, 488.

Fujino, M., Yamazaki, I., Kobayashi, S., Fukuda, T., Shinagawa, S., Nakayama, R., White, W. F., and Rippel, R. H. (1974a). *Biochem. Biophys. Res. Commun.* **57**, 1248.

Fujino, M., Fukuda, T., Shinagawa, S., Kobayashi, S., Yamazaki, I., Nakayama, R., Seely, J. H., White, W. F., and Rippel, R. H. (1974b). *Biochem. Biophys. Res. Commun.* **60**, 406.

Geiger, R., Wissman, H., Konig, W., Sandow, J., Schally, A. V., Redding, T. W., Debeljuk, L., and Arimura, A. (1972). *Biochem. Biophys. Res. Commun.* **49**, 1467.

Geiger, R., Konig, W., Sandow, J., and Schally, A. V. (1974). *Hoppe-Seyler's Z. Physiol. Chem.* **355**, 1526.

Gemzell, C., and Roos, P. (1966). *In* "The Pituitary Gland" (G. W. Harris and B. T. Donovan, eds.), p. 492. Butterworth, London.

Gonzalez-Barcena, D., Kastin, A. J., Coy, D. H., Schalch, D. S., Miller, M. C., III, Escalante-Herrera, A., and Schally, A. V. (1975). *Cancet* **2**, 1126.

Gonzalez-Barcena, D., Kastin, A. J., Schalch, D. S., Coy, D. H., and Schally, A. V. (1976). *Fertil. Steril.* **27**, 1246.

Gonzalez-Barcena, D., Kastin, A. J., Coy, D. H., Trevino-Ortiz, H., Gordon, F., Nikolics, K., and Schally, A. V. (1977). *Lancet* **2**, 997.

Gonzalez-Barcena, D., Kastin, A. J., Schally, A. V., Coy, D. H., Vilchez-Martinez, J. A., Pedroza, E., Nikolics, K., and Seprodi, J. (1978). *Fertil. Steril.* **29**, 246.

Gonzalez-Barcena, D., Kastin, A. J., Coy, D. H., and Schally, A. V. (1980). *Int. J. Fertil.* **25**, 185.

Goodfriend, T. L., Levine, L., and Fasman, G. L. (1964). *Science* **144**, 1344.

Gosselin, R. E., Fuller, G. B., Coy, D. H., Schally, A. V., and Hobson, W. C. (1979). *Proc. Soc. Expl. Biol. Med.* **161**, 21.

Guitelman, A., Mancini, A., Levalle, O., Aparicio, N., Comaru-Schally, A. M., and Schally, A. V. (1980). *World Cong. Fertil. Ster. Madrid 1980* **10**, Abst. 157.

Hagino, N., Coy, D. H., Schally, A. V., and Arimura, A. (1977). *Horm. Metab. Res.* **9**, 247.

Hanker, J. P., Bohnet, H. G., Mohlenstedt, D., Nowack, C., and Schneider, H. P. G. (1978). *Acta Endocrinol. (Copenhagen)* **89**, 625.

Happ, J., Kollman, F., Krawehl, C., Neubauer, M., Krause, U., Demisch, K., Sandow, J. von Rechenberg, W., and Beyer, J. (1978a). *Fertil. Steril.* **29**, 546.

Happ, J., Weber, T., Callensee, W., Ermert, J. A., Eshkol. A., and Beyer, J. (1978b). *Fertil. Steril.* **29**, 552.

Happ, J., Hartmann, V., Weber, T., Cordes, V., and Beyer, J. (1978c). *Fertil. Steril.* **30**, 666.

Happ, J., Scholz, P., Weber, T. H., Cordes, U., Schramm, P., Neubauer, M., and Beyer, J. (1978d). *Fertil. Steril.* **30**, 674.

Hearn, J. P., Hodges, J. K., Coy, D. H., and Schally, A. V. (1980). *J. Reprod. Fertil.* (in press).

Heber, D., and Odell, W. D. (1978). *Biochem. Biophys. Res. Commun.* **82**, 67.

Heber, D., Marshall, J. C., and Odell, W. D. (1978). *Am. J. Physiol.* **235**, E227.

Hirotsu, Y., Coy, D. H., Coy, E. J., and Schally, A. V. (1974). *Biochem. Biophys. Res. Commun.* **59**, 277.

Hodges, J. K., and Hearn, J. P. (1977). *Nature (London)* **265**, 746.

Hökfelt, T., Elde, R., Johansson, D., Ljungdahl, A., Nilsson, G., and Jeffcoate, S. L. (1978). *In* "Centrally Acting Peptides" (J. Hughes, ed.), p. 17. University Park Press, Baltimore, Maryland.

Hsueh, A. J. W., and Erickson, G. F. (1979a). *Science* **204**, 855.

Hsueh, A. J. W., and Erickson, G. F. (1979b). *Nature (London)* **281**, 66.

Hsueh, A. J. W., Dufau, M. L., and Catt, K. J. (1976). *Biochem. Biophys. Res. Commun.* **72**, 1145.

Hsueh, A. J. W., Dufau, M. L., and Catt, K. J. (1977). *Proc. Natl. Acad. Sci. U.S.A.* **74**, 592.

Humphrey, R. R., Windsor, B. L., Bousley, F. G., and Edgren, R. A. (1976). *Contraception* **14**, 625.

Humphrey, R. R., Windsor, B. L. Reed, J. R., and Edgren, R. A. (1977). *Biol. Reprod.* **16**, 614.

Humphrey, R. R., Redd, J. R., and Edgren, R. A. (1978). *Biol. Reprod.* **19**, 84.

Humphries, J., Wan, J., Folkers, K., and Bowers, C. Y. (1976). *Biochem. Biophys. Res. Commun.* **72**, 939.

Illig, R., Kollman, F., Borkenstein, M., Kuber, W., Exner, G. U., Kellerer, K., Lunglmayr, L., and Prader, A. (1977). *Lancet* **2**, 518.

Jaramillo-Jaramillo, C., Perez-Infante, V., Lopez-Macia, A., Charro-Salgado, A., Coy, D. H., and Schally, A. V. (1977). *Int. J. Fertil.* **22**, 77.

Jaramillo-Jaramillo, C., Charro-Salgado, A., Perez-Infante, V., Puenta-Cueva, M., Botella-Llusia, J., Coy, D. H., and Schally, A. V. (1978a). *Fertil. Steril.* **29**, 153.

Jaramillo-Jaramillo, C., Charro-Salgado, A., Perez-Infante, V., Lopez del Campo, G., Botella-Llusia, J., Coy, D. H., and Schally, A. V. (1978b). *Fertil. Steril.* **29**, 418.

Jaramillo-Jaramillo, C., Charro-Salgado, A., Perez-Infante, V., Bordiu Obanza, E., Cano Iglesias, R., Fernandez-Cruz, A., Coy, D. H., and Schally, A. V. (1978c). *Fertil. Steril.* **30**, 430.

Jeffcoate, S. L., Greenwood, R. M., and Holland, D. T. (1974). *J. Endocrinol.* **60**, 305.

Johnson, E., Gendrich, R. L., and White, W. F. (1976). *Fertil. Steril.* **27**, 853.

Jonas, H. A., Burger, H. G., Cummig, I. A., Findlay, J. K., and de Krestser, D. M. (1975). *Endocrinology* **96**, 384.

Jutisz, M., and Kerdelhué, B. (1973). *In* "Hypothalamic Hypophysiotropic Hormones" (C. Gual and E. Rosenberg, eds.), p. 98. Excerpta Med. Found.; Amsterdam.

Katzorke, T., Propping, D., Tauber, F. P., and Ludwig, H. (1978). *1978 Abstr. Eur. Congr. Steril. Fertil. 5th, 1978.*

Katzorke, T., Propping, D., von der Ohe, M., and Tauber, P. (1980). *Fertil. Steril.* (in press).

Kerdelhué, B., Catin, S., Kordon, C., and Jutisz, M. (1976). *Endocrinology* **98**, 1539.

Keyes, P. L., and Nalbandov, A. V. (1968). *J. Reprod. Fertil.* **17**, 183.

Kledzik, G. S., Cusan, L., Auclair, C., Kelly, P. A., and Labrie, F. (1978a). *Fertil. Steril.* **29**, 560.

Kledzik, G. S., Cusan, L., Auclair, C., Kelly, P. A., and Labrie, F. (1978b). *Fertil. Steril.* **30**, 348.

Koch, Y., Wilchek, M., Fridkin, M., Chobsieng, P., Zor, U., and Lindner, H. R. (1973a). *Biochem. Biophys. Res. Commun.* **55**, 616.

Koch, Y., Chobsieng, P., Zor, U., Fridkin, M., and Lindner, H. R. (1973b). *Biochem. Biophys. Res. Commun.* **55**, 623.

Koch, Y., Baram, T., Hazum, E., and Fridkin, M. (1977). *Biochem. Biophys. Res. Commun.* **74**, 488.

König, W., Sandow, J., and Geiger, R. (1975). *In* "Peptides: Chemistry, Structure and Biology" (W. Rand and J. Meienhofer, eds.), p. 883. Ann Arbor Sci. Publ., Ann Arbor, Michigan.

Koyama, T., Ohkura, T., Kumasaka, T., and Saito, M. (1978). *Fertil. Steril.* **30**, 549.

Labrie, F., Pelletier, G., Crouin, J., Bélanger, A., Ferland, L., Lemay, A., Lemaire, S., and Beaulieu, M. (1976a). *In* "Basic Applications and Clinical Uses of Hypothalamic Hormones" (A. Charro-Salgado, R. Fernandez-D., and J. G. Lopez del Campo, eds.), p. 100. Excerpta Med. Found., Amsterdam.

Labrie, F., Savary, M., Coy, D. H., Coy, E. J., and Schally, A. V. (1976b). *Endocrinology* **98**, 289.

Lemay, A., Labrie, F., Azadian-Boulanger, G., and Raynaud, J. P. (1978). *C. R. Hebd. Seances Acad. Sci., Ser. D* **286**, 527.

Lemay, A., Labrie, F., Ferland, L., and Raynaud, J. P. (1979). *Fertil. Steril.* **31**, 29.

Lemay, A., Labrie, F., Auclair, C., Kelly, P. A., Seguin, C., Cusan, L., Kledzik, G., and Raynaud, J. P. (1980). *Int. J. Fertil.* **25**, 203.

Liu, T. C., and Jackson, G. L. (1969). *Endocrinology* **104**, 962.

McCormack, J. I., Plant, T. M., Hess, D. L., and Knobil, E. (1977). *Endocrinology* **100**, 663.

Macdonald, C. J., Tashjian, A. H., and Greep, R. O. (1970). *Biol. Reprod.* **2**, 202.

Malacara, J., Seyler, L. E., Jr., and Reichlin, S. (1972). *J. Clin. Endocrinol. Metab.* **34**, 271.

Marks, N., and Stern, F. (1974). *Biochem. Biophys. Res. Commun.* **61**, 1458.

Mastroianni, L. (1978). *Fed. Proc., Fed. Am. Soc. Exp. Biol.* **37**, 2664.

Matsuo, H., Baba, Y., Nair, R. M. G., Arimura, A., and Schally, A. V. (1971a). *Biochem. Biophys. Res. Commun.* **43**, 1334.

Matsuo, H., Arimura, A., Nair, R. M. G., and Schally, A. V. (1971b). *Biochem. Biophys. Res. Commun.* **45**, 822.

Mayar, M. Q., Tarnavsky, G. K., and Reeves, J. J. (1979). *Proc. Soc. Exp. Biol. Med.* **161**, 216.

Maynard, P. V., and Nicholson, R. I. (1979). *Br. J. Cancer* **39**, 274.

Means, A. R. (1975). *In* "Handbook of Physiology" Sect. 7, (R. O. Greep and E. B. Astwood, eds.), Vol. V, p. 203. Am. Physiol. Soc., Washington, D.C.

Momany, F. A. (1978). *J. Med. Chem.* **21**, 63.

Monahan, M. W., Amoss, M. S., Anderson, H. A., and Vale, W. (1973). *Biochemistry* **12**, 4616.

Mortimer, C. H., McNeilly, A. S., Fisher, R. A., Murray, M. A. F., and Besser, G. M. (1974). *Br. Med. J.* **4**, 617.

Nakano, H., Fawcett, C. P., Kimura, F., and McCann, S. M. (1978). *Endocrinology* **103**, 1527.

Naor, Z., Zor, U., Meidan, R., and Koch, Y. (1978). *Am. J. Physiol.* **235**, 37.

Nett, T. M., and Niswender, G. D. (1979). *In* "Methods of Hormone Radioimmunoassay" (B. M. Jaffe and H. R. Behrman, eds.), p. 57. Academic Press, New York.

Nett, T. M., Akbar, A. M., Niswender, G. D., Hedlund, M. T., and White, W. F. (1973). *J. Clin. Endocrinol. Metab.* **36**, 880.

Neves-e-Castro, M., and Reis-Valle, A. (1975). *J. Steroid Biochem.* **7**, 701.

Neves-e-Castro, M., Lucio, A., Silva, L. A., and Reis-Valle, A. (1974). *Reproduccion* **1**, 393.

Nikolics, K., Coy, D. H., Vilchez-Martinez, J. A., Coy, E. J., and Schally, A. V. (1977). *Int. J. Pept. Protein Res.* **8**, 57.

Nillius, S. J., and Wide, L. (1975). *Br. Med. J.* **187**, 405.

Nillius, S. J., and Wide, L. (1977). *Upsala J. Med. Sci.* **82**, 21.

Nillius, S. J., Bergquist, C. H., and Wide, L. (1978). *Contraception* **17**, 537.

Nillius, S. J., Bergquist, C., and Wide, L. (1980). *Int. J. Fertil.* **25**, 239.

Nishi, N., Arimura, A., de la Cruz, K. G., and Schally, A. V. (1976a). *Endocrinology* **98**, 1024.

Nishi, N., Coy, D. H., Coy, E. J., Arimura, A., and Schally, A. V. (1976b). *J. Reprod. Fertil.* **48**, 119.

Niswender, G. D., and Midgley, A. R., Jr. (1970). *In* "Immunologic Methods in Steroid Determination" (F. G. Peron and B. V. Galdwell, eds.), p. 149.

Pedroza, E., Vilchez-Martinez, J. A., Fishback, J., Arimura, A., and Schally, A. V. (1977a). *Biochem. Biophys. Res. Commun.* **79**, 234.

Pedroza, E., Vilchez-Martinez, J. A., and Hoffman, E. O. (1977b). *59th Annu. Meet. Endocr. Soc.* Abstract No. 167, p. 140.

Pedroza, E., Vilchez-Martinez, J. A., Coy, D. H., Arimura, A., and Schally, A. V. (1978). *Int. J. Fertil.* **23**, 294.

Pelletier, G., Cusan, L., Auclair, C., Kelly, P. A., Desy, L., and Labrie, F. (1978). *Endocrinology* **103**, 641.

Phelps, C. P., Coy, D. H., Schally, A. V., and Sawyer, C. H. (1977). *Endocrinology* **100**, 1526.

Potashnik, G., Homburg, R., Eshkol, A., Insler, V., and Lunenfeld, B. (1978). *Fertil. Steril.* **29**, 148.

Ramirez, V. D., and McCann, S. M. (1963). *Endocrinology* **73**, 193.

Redding, T. W., Kastin, A. J., Gonzalez-Barcena, D., Coy, D. H., Schalch, D. S., and Schally, A. V. (1973). *J. Clin. Endocrinol. Metab.* **37**, 626.

Rees, R. W. A., Foell, T. J., Chai, S. Y., and Grant, N. (1974). *J. Med. Chem.* **17**, 1016.

Reeves, J. J., Tarnavsky, G. K., Becker, S. R., Coy, D. H., and Schally, A. V. (1977). *Endocrinology* **101**, 540.

Rippel, R. H., and Johnson, E. S. (1976a). *Proc. Soc. Exp. Biol. Med.* **152**, 29.

Rippel, R. H., and Johnson, E. S. (1976b). *Proc. Soc. Exp. Biol. Med.* **152**, 432.

Rippel, R. H., Johnson, E. S., White, W. F., Fujino, M., Fukuda, T., and Kobayashi, S. (1975). *Proc. Exp. Biol. Med.* **148**, 1193.

Rivier, C., Rivier, J., and Vale, W. (1978). *Endocrinology* **103**, 2299.

Rivier, C., Rivier, J., Lasley, B., and Vale, W. (1980). *Int. J. Fertil.* **25**, 145.

Rivier, J., and Vale, W. (1978). *Life Sci* **23**, 869.

Rivier, J., Monahan, M., Vale, W., Grant, G., Amoss, M., Blackwell, R., Guillemin, R., and Burgus, R. (1972). *Chimia* **26**, 300.

Rothchild, I. I., and Schwartz, N. B. (1965). *Acta Endocrinol. (Copenhagen)* **49**, 120.

Saffran, M., and Schally, A. V. (1955). *Can. J. Biochem. Physiol.* **33**, 408.

Saito, M., Kumasaka, T., Yaoi, Y., Nishi, N., Arimura, A., Coy, D. H., and Schally, A. V. (1977). *Fertil. Steril.* **28**, 240.

Sandow, J. (1976). *In* "Basic Applications and Clinical Uses of Hypothalamic Hormones" (A. Charro-Salgado, R. Fernandez-Durango, and J. G. Lopez del Campo, eds.), p. 113. Excerpta Med. Found., Amsterdam.

Sandow, J., and König, W. (1979). *J. Endocrinol.* **81**, 111.

Sandow, J., von Rechenberg, W., Jerzabek, G., and Stoll, W. (1978a). *Fertil. Steril.* **30**, 205.

Sandow, J., von Rechenberg, W., König, W., Hahn, M., Jezabek, G., and Fraser, H. (1978b). *In* "Hypothalamic Hormones—Chemistry, Physiology and Clinical Applications" (D. Gupta and W. Voelters, eds.), p. 307. Verlag Chemie, Weinhelm.

Sarkar, D. K., Chippa, S. A., Fink, G., and Sherwood, N. M. (1976) *Nature (London)* **264**, 461.

Schally, A. V., and Coy, D. H. (1977). *In* "Hypothalamic Peptide Hormones and Pituitary Regulation" (J. C. Porter, ed.), p. 99. Plenum, New York.

Schally, A. V., and Kastin, A. J. (1971). *Drug Ther.* **1**, 29.

Schally, A. V., Arimura, A., Baba, Y., Nair, R. M. G., Matsuo, H., Redding, T. W., Debeljuk, L., and White, W. F. (1971a). *Biochem. Biophys. Res. Commun.* **43**, 393.

Schally, A. V. Arimura, A., Kastin, A. J., Matsuo, H., Baba, Y., Redding, T. W., Nair, R. M. G., Debeljuk, L., and White, W. F. (1971b). *Science* **173**, 1036.

Schally, A. V., Kastin, A. J., and Arimura, A. (1971c). *Fertil. Steril.* **22**, 703.

Schally, A. V., Nair, R. M. G., Redding, T. W., and Arimura, A. (1971d). *J. Biol. Chem.* **246**, 7230.

Schally, A. V., Arimura, A., Carter, W. H., Redding, T. W., Geiger, R., Konig, W., Wissman, H., Jaeger, G., Sandow, J., Yanaihara, N., Hashimoto, T., and Sakagami, M. (1972a). *Biochem. Biophys. Res. Commun.* **48**, 366.

Schally, A. V., Redding, T. W., Matsuo, H., and Arimura, A. (1972b). *Endocrinology* **90,** 1561.

Schally, A. V., Arimura, A., and Kastin, A. J. (1973a). *Science* **179,** 341.

Schally, A. V., Kastin, A. J., Arimura, A., Coy, D. H., Coy, E. J., Debeljuk, L., and Redding, T. W. (1973b). *J. Reprod. Fertil.* **22,** 119.

Schally, A. V., Redding, T. W., and Arimura, A. (1973c). *Endocrinology* **93,** 893.

Schally, A. V., Kastin, A. J., and Coy, D. H. (1976). *Int. J. Fertil.* **21,** 1.

Schally, A. V., Coy, D. H., and Meyers, C. A. (1978). *Annu. Rev. Biochem.* **47,** 89.

Schally, A. V., Comaru-Schally, A. M., Kastin, A. J., and Gonzalez-Barcena, D. (1979a). *Proc. Int. Symp. Clin. Psycho-Neuroendocrinol, Reprod., 2nd, 1979* Abstracts, p. 1.

Schally, A. V., Comaru-Schally, A. M., Zadina, J., and Kastin, A. J. (1979b). *Proc. Int. Symp. Clin. Psycho-Neuroendocrinol. Reprod. 2nd, 1979* p. 9.

Schwarzstein, L., Aparicio, N. J., Turner, D., Calamera, J. C., Mancini, R., and Schally, A. V. (1975). *Fertil. Steril.* **26,** 331.

Seprodi, J., Coy, D. H., Vilchez-Martinez, J. A., Pedroza, E., and Schally, A. V. (1978a). *J. Med. Chem.* **21,** 276.

Seprodi, J., Coy, D. H., Vilchez-Martinez, J. A., Pedroza, E., Huang, W. Y., and Schally, A. V. (1978b). *J. Med. Chem.* **21,** 993.

Setalo, G., Flerko, B., Arimura, A., and Schally, A. V. (1978). *Int. Rev. Cytol. Suppl.* **7,** 2.

Short, R. V. (1974). *In* "Physiology and Genetics of Reproduction" (E. Coutinho and F. Fuchs, eds.), Vol. 4, Part A, p. 3. Plenum, New York.

Soria, J., Zarate, A., Canales, E. S., Ayala, A., Schally, A. V., Coy, D. H., Coy, E. J., and Kastin, A. J. (1975). *Am. J. Obstet. Gynecol.* **123,** 145.

Spies, H. G., Coon, L. L., and Gier, M. T. (1966). *Endocrinology* **78,** 67.

Spies, H. G., Arimura, A., Coy, D. H., and Schally, A. V. (1980). In preparation.

Spona, J. (1974). *FEBS Lett.* **48,** 88.

Takahashi, M., Ford, J. J., Yoshinaga, K., and Greep, R. O. (1978). *Biol. Reprod.* **18,** 754.

Tamada, T., and Matsumoto, S. (1969). *Fertil. Steril.* **20,** 840.

Teuwissen, B., Thomas, K., and Ferin, J. (1976). *FEBS Lett.* **72,** 341.

Tharandt, L., Shulte, H., Benker, G., Hackenberg, K., and Reinwein, D. (1977). *Neuroendocrinology* **24,** 195.

Theoleyre, M., Berault, A., Garnier, J., and Jutisz, M. (1976). *Mol. Cell. Endocrinol.* **5,** 365.

Vale, W., Grant, G., Amoss, M., Blackwell, R., and Guillemin, R. (1972a). *Endocrinology* **91,** 562.

Vale, W., Grant, G., Rivier, J., Monahan, M., Amoss, M., Blackwell, R., Burgus, R., and Guillemin, R. (1972b). *Science* **176,** 933.

Vale, W., Rivier, C., Brown, M., and Rivier, J. (1977). *In* "Hypothalamic Peptide Hormones and Pituitary Regulation" (J. C. Porter, ed.), p. 123. Plenum, New York.

Van Loon, G. R., and Brown, G. M. (1975). *J. Clin. Endocrinol. Metab.* **41,** 640.

Vilchez-Martinez, J. A., and Pedroza, E. (1978). *Abstr. 60th Annu. Meet. Endocr. Soc.* Abstract No. 200, p. 174.

Vilchez-Martinez, J. A., Coy, D. H., Arimura, A., Coy, E. J., Hirotsu, Y., and Schally, A. V. (1974a). *Biochem. Biophys. Res. Commun.* **59,** 1226.

Vilchez-Martinez, J. A., Schally, A. V., Coy, D. H., Coy, E. J., Debeljuk, L., and Arimura, A. (1974b). *Endocrinology* **95,** 213.

Vilchez-Martinez, J. A., Coy, D. H., Coy, E. J., Schally, A. V., and Arimura, A. (1975a). *Fertil. Steril.* **26,** 554.

Vilchez-Martinez, J. A., Schally, A. V., Coy, D. H., Coy, E. J., Miller, C. M., III, and Arimura, A. (1975b). *Endocrinology* **96,** 1130.

Vilchez-Martinez, J. A., Coy, D. H., Coy, E. J., Arimura, A., and Schally, A. V. (1976a). *Endocr. Res. Commun.* **3**, 231.

Vilchez-Martinez, J. A., Coy, D. H., Coy, E. J., Arimura, A., and Schally, A. V. (1976b). *Fertil. Steril.* **27**, 628.

Vilchez-Martinez, J. A., Pedroza, E., Coy, D. H., Arimura, A., and Schally, A. V. (1978). *Proc. Soc. Exp. Biol. Med.* **159**, 161.

Vilchez-Martinez, J. A., Pedroza, E., Arimura, A., and Schally, A. V. (1979). *Fertil. Steril.* **31**, 677.

Wass, J. A. H., Besser, G. M., Gomez-Pan, A., Scanlon, M. F., Hall, R., Kastin, A. J., Coy, D. H., and Schally, A. V. (1979). *Clin. Endocrinol. (Oxford)* **10**, 419.

Wiegelmann, W., Solbach, H. G., Kley, H. K., Nieschlag, E., Rudorff, K. H., and Kruskemper, H. L. (1976). *Horm. Res.* **7**, 1.

Wiegelmann, W., Solbach, H. G., Kley, H. K., and Kruskemper, H. L. (1977). *Horm. Metab. Res.* **9**, 521.

Worobec, R. B., Wallace, J. H., and Huggins, C. G. (1972). *Immunochemistry* **9**, 229.

Yanaihara, N., Tsuji, K., Yanaihara, C., Hashimoto, T., Kaneko, T., Oka, H., Arimura, A., and Schally, A. V. (1973a). *Biochem. Biophys. Res. Commun.* **51**, 165.

Yanaihara, N., Hashimoto, T., Yanaihara, C., Tsuji, K., Kenmochi, Y., Ashizawa, F., Kaneko, T., Oka, H., Arimura, A., and Schally, A. V. (1973b). *Biochem. Biophys. Res. Commun.* **52**, 64.

Yang, W. H., and Chang, M. C. (1968). *Endocrinology* **83**, 217.

Yardley, J. P., Foell, T. J., Beattie, C. W., and Grant, N. H. (1975). *J. Med. Chem.* **18**, 1244.

Ying, S.-Y. and Guillemin, R. (1979). *Nature (London)* **280**, 593.

Yoshinaga, K. (1979). *In* "Follicular and Corpus Luteum Function of the Ovary" (C. P. Channing, J. March, and W. A. Sadler, eds.), p. 729. Plenum, New York.

Zanartu, J., Dabacens, A., Kastin, A. J., and Schally, A. V. (1974). *Fertil. Steril.* **25**, 169.

Zanartu, J., Rosner, J. M., Guiloff, E., Ibarra-Polo, A. A., Croxatto, H. D., Croxatto, H. B., Aguilera, E., Coy, D. H., and Schally, A. V. (1975). *Br. Med. J.* **2**, 527.

Zanartu, J., Guerrero, R., Coy, D. H., and Schally, A. V. (1979). *Proc. Int. Symp. Clin. Psycho-Neuroendocrinol. Reprod. 2nd, 1979*, p. 307.

Zarate, A., Canales, E. S., Soria, J., Gonzalez, A., Schally, A. V., and Kastin, A. J. (1974). *Fert. Steril.* **25**, 3.

Zimmerman, E. (1976). *In* "Frontiers in Neuroendocrinology" (L. Martini and W. F. Ganong, eds.), Vol. 4, p. 25. Raven, New York.

VITAMINS AND HORMONES, VOL. 38

Sexual Differentiation of the Brain

GÜNTER DÖRNER

*Institute of Experimental Endocrinology, Humboldt University, Berlin,
German Democratic Republic*

I. NEUROENDOCRINE CONTROL OF REPRODUCTION

A. GONADOTROPIN SECRETION

The first outstanding experiment in sexual endocrinology was done by Berthold (1849). Castration of roosters resulted in atrophy of the genital organs and decrease of sexual activity, which could be prevented by reimplantation of testes. It was therefore suggested that a substance produced by the testes was responsible for the development and function of the sex organs and also for the control of sexual behavior.

The gonadotropic function of the pituitary gland was demonstrated by Aschner (1912), who observed gonadal atrophy in dogs after hypophysectomy Subsequently, the gonadotropins (FSH, LH, hCG) were discovered by Aschheim and Zondek (1927) (in our laboratories) and simultaneously by Smith and Engle (1927) in America.

In 1932, Hohlweg and Junkmann envisaged the central nervous system as controller of the hypophysial gonadotropic functions, and later Barraclough and Gorski (1961) distinguished, in rats, a rostral "cyclic sex center" located in the preoptic anterior hypothalamic region that regulates cyclic gonadotropin secretion in females and a caudal "tonic sex center" located in the hypothalamic ventromedial arcuate region that is responsible for tonic gonadotropin secretion in both sexes. More recent data suggest that structures of the limbic system, especially of the amygdala, are also responsible for cyclic gonadotropin release in females (Kawakami and Terasawa, 1974; Döcke et al., 1975).

Present day knowledge regarding the hypothalamic-hypophysial gonadal system may be summarized in the following manner: In the medial basal hypothalamus a gonadotropin releasing hormone (Schally et al., 1971, 1978) is secreted under the influence of neurotransmitters (Kamberi, 1974; Sawyer, 1979). It is transported by the hypothalamic-hypophysial portal vessels to the anterior pituitary, where it stimulates the secretion of gonadotropins. In females, an additional so-called cyclic sex center is responsible for a cyclically increased liberation of this gonadotropin releaser. In consequence, a periodic overrelease of hypophysial gonadotropins occurs, which promotes the induction of ovulation.

The hypophysial gonadotropic hormones control the generative functions as well as the secretion of the gonadal hormones. The sex hormones, in turn, exert either only an inhibitory (negative) or also a stimulatory (positive) feedback effect on gonadotropin secretion depending on sex hormone concentrations during the critical hypothalamic differentiation period and the postpubertal activation period as well (Dörner, 1976).

B. Sexual Behavior

The neuroendocrine control of sexual behavior was investigated by means of stereotactic lesions or deafferentations in discrete brain regions, implantations of sex hormones in specific brain areas, electrical stimulations within specific brain regions, or administration of psychotropic drugs that affect neurotransmitter metabolism in the brain.

1. Stereotactic Lesions and Deafferentations

a. Findings in Genetic Females. Brookhart et al. (1940, 1941) were the first to demonstrate by means of intrahypothalamic lesions a so-called mating center in the brain. Lesions located in the middle hypothalamus, i.e., at the posterior boundary of the optic chiasma, resulted in reduced female mating activity in intact female guinea pigs. A similar finding was then obtained by Goy and Phoenix (1963) in ovariectomized guinea pigs with sex hormone replacement.

In 1942, Clark described some decrease of female sexual behavior in female rats with anterior hypothalamic lesions. By contrast, Law and

Meagher (1958) found even a slight increase of female mating behavior in ovariectomized and sex hormone-treated rats after lesions of the anterior hypothalamus, whereas in ovariectomized animals with lesions located at the posterior boundary of the optic chiasm a clear loss of female lordotic behavior was observed. Kennedy (1964) then described a blockade of female sexual behavior without interruption of ovarian cycles in intact female rats after ablation of the hypothalamic ventromedial nucleus.

In 1968 and 1969, we first studied the effects of hypothalamic lesions on female and male behavior in castrated rats replaced with sex hormones. In these experiments, we found a significant decrease of female lordotic behavior toward vigorous males associated with a simultaneous significant increase of male mounting behavior toward estrous females after bilateral or even unilateral lesions of the ventromedial nuclear region (Dörner et al., 1968a, 1969, 1975a). Hence, we hypothesized that different brain regions may be responsible for the control of female and male behavior and that there may be some antagonistic interactions between female and male mating centers in the brain.

This hypothesis was strongly supported by Nance et al. (1977), who also described· a significant reduction of female behavior associated with a dramatic increase of male copulatory behavior after ventromedial nucleus lesions in female rats. On the other hand, lesions in the preoptic area produced a significant increase in lordotic behavior and virtual elimination of male sex behavior. Similar data were obtained by Powers and Valenstein (1972).

In 1970, Kalra and Sawyer reported that stereotactic deafferentation cuts located immediately behind the suprachiasmatic nuclei interfered with female sexual behavior in rats. Malsbury et al. (1978) performed half-cylinder cuts anterolateral to the ventromedial nuclei that reduced female mating activity in golden hamsters. Most recently, we observed significantly decreased female lordotic behavior associated with markedly increased male mounting behavior after anterolateral cuts to the ventromedial nuclei in ovariectomized rats treated with androgens (Dörner et al., 1979).

b. Findings in Genetic Males. Brookhart and Dey (1941) were also the first to demonstrate decreased male mounting behavior after anterior hypothalamic lesions in male guinea pigs. Stereotactic lesions located in the preoptic anterior hypothalamic region were found to reduce male sexual behavior in frogs (Noble and Aronson, 1945) as well as in rats (Soulairac, 1963; Larsson and Heimer, 1964; Heimer and Larsson, 1967; Dörner et al., 1969). Furthermore, septal lesions resulted in increased heterotypical (female-like) behavior in male rats treated with estrogen (Nance *et al.,* 1974). A similar effect was described after removal of dorsal inputs to the preoptic and hypothalamic area (Yamomachi and Arai, 1975).

On the other hand, ventromedial nucleus lesions produced homotypical hypersexuality in male rats (Dörner *et al.,* 1969). This finding was later confirmed by Christensen *et al.* (1977).

Furthermore, predominantly heterotypical behavior (termed homosexual by our group) observed in male rats castrated on the first day of life and implanted with testes in adulthood could be suppressed by means of stereotactic lesions in the hypothalamic ventromedial nuclear region (Dörner *et al.,* 1968a). Meanwhile, it was concluded that pedophilic homosexual men displayed clearly decreased homosexual and increased heterosexual behavior after lesions of the hypothalamic ventromedial nucleus (Müller *et al.,* 1974; Dieckmann and Hassler, 1975).

In heterosexual males suffering from uncontrolled hypersexuality, pedophilia, or exhibitionism, a significant reduction of the sexual drive was reported to occur after lesions of the preoptic area (Müller *et al.,* 1974; Dieckmann and Hassler, 1975). Hence, male and female sexual behavior may be open to a relatively selective influence by means of stereotactic operations.

However, I believe that psychosurgery should be taken into consideration only as a last resort after fruitless attempts with other therapeutic methods.

2. *Sex Hormone Implantations in the Brain*

Since brain lesions may affect sexual behavior by destroying neurons as well as afferent or efferent neural pathways, attempts were made to provide direct evidence for the existence of sex hormone-sensitive neurons responsible for the regulation of sexual behavior by use of sex hormone implantations.

In ovariectomized cats, Harris *et al.* (1958) found that estrogen implants located in the posterior hypothalamus induced estrous behavior. In the same species, Sawyer (1963) then observed increased female sexual activity after implantation of estradiol benzoate into the anterior hypothalamus, whereas implants located in the posterior hypothalamus were ineffective. In female rabbits, on the other hand, Palka and Sawyer (1964, 1966) found that estrogen implants located in the middle hypothalamus induced female mating behavior as early as 1 or 2 days afterward.

In castrated female rats, Lisk (1962) described lordosis reflexes 3–5 days after estrogen implantation into the medial preoptic-anterior hypothalamic region. However, the quantity of the implanted estrogen was not exactly defined. Furthermore, estrogen or estrogen plus progesterone implants, when placed in the middle hypothalamus, also induced estrous behavior in ovariectomized rats (Lisk, 1967; Lisk and Suydam, 1967).

In our own experiments (Dörner *et al.*, 1968b, c), precisely defined quantities of crystalline estradiol benzoate (EB) were implanted into the anterior or middle hypothalamus of spayed female rats, and tests for male as well as female sexual behavior were performed.

The following results were obtained (Fig. 1): Implantation of 1 μg of EB into the medial preoptic-anterior hypothalamic region of spayed female rats elicited receptive female behavior (lordosis reflexes) in only one out of nine animals when exposed to active males. On the other hand, the majority of these rats showed some male behavior

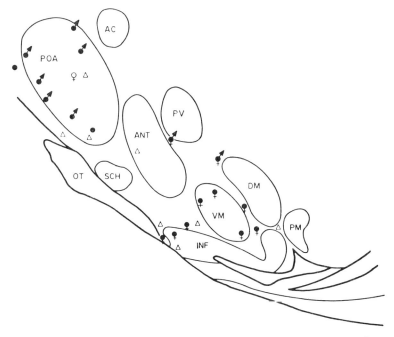

FIG. 1. Parasagittal diagram of the rat hypothalamus. Sites of estradiol implants that induced lordosis reflexes (♀) or trials of mountings (♂) in postpubertally spayed females. Triangles represent sites of cholesterol implants. AC, anterior commissure; ANT, anterior hypothalamic nucleus; DM, dorsomedial nucleus; INF, infundibular (arcuate) nucleus; PM, premamillary nucleus; POA, preoptic area; PV, paraventricular nucleus; SCH, suprachiasmatic nucleus; VM, ventromedial nucleus. From Dörner (1972, 1976).

(trials of mounting) when placed together with estrous females. In contrast, implantation of 1 μg of EB in the middle hypothalamus resulted in distinct female behavior in all rats, whereas these implants were relatively ineffective in activating male behavior.

Furthermore, predominantly female, i.e., heterosexual, behavior, was observed in spayed female rats implanted with testosterone propionate (TP) in the middle hypothalamus. In contrast, after TP implantations into the preoptic-anterior hypothalamic region, predominantly male, i.e., "homosexual" behavior, was observed in these females (Dörner et al., 1968b).

We drew the following conclusion from these findings: There are sex hormone-sensitive neural structures within the middle hypothalamus, especially in the ventromedial nuclear region, responsible for the activation of female behavior. In the medial preoptic-anterior hypothalamic area, on the other hand, sex hormone-sensitive neural structures are located that are responsible for the activation of male behavior (Dörner, 1972).

Most recently, Davis and Barfield (1979a, b) published similar findings obtained in male rats. Estradiol benzoate implants located in the medial preoptic-anterior hypothalamic area stimulated male sexual behavior, whereas EB implants located in the region of the ventromedial hypothalamic nucleus activated female behavior.

Moreover, in our own experiments, intracerebral implantations of estrogen were significantly more effective than implantations of androgen in activating male as well as female behavior in ovariectomized rats. Thus 0.001 mg of estradiol benzoate (EB) induced male behavior when implanted into the medial preoptic area, but female behavior when implanted into the ventromedial nuclear region, whereas 0.05 mg of TP, i.e., a 50-fold higher dose of TP as compared to EB, was completely ineffective in both cases (Dörner et al., 1968a, b). In view of these findings, estrogen appeared to be the most important sex hormone for activation of male and female sexual behavior in rats.

In contrast, androgen appears to be the most important sex hormone for activation of male and even female sexual behavior in primates. Thus, female sexual behavior is maintained in women—in contrast to rats—after ovariectomy. After adrenalectomy in addition, however, an absolute loss of female sexuality has been observed in women (Waxenberg et al., 1959). Furthermore, libido in women can be stimulated much better by androgen than by estrogen (Salmon and Geist, 1943; Foss, 1951; Persky, 1978). These findings suggest that female sexual behavior in women, in clear contrast to that in rats, is less activated by ovarian estrogens than by adrenal and ovarian androgens.

In 1974, Christensen and Clemens reported that intracerebral implantations of estrogen into orchidectomized rats were also much more effective in activating male sexual behavior than similar implantations of androgen. In this context it should be mentioned that testosterone can be aromatized in the brain to estrogen (Naftolin et al., 1976). A blockade of testosterone-induced mounting behavior could be prevented in male rats by aromatization inhibitors (Christensen and Clemens, 1975; Moralli et al., 1977). Furthermore, the nonaromatizable androgen 5α-dihydrotestosterone failed to initiate sexual behavior in the orchidectomized rat when administered alone (McDonald et al., 1970). Some facilitation of mounting behavior by 5α-dihydrotestosterone was found, however, in estrogen-treated orchidectomized rats (Lodder and Baum, 1977). In view of these findings, the stimulating effect of testosterone on male sexual behavior in rats is mediated, at least to a great extent, by conversion to estrogen.

This mechanism, however, does not appear to play an essential role in primates, particularly in men. In our experience, male sexual behavior cannot be stimulated by estrogen in orchidectomized men (with prostatic cancer) in contrast to orchidectomized rats. Furthermore, 5α-dihydrotestosterone can clearly stimulate male sexual behavior in orchidectomized primates, even when administered alone (Phoenix, 1974).

3. Electrical Stimulation of Brain Regions

Activation of male sexual behavior after electrical stimulation of the preoptic and/or anterior hypothalamic region has been observed by several authors (Hillarp et al., 1954; Vaughan and Fisher, 1962; Malsbury, 1971; Merari and Ginton, 1975). On the other hand, activation of female behavior has been produced by electrical stimulation of the ventromedial hypothalamic nucleus (Pfaff and Sakuma, 1979).

4. Neurotransmitters and Luteinizing Hormone-Releasing Hormone (LH-RH)

In recent years, several drugs have been described that can stimulate or inhibit sexual behavior by direct interaction with neurotransmitters; i.e., sexual behavior appears to be under the control of sex hormones and neurotransmitters as well.

Meyerson (1964, 1966, 1968) was the first to describe an increase of female receptive behavior by application of reserpine and tetrabenazine, which decrease the cerebral content of monoamines, especially of serotonin. For example, reserpine or tetrabenazine administered to estrogen-treated female rats can activate sexual receptivity by replacing the synergistic action of progesterone and estrogen (Meyerson, 1964). Further studies in which serotonin levels were reduced by more specific methods have confirmed that such procedures potentiate estrous behavior (Meyerson and Lewander, 1970; Zemlan et al., 1973; Södersten et al., 1976).

Herbert (1974) observed that p-chlorophenylalanine, a drug that depletes serotonin, can restore sexual receptivity in dexamethasone-treated monkeys, thus mimicking the effect of androgens. In male rats, reserpine and p-chlorophenylalanine were also reported to increase sexual activity (Dewsbury and Davis, 1970; Gawienowski et al., 1973).

But the cholinergic system and the catecholaminergic system also appear to play a role in regulating sexual activity (Lindstrom and Meyerson, 1966; Soulairac and Soulairac, 1970; Gessa and Tagliamonte, 1975). To summarize some influences of neurotransmitters on sexual behavior:

1. The cholinergic system can stimulate male and female behavior (Bignani, 1966; Soulairac and Soulairac, 1975; Fuxe et al., 1977).
2. The serotonergic system can inhibit male and female behavior (Crowley et al., 1975, 1976; Foreman and Moss, 1978).
3. The β-adrenergic system appears to stimulate, whereas the α-adrenergic system appears to inhibit, male and female sexual behavior (Crowley et al., 1975, 1976; Soulairac and Soulairac, 1975; Foreman and Moss, 1978).

Furthermore, synthetic LH-RH has been described as a possible potentiator of sexual behavior in rats (Moss and McCann, 1973). Ovariectomized rats treated with estrogen in dosages too low to provoke estrous behavior, displayed this behavior when given an s.c. injection of LH-RH. Estrogen-primed ovariectomized rats infused with LH-RH through cannulas placed in the preoptic area or ventromedial-arcuate complex also showed more lordotic behavior than saline-treated animals. In the castrated and testosterone-primed male rat, LH-RH enhanced mating behavior as measured by a significant decrease in time to the first intromission and to subsequent ejaculation. The LH-RH may act on sexual behavior by modulating neurotransmission, particularly through effects on α- and β-adrenergic receptors (Foreman and Moss, 1978). However, no mating behavior was observed in castrated female or male rats treated with LH-RH alone (Moss et al., 1975).

Finally, estrogen was found to affect specific enzyme activities (e.g., choline acetyltransferase, tyrosine hydroxylase, monoamine oxidase, or catechol-o-methyltransferase) in discrete brain regions (McEwen *et al.,* 1978; Breuer *et al.,* 1978). Hence, sex hormones may activate sexual behavior, at least in part, by changing neurotransmitter metabolism in the brain.

5. *Influence of Sexual Stimuli and Stressful Situations on Sex Hormone Secretion*

Sex hormones not only affect sexual behavior, but behavior can also alter gonadotropin and sex hormone secretion. For example, it seems that sexual stimuli are able to increase the testosterone level in males. Thus, the testes of male rhesus monkeys were reactivated during the nonbreeding season if the males were placed together with estrogen-treated females (Vandenburgh, 1969). Moreover, testicular reactivation was observed even when the males were only exposed to the sight or sound of breeding females (Gordon and Bernstein, 1973). In men, testosterone levels may be raised also by sexual activity or anticipation of it (Annonymous, 1970).

In females, too, mating behavior can affect gonadotropin and sex hormone secretion. For example, copulation can provoke an ovulation-inducing increase of LH secretion, especially in reflex ovulators. All these data indicate that brain regions involved in the expression of sexual behavior as well as those concerned with the secretion of gonadotropins may exert some functional interactions.

Finally, it may be mentioned that the testosterone level in male monkeys as well as in men is significantly decreased by stressful situations (Kreuz *et al.,* 1972; Nakashima *et al.,* 1975).

II. Sexual Differentiation of the Brain

A. Gonadotropin Secretion

1. *The Significance of the Gonads for the Differentiation of Cyclic or Tonic Gonadotropin Secretion*

Female mammals are characterized by cyclic hypophysial gonadotropin secretion during sexual maturity, whereas male mammals display a tonic release of gonadotropins. Cyclic gonadotropin secretion can be demonstrated indirectly by the presence of corpora lutea in the ovaries or by cyclic changes of the vaginal epithelium. For example, infantile ovaries transplanted into postpubertally castrated female rats formed corpora lutea, and the vaginas of these animals showed cyclic alterations of the epithelium (Goodman, 1934). On the other hand, ovaries transplanted into postpubertally castrated or intact male rodents failed to develop corpora lutea (Goodman, 1934; Harris, 1964; Gorski and Wagner, 1965). Furthermore, vaginas transplanted in addition to the ovaries into male rats exhibited persistent estrus (Yazaki, 1960).

The crucial experiment on sex-specific differentiation of cyclic or tonic gonadotropin secretion was done by Pfeiffer (1936). He castrated newborn female rats and implanted ovaries in adulthood. These animals showed normal vaginal cycles, and fresh corpora lutea were found in the ovaries. If, however, testicular tissue was implanted into the neonatally spayed females immediately after castration, corpora lutea did not develop in the ovaries transplanted during adulthood. These animals were found to be sterile and in persistent estrus. In contrast, corpora lutea were observed in ovaries transplanted into adult male rats that had been orchidectomized during the first days of life, but not later. These findings were confirmed by several authors (Harris, 1963; Döcke and Dörner, 1966; Gorski, 1967).

Hence, male and female rats are born with the latent capacity of cyclic gonadotropin secretion. If testes are present during the first days of life, a male differentiation will take place that gives rise to tonic gonadotropin secretion in adult life. The absence of testes during this critical developmental period, on the other hand, leads to female differentiation, irrespective of the presence or absence of ovaries.

2. *Androgen-Dependent Differentiation of Gonadotropin Secretion*

Shay and co-workers (1939) observed permanent sterility in female rats treated with testosterone during early postnatal life. This finding was soon confirmed by Bradbury (1941) and Wilson (1943). The ovaries of postnatally androgenized females did not contain any corpora lutea and the vaginas showed persistent estrus.

In later experiments, different quantities of androgens were administered to female mice and rats during different periods of pre- and/or postnatal life (Barraclough and Leathem, 1954, 1959; Harris and Levine, 1962; Levine and Mullins, 1966; Barraclough, 1967). Barraclough (1955, 1961) injected 1.25 mg of testosterone propionate (TP) on day 2, 5, 10, or 20 of life. The ovaries of all animals that had received the injection on day 2 or 5 of life failed to develop corpora lutea and showed some cystic follicles. These ovarian changes were found in only 40% of the females androgenized on day 10 of life, but they were completely missing in the animals androgenized on day 20. Therefore, the conclusion was drawn that a critical steroid-sensitive period does exist in female mice and rats between birth and day 10 of life. Androgen administration during this period results in permanent sterility. By injecting different doses of TP into female rats on day 5 of life, Barraclough (1967) achieved permanent sterility in 99.8% after 1.25 mg, in 70.6% after 10 μg, in 44% after 5 μg, and in 30% after 1 μg of TP.

Swanson and van der Werff ten Bosch (1964) injected 5 and 10 μg of TP as early as day 3 of life and did not find any corpora lutea in the ovaries of these animals during adulthood. When 2.5 mg of TP, on the other hand, were injected into pregnant rats during the last days of the gestation period, the female offspring exhibited normal ovarian function in adulthood (Swanson and van der Werff ten Bosch, 1964). Hence, it was assumed that the critical androgen-dependent differentiation period for cyclic or tonic gonadotropin secretion is timed during the first days of life in rats and mice as well as in hamsters (Swanson, 1966, 1970; Alleva et al., 1969).

However, Flerkó and co-workers (1967), who administered still higher doses of TP (5-16 mg) to pregnant female rats during the last days of gestation, induced anovulatory and polyfollicular ovaries in the female offspring associated with persistent estrus. Similar results were obtained by Kobayashi (1967). These data suggest that the androgen-dependent critical differentiation period for cyclic or tonic gonadotropin secretion in rats begins already prenatally.

In male rats, castration carried out during the first 3 days of life led to cyclic gonadotropin secretion (Pfeiffer, 1936; Kawashima, 1960; Yazaki, 1960; Harris, 1964). A similar effect was reached by perinatal administration of cyproterone acetate (Neumann and Elger, 1965, 1966; Neumann et al., 1966). In this case, the masculinizing effect of endogenous testosterone was competitively inhibited by this antiandrogenic substance. Finally, the masculinizing effect of exogenous testosterone on brain differentiation in newborn female rats could be prevented, at least in part, by simultaneous administration of cyproterone acetate (Neumann and Kramer, 1966; Wollman and Hamilton, 1967; Dörner and Fatschel, 1970).

Moreover, the following effects were observed in neonatally androgenized female rats:

1. Administration of TP during the first 3 days of life gives rise to inhibition or delay of vaginal opening (Swanson and van der Werff ten Bosch, 1963a; Wrenn et al., 1969; Dörner and Fatschel, 1970). In contrast, androgen administered during the following days can provoke even precocious vaginal opening (Harris and Levine, 1965; Barraclough, 1966; Feder, 1967).

2. The hypophysial gonadotropin content and gonadotropin secre-

tion are decreased in highly androgenized females (Matsuyama *et al.*, 1966; Dörner, 1969; Kurcz *et al.*, 1969b).

3. The estradiol uptake in the hypothalamus is significantly reduced in androgenized female rats (Flerkó *et al.*, 1969; Poppe *et al.*, 1975; Vértes *et al.*, 1977; Whalen and Olsen, 1978).

4. Ovulations can be induced in androgenized female rats by the administration of gonadotropins (Segal and Johnson, 1959; Dörner, 1962; Schuetz and Meyer, 1963). A similar effect was achieved by electrical stimulation of the hypothalamus (Barraclough and Gorski, 1961). Ovarian luteinization was also obtained in androgenized females after the removal of both ovaries and reimplantation of half an ovary (Swanson and van der Werff ten Bosch, 1963a).

5. Neonatally androgenized female rats show increased body growth (Swanson and van der Werff ten Bosch, 1963b; Harris, 1964; Dörner and Fatschel, 1970), and the hypophysial content of STH was significantly increased in these animals (Kurcz *et al.*, 1969a; Somana *et al.*, 1978).

6. Enzyme activities in the liver catalyzing steroid metabolism (e.g., 5α-reductase or 15β-hydroxylase) also underlie a sex-specific development in dependence on the androgen level occurring during a critical differentiation period (Schriefers *et al.*, 1979). Some sexual differences in hepatic steroid-metabolizing enzymes disappear not only after neonatal orchidectomy but also after adult hypophysectomy, which suggests that they are mediated by androgen-induced differentiation of the pituitary (Denef, 1972; Gustafsson and Stenberg, 1974). A feminizing factor called "feminotropin" was extracted from pituitary tissue and partially characterized (Mode *et al.*, 1978). However, some experimental results suggest that this factor is prolactin (Lax *et al.*, 1976; Schriefers *et al.*, 1979). The secretion of "feminotropin" is controlled by a release-inhibiting factor produced by a hypothalamic control center, which is assumed to be "turned on" by testicular androgen during brain differentiation.

3. Androgen-Dependent Differentiation of the Pituitary or Hypothalamus

Pfeiffer (1936) first assumed that the pituitary gland may be the site of action for the testicular hormone differentiating the sex-specific gonadotropin secretion. This hypothesis was disproved, however, by investigations of Harris and Jacobsohn (1951) and Martinez and Bittner (1956). They demonstrated that pituitaries of males transplanted under the hypothalamus of hypophysectomized females did not prevent normal ovarian cycles, ovulations, pregnancy, and delivery of normal litters. These findings suggest that the differences of the hypophysial gonadotropin secretion between males and females are based on different brain functions.

Moreover, Segal and Johnson (1959) implanted pituitaries of androgen-sterilized female rats into the sella turcica of hypophysectomized normal females and observed normal cycles and pregnancies in these animals. Finally, Nadler (1966) and Wagner *et al.* (1966) achieved permanent anovulatory sterility by intrahypothalamic implantation of minimal testosterone doses, which were ineffective when implanted systemically.

4. *Influence of Ovaries and Ovarian Hormones on Differentiation of Gonadotropin Secretion*

Pfeiffer (1936) was the first to observe that not the presence of ovaries, but the absence of testes, during a critical organization period is responsible for the differentiation of cyclic gonadotropin secretion. This independence of sex-specific brain differentiation from the ovaries has been repeatedly confirmed (Smith, 1967; Swanson, 1970; Yazaki, 1970).

Unphysiologically high estrogen doses are capable even of imitating the masculinizing differentiation effect of androgens on the brain of rodents. Thus, estrogen administration in newborn female rats or mice led to anovulatory sterility and persistent estrus (Turner, 1940; Wilson, 1943; Hale, 1944; Takasugi, 1963; Kikuyama, 1963; Gorski, 1963).

On the other hand, progestagens exert an antagonistic effect against androgens and estrogens on brain differentiation. Permanent changes of gonadotropin secretion caused by neonatal androgen or estrogen administration could be prevented, at least to a certain extent, by simultaneous injections of high doses of progesterone (Kincl and Maqueo, 1965; Dorfman, 1967). Hence, progestagens appear to possess some protective action on sex-specific brain differentiation. A similar effect was then achieved with the synthetic progestagen cyproterone acetate (Neumann and Kramer, 1966; Dörner and Fatschel, 1970).

5. *Action of Psychotropic Drugs and Inhibitors of DNA, RNA, and Protein Synthesis on Sex Hormone-Dependent Brain Differentiation*

a. Psychotropic Drugs. Kikuyama (1961) reported that the effects of androgens and estrogens on male-type brain differentiation in female rats could be prevented by simultaneous administration of reserpine. However, Simmons and Lusk (1969) were not able to confirm these observations in full.

In male rats, Kawashima (1964) administered reserpine during the hypothalamic differentiation phase and found corpus luteum development in ovaries that were implanted into these male animals during adulthood. Similar effects were obtained in guinea pigs and rabbits (Mitskevich and Borisova, 1974).

In female rats, Arai and Gorski (1968) demonstrated some protective actions of barbitals against the permanent sterilizing effect of androgens.

b. *Inhibitors of DNA, RNA, and Protein Synthesis.* Kobayashi and Gorski (1970) observed that actinomycin D and puromycin, inhibitors of RNA or protein synthesis, exerted some antagonism against the effect of androgen on hypothalamic differentiation. In female rats, 30 μg of TP were injected on day 5 of life together or without these inhibitors of RNA or protein synthesis. On day 45 of life, the animals treated with the combination showed significantly more corpus luteum development than those treated with androgen alone.

Salaman (1974) then reported that inhibitors of protein synthesis, puromycin and 5-fluorouracil, were effective only against a low dose of TP (30 μg) with respect to the differentiation of brain centers regulating gonadotropin secretion. On the other hand, the inhibitor of nucleoplasmic RNA synthesis, α-amanitin, gave almost complete protection against low and moderate doses of TP (30 and 80 μg) and considerable protection against a high dose of TP (200 μg). The inhibitor of DNA synthesis, hydroxyurea, was equally effective against moderate and high doses of TP.

These findings suggest a mode of androgen action on brain differentiation at the level of gene transcription initiating a sequence of selective mRNA and protein synthesis.

B. Sexual Behavior

1. *Findings in Genetic Females*

In 1938, a remarkable observation was reported by Vera Dantchakoff. Female guinea pigs, prenatally androgenized, exhibited strong male sexual behavior when the androgen treatment was repeated in adulthood.

Wilson et al. (1940) treated female rats with testosterone propionate (TP) during perinatal life and studied their sexual behavior in adulthood. The female mating activity of animals androgenized during the early postnatal life remained permanently inhibited and could not be elicited even by the administration of estrogens, whereas females androgenized prenatally (on days 14–16 of pregnancy) exhibited lordosis reflexes in adulthood. These findings indicated that in rats, in contrast to guinea pigs, the critical period for differentiation of sexual behavior is mainly timed during early postnatal life. Finally, androgen administration was begun on different days of postnatal life (Wilson et al., 1941a). Female rats treated with androgens from day 5 or 10 of life showed a clear-cut decrease of spontaneous estrus behavior, whereas the rats treated from day 15 of life exhibited normal female behavior.

On the other hand, female rats ovariectomized as early as on the first day of life were found to display normal female sexuality after sex hormone replacement in adulthood (Wilson et al., 1941b). Furthermore, Wilson (1943) reported that a permanent suppression of female sexual behavior can be achieved in female rats by estrogen if it is administered during early postnatal life. Finally, Koster (1943) found a considerable increase of male sexual behavior in adult female rats estrogenized postnatally.

During the last two decades, more precise quantitative studies have been carried out in order to evaluate sexual behavior of pre- and/or postnatally androgenized rodents. In female guinea pigs, prenatal androgen administration caused a permanent strong suppression of female sexual activity (Phoenix et al., 1959; Goy et al., 1964, 1967). These prenatally androgenized females were pseudohermaphrodites as a rule, presenting considerable masculinization of their genitalia. However, some androgenized females with more of less normal genitalia but impaired sexual behavior were also observed. Data obtained by Goy et al. (1964) suggested that in guinea pigs the androgen-sensitive phase for differentiation of sexual behavior may be timed between day 30 and 35 of prenatal life.

Gerall and Ward (1966) also observed inhibition of female sexuality in female rats androgenized prenatally, but Revesz et al. (1963) and Whalen et al. (1966) did not. On the other hand, in female rats androgenized during the first days of postnatal life, a permanent suppression of female sexual behavior has been reported by several authors (Barraclough and Gorski, 1962; Ericsson and Baker, 1966; Nadler, 1966; Dörner and Fatschel, 1970).

Pre- and/or early postnatal androgen treatment led not only to decreased female, but also to increased male, sexual behavior, e.g., in female guinea pigs (Phoenix et al., 1959; Goy et al., 1964; Gerall, 1966), rats (Harris and Levine, 1962, 1965; Gerall and Ward, 1966; Nadler, 1966; Dörner and Fatschel, 1970), hamsters (Swanson, 1970; Swanson et al., 1974), and monkeys (Young et al., 1964; Goy et al.,

1977). Finally, perinatally androgenized animals also showed increased aggressiveness in adult life (Feder, 1967; Gerall, 1967; Bronson and Desjardin, 1969; Swanson et al., 1974).

In view of these findings, it can be concluded that androgens can induce a male-type differentiation of central nervous regions responsible for sexual behavior, irrespective of the genetic sex. On the other hand, ovarian hormones are not necessary for the differentiation of central nervous regions that regulate female sexual behavior (Whalen and Edwards, 1967).

Unphysiologically high estrogen doses administered during brain differentiation are able even to imitate the effect of androgens and to suppress female sexual behavior for the entire life (Whalen and Nadler, 1963; Gerall, 1967). After androgen administration in adulthood, male behavior increased significantly in such neonatally estrogenized females (Levine and Mullins, 1964; Dörner et al., 1971a).

2. Findings in Genetic Males

Several authors have reported increased female sexual behavior in male rats that had been orchidectomized immediately after birth and treated with estrogen and progestagen during adulthood (Grady and Phoenix, 1963; Harris, 1964; Feder and Whalen, 1965; Grady et al., 1965; Whalen and Edwards, 1966, 1967). After androgen replacement in adult life, neonatally orchidectomized males showed less male sexual activity than males castrated later (Beach and Holz, 1946; Harris, 1964; Whalen and Edwards, 1967; Larsson, 1966, 1967). In male hamsters orchidectomized during the first 2 days of life, male sexual behavior was completely missing even after androgen substitution in adult life (Swanson, 1970).

Neumann and Elger (1966) achieved partial feminization of sexual behavior in male rats by injecting the antiandrogen cyproterone acetate during the last week of prenatal life and the first 3 weeks of postnatal life. After castration and implantation of ovaries, these feminized genetic males (male pseudohermaphrodites) exhibited some female sexual behavior, associated with prolonged vaginal cycles.

Neumann et al. (1967) also examined the sexual behavior of male rats treated with cyproterone acetate only during the first 2 weeks of postnatal life. After orchidectomy and implantation of ovaries, they showed some increased female behavior although they possessed male genitalia. Without castration and implantation of ovaries, however, these animals exhibited atypical male behavior. These findings suggested that a partial inhibition of male brain differentiation can be achieved by antiandrogens administered during the critical period of brain organization.

III. Animal Experiments in Our Laboratory on Sex Hormone-Dependent Brain Development

In our laboratory, parallel testing of sexual behavior in rats of both sexes was generally carried out with both female and male partners, i.e., observing behavior toward partners of the same and the opposite sex. This method permitted an evaluation of sexual preference for partners of the same or opposite sex (Dörner, 1967, 1976).

A significant predominance of heterotypical behavior, i.e., sexual behavior contrary to the genetic, gonadal, and somatophenotypic sex, was defined by our group as homosexuality. In such case, sexual activities toward partners of the same sex occurred significantly more often than those toward partners of the opposite sex. In other words, these animals were sexually stimulated preferentially by partners of the same sex. When hetero- and homotypical behavioral responses were equally frequent, these animals were termed bisexual. Heterosexuality was defined by a significant predominance of homotypical behavior, i.e., of sexual behavior in accordance with the genetic, gonadal, and somatophenotypic sex. In this case, sexual activities toward partners of the opposite sex occurred significantly more often than those toward partners of the same sex.

Such differentiation between homo-, bi-, and heterosexual behavior (Dörner, 1967, 1976) had not been attempted before; previous studies were confined to tests of behavior toward female or male partners after androgen and estrogen treatment, respectively. After androgen treatment in adult life, neonatally castrated males or androgenized females had been tested only with female partners, whereas after estrogen (with or without progestagen) treatment in adult life they had been tested only with male partners (Harris and Levine, 1962, 1965; Grady and Phoenix, 1963; Whalen and Nadler, 1963; Harris, 1964; Levine and Mullins, 1964; Feder and Whalen, 1965; Grady *et al.*, 1965; Larsson, 1966, 1967; Whalen and Edwards, 1966, 1967; Gerall and Ward, 1966; Goy *et al.*, 1967).

1. *Findings in Females*

a. Effects of Androgens on Brain Differentiation. Female rats androgenized with 1.25 mg of TP on day 3 of postnatal life showed persistent estrus, polycystic ovaries without corpora lutea, infertility, and reduced heterosexual behavior in adulthood. After postpubertal ovariectomy plus androgen treatment, predominantly heterotypical, i.e., "homosexual" behavior, was observed. By contrast, females treated with 1.25 mg of TP on day 15 or neonatally untreated and postpubertally equally treated females exhibited predominantly homotypical, i.e., heterosexual, behavior (Dörner, 1968, 1976; Dörner and Fatschel, 1970).

In female rats androgenized with 1.25 mg of TP on day 10 of life, cyclic gonadotropin secretion, as indicated by ovulations and vaginal cycles, was found. Nevertheless, these animals also showed "homosexual" behavior after ovariectomy plus androgen administration in adult life. This finding suggests a time-dependent partial dissociation between the differentiation of sex and mating centers in the brain, that are responsible for the control of gonadotropin secretion and sexual behavior, respectively.

Adult female rats androgenized with 0.02 mg of TP on day 3 of life had polyfollicular ovaries with some corpora lutea. These animals were found to be subfertile. Postpubertal ovariectomy plus androgen treatment resulted in bisexual behavior. Such permanent effects on ovarian functions and sexual behavior produced by 0.02 mg of TP when administered on day 3 could be prevented by simultaneous administration of the antiandrogen cyproterone acetate (Dörner and Fatschel, 1970; Dörner, 1976).

b. *Complete Inversion of Sexual Behavior.* In a further experiment, rats of both sexes were highly androgenized during late prenatal and early postnatal life (Dörner, 1968). Five milligrams of TP were administered s.c. to the mother animals on days 17, 19, and 21 of gestation. Cesarean section was performed on day 22 of gestation, and 0.5 mg of TP plus 2 mg of testosterone phenylpropionate were injected on day 2 of postnatal life. When adult, the animals were castrated and received daily injections of 1 mg of TP for 10 days and 0.25 mg of TP for the following 18 days.

Androgen administration to female rats during the late prenatal plus early postnatal life produced a complete male differentiation of the brain. With regard to their sexual behavior, the perinatally androgenized females could not be distinguished from equally treated male littermates. Female activity was completely abolished. After androgen treatment in adulthood the frequency of mountings and ejaculatory-type patterns as well as the refractory periods between the ejaculatory-type activities did not differ significantly between the genetic females and males. The perinatally androgenized females mounted and showed ejaculatory-type behavioral patterns, when exposed to females or even to neonatally castrated males that reacted with lordosis responses (Fig. 2). Hence a complete inversion of sexual behavior was achieved by alterations of the androgen level during the period of brain differentiation plus androgen administration during the postpubertal activation period. These findings suggested that the direction of sex drive is determined—independently of genetic sex—by the androgen level during a critical differentiation phase of the brain.

c. *Androgen-Dependent Brain Differentiation and Life-Span.* Neonatal androgen treatment in female rats (1.25 mg of TP on the first day of life) resulted in a significantly shorter life-span than that of untreated controls. In male rats, on the other hand, orchidectomy on the first day of life resulted in a significantly longer life than that of intact males (Dörner, 1973) and of males orchidectomized on day 75 of life (Dörner and Hinz, 1975).

These findings indicate a negative correlation between the androgen level during brain differentiation and duration of life. Independently of

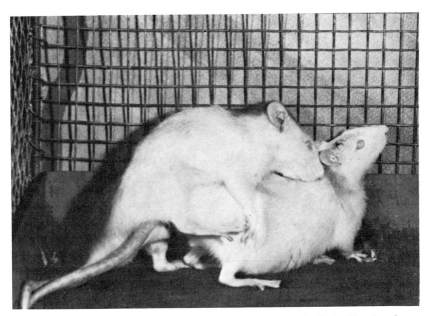

FIG. 2. Female rat mounting a male rat that is showing lordosis. The female was perinatally and postpubertally treated with testosterone propionate, and the male was castrated neonatally and substituted with androgen during adulthood. A total sex hormone-dependent inversion of sexual behavior is demonstrated. From Dörner (1972, 1976).

genetic sex, a low androgen level during brain differentiation appears to be correlated with a relatively long duration of life, and vice versa.

d. *"Paradoxical Effects" of Estrogen on Brain Differentiation.* Anovulatory sterility with polycystic ovaries as well as diminished female and in some cases enhanced male sexual activity were observed in female rats after high doses of estrogen administered during brain differentiation (Wilson, 1943; Takewaki, 1962; Gorski, 1963; Whalen and Nadler, 1963; Levine and Mullins, 1964). These data, which suggested paradoxical, i.e., androgen-like effects of estrogen on brain differentiation, were reinvestigated. Furthermore, the influence of early postnatal estrogen treatment on the postpubertal evocability of a positive estrogen-feedback effect was examined (Dörner *et al.,* 1971a).

In female rats treated with 100 μg of estradiol benzoate (EB) on the first day of life, the following data were obtained in adult or juvenile life: Predominance of persistent vaginal estrus, significantly enhanced male and completely suppressed female sexual behavior associated with an increased attractiveness to male test partners, hypogonadotropic hypogonadism, sterility, a significant increase of postpubertal body growth, and nonevocability of a positive estrogen feedback effect on LH secretion. A paradoxical, androgen-like influence of estrogen on brain differentiation was offered as an explanation of these findings.

Moreover, persistent vaginal estrus and anovulatory ovaries were found in adult rats that had been implanted with paraffin micropellets containing 0.5% EB into the mediobasal hypothalamus on day 4 of life, in contrast to the absence of these effects in experimental controls that had received intrahypothalamic paraffin pellets or EB-paraffin implants located subcutaneously or in other brain regions (Döcke and Dörner, 1975). This finding suggested that the mediobasal hypothalamus is a site of estrogen action on sex-specific brain differentiation.

More recently, Christensen and Gorski (1978) reported that there appear to be specific neuronal sites where implantation of testosterone (T) or estradiol (E) produces independent masculinization of gonadotropin secretion and sexual behavior. The ventromedial hypothalamus was found to be the only area in which neonatal implants of T or E produced acyclic gonadotropin secretion in adults. On the other hand, neonatal implants of T or E in the dorsal preoptic area increased the amount of male sexual behavior in adult life.

e. *Androgen-Dependent Brain Differentiation Mediated by Conversion of Androgens to Estrogens.* As described before, the androgen-like effects of estrogen on brain differentiation were produced even by estrogen doses that were much lower than effective androgen doses. This finding indicated that androgens may be aromatized to estrogens in the brain for sex-specific differentiation processes. The presence of aromatizing enzymes in the brain has been demonstrated by several investigators (Knapstein et al., 1968; Naftolin et al., 1971; Weisz and Gibbs, 1974; Lieberburg and McEwen, 1975; McEwen et al., 1977).

Furthermore, neonatal treatment with a nonaromatizable androgen, such as dihydrotestosterone (DHT), was found to be ineffective (Luttge and Whalen, 1970; McDonald et al., 1970; McDonald and Doughty, 1974) or only partially effective (Gerall et al., 1975, 1976) with respect to sex-specific brain differentiation. On the other hand, testosterone-induced masculinization (Vreeburg et al., 1977; McEwen et al., 1978) as well as estrogen-induced masculinization of the brain (Södersten, 1978a, b) could be prevented, at least in part, by antiestrogens, which compete with estradiol for the receptor sites in the brain. Attenuation of the masculinizing effects of both endogenous and exogenous testosterone on brain differentiation was also achieved by inhibitors of aromatizing enzymes, which block the conversion of testosterone to estradiol (Booth, 1978; McEwen et al., 1977; Vreeburg et al., 1977).

Target cells of the brain that concentrate estrogens were demonstrated by ^{3}H-labeled steroid autoradiography in the hypothalamus, preoptic area, or limbic system in 2-day-old neonatal rats (Sheridan et al., 1975) as well as in 16-day-old fetal mice (Stumpf and Sar, 1978).

It is assumed that the fetal and neonatal female brain of rodents is protected, at least in part, from masculinization by circulating endogenous estrogens through functional inactivation by an estrogen-binding α-fetoprotein (Nunez et al., 1971; Raynaud, 1973; Puig-Duran et al., 1979). Testosterone, on the other hand, which is not bound by α-fetoprotein, has free access to specific androgen-binding receptors (Lieberburg et al., 1978) in the neonatal brain, where it appears to be partially aromatized to estradiol.

All these findings support the hypothesis that androgen-dependent sex-specific brain differentiation in rodents may be mediated, at least in part, by the conversion of androgens to estrogens.

However, testosterone is also irreversibly metabolized to 5α-dihydrotestosterone in the brain (Jaffe, 1969; Kniewald et al., 1971; Poppe et al., 1974; Martini, 1978). In this context, it should be noted that the nonaromatizable 5α-dihydrotestosterone and the aromatizable testosterone were equally capable of imparting male psychological traits, particularly male-like mounting behavior, to genetic female rhesus monkeys treated prenatally with one of these androgens (Goy et al., 1977). On the other hand, domestic pigs exposed prenatally to high estrogen doses displayed no increase, but instead a significant decrease, of male-like mounting behavior in adult life, even after castration and androgen treatment (Dörner *et al.*, 1977a).

Although in rats estrogens converted from androgens within the brain appear to be most important for sexual differentiation of the brain, in other mammals, particularly in primates, androgens themselves may be responsible for sexual differentiation of the brain. This hypothesis would be consistent with the observation that estrogens are bound by α-fetoprotein in fetal and neonatal rats, but not in fetal and neonatal primates (Swartz and Soloff, 1974).

2. Findings in Males

a. *"Homosexual" Behavior of Neonatally Orchidectomized Males Substituted with Estrogen plus Progestagen or Androgen in Adulthood.* Several authors have reported on strong female (heterotypical) sexual behavior in male rats orchidectomized shortly after birth and treated with estrogen plus progestagen in adulthood (Grady and Phoenix, 1963; Harris, 1964; Feder and Whalen, 1965; Grady *et al.*, 1965; Whalen and Edwards, 1966, 1967).

In homosexual men, however, a normal or approximately normal androgen level is found in adult life (Kinsey, 1941; Dörner *et al.*, 1975b). Hence, human male homosexuality can be explained only by a neuroendocrine predisposition, if homosexual, i.e., predominantly heterotypical sexual, behavior can also be induced by androgens in adult life in genetic and phenotypic males. Therefore, investigations were carried out to see whether such an experimental model could be produced in rats (Dörner, 1967; Dörner and Hinz, 1967).

The following findings were obtained: Genotypic and phenotypic males orchidectomized on the day of birth showed predominantly heterotypical (female) sexual behavior after androgen substitution in adulthood. The percentage of tests with female (heterotypical) sexual behavior toward normal males was significantly higher than the percentage of tests with male (homotypical) behavior toward estrous females. Hence, we believe that male "homosexuality" was produced in these animals, which were sexually more stimulated by males than by females.

In contrast, this "homosexual" behavior was observed neither in intact males nor males castrated between day 14 and 22 of postnatal life and substituted with androgen in adulthood. These animals did not exhibit any lordosis reflexes when mounted by vigorous male test partners. They showed either apathetic behavior or rejected their isosexual (male) test partners. Some bisexual behavior was observed in only one out of 20 intact male rats. Besides male sexual activity toward estrous females, a few lordosis reflexes toward vigorous males were seen in this one male.

In another experiment, male "homosexuality" was produced in male rats orchidectomized on the day of birth when testes were implanted during adulthood (Dörner *et al.*, 1968a).

In view of these experimental data the following hypothesis was advanced: In genetic males, androgen deficiency during a critical period of brain differentiation can lead to a female organization of specific brain regions. During the postpubertal activation phase, testosterone then stimulates the female-differentiated brain. As a result, homosexuality in genetic and somatophenotypic males can occur.

b. Prevention of Experimental "Homosexuality" in Male Rats by Testosterone Administered during Brain Differentiation. In another experiment, we investigated whether and to what extent male "homosexuality" observed in neonatally castrated and later androgen-substituted males can be prevented by androgen administered during brain differentiation (Dörner and Hinz, 1968). Therefore, male rats orchidectomized on the day of birth were injected s.c. with 1.25 mg of testosterone propionate (TP) on day 3 of life. In adulthood, these animals received daily s.c. injections of 1.0 mg TP for 12 days followed by daily injections of 0.25 mg of TP for 18 days. After this treatment they exhibited clear heterosexual behavior. This finding suggests that male "homosexuality" in rats based on androgen deficiency during brain differentiation can be prevented once and for all by androgen administered during the critical differentiation period.

c. Primary Male Hypo-, Bi-, and Homosexuality in Rats as an Expression of Different Degrees of Androgen Deficiency during Sex-Specific Brain Differentiation. A positive correlation was found between the androgen level during brain differentiation and male sexual behavior during the postpubertal activation period. Simultaneously, a negative correlation was observed between the androgen level during brain differentiation and female sexual behavior during the postpubertal activation phase (Dörner, 1969). In view of these results, the conclusion was drawn that neuroendocrine conditioned primary hypo-, bi-, and homosexuality can be caused by different degrees of androgen deficiency during sex-specific brain differentiation in genetic males.

On the other hand, when unphysiologically high androgen doses were administered to male or even female rats during the critical (perinatal) differentiation period, clearly more male sexual activity was observed in these animals after postpubertal castration and androgen treatment than in perinatally untreated, but postpubertally equally treated males. This finding indicates that primary male hypersexuality can be based on temporary hyperandrogenicity during brain differentiation (Dörner, 1969; Götz et al., 1974).

Finally, male rats were castrated on day 14 of life and substituted with androgens during adulthood. In these animals, male sexual behavior was permanently reduced and atrophy of accessory sex organs occurred, despite prolonged androgen replacement in doses that proved to be fully sufficient to restore normal sexual behavior and normal weight of accessory sex organs in males castrated at puberty, i.e., at the end of the prepubertal maturation phase (Götz and Dörner, 1976). These findings suggest that in genetic males a specific androgen level is necessary not only during the differentiation phase, but also during the maturation phase, in order to obtain normal responsiveness of androgen-dependent organs, in particular of the brain.

   d. *Sex-Specific Brain Differentiation and the Evocability of a Positive Estrogen Feedback.* My teacher Hohlweg (1934) was the first to demonstrate a positive estrogen feedback. Administration of estrogen to intact juvenile rats led to corpus luteum formation. On the other hand, corpus luteum formation could not be induced by estrogen in hypophysectomized animals (Hohlweg and Chamorro, 1937). Hence, it was concluded that estrogen administered in intact female rats results in increased secretion of hypophysial LH. Meanwhile, this so-called "Hohlweg effect" was observed in females of several species, and numerous investigations speak in favor of the idea that the positive estrogen feedback also plays a decisive role in the regulation of cyclic gonadotropin secretion and ovarian function in women.

   Therefore, we carried out experimental studies to investigate the significance of sex hormone-dependent brain differentiation for the evocability of a positive estrogen feedback effect (Dörner and Döcke, 1964a, b; Döcke and Dörner, 1966). In a first experiment, infantile ovaries were implanted under the kidney capsule of juvenile female or male rats followed by castration and s.c. injection of 30 μg of estradiol benzoate (EB). Four days later, corpus luteum formation was observed in the ovarian implants of female host animals. In contrast, male host animals as well as neonatally androgenized female host animals failed to develop any corpora lutea in the implanted ovaries after estrogen administration.

   In a second experiment, male rats were orchidectomized on day 1 or 5 of life. One infantile ovary was implanted immediately after castration and a second one on day 21, the female donor animals always being of the same age as the male host animals. On day 24 the male host animals were injected s.c. with 30 μg of EB. In 15 out of 20 male host animals orchidectomized on the first postnatal day, corpus luteum formation was induced by estrogen administration. In contrast, 14 out of 15 male host animals orchidectomized on day 5 failed to develop any corpora lutea after estrogen treatment.

These findings suggested that the evocability of a corpus luteum-inducing positive estrogen-feedback is dependent on the androgen level during a critical period of sex-specific brain differentiation. The higher the androgen level during this period, the lower appears to be the evocability of a positive estrogen-feedback in later life. Meanwhile, surges of LH secretion after estrogen administration were also described in female rats, in contrast to males or neonatally androgenized females (Neill, 1972; Mennin and Gorski, 1975).

Similar sex-specific differences were first obtained in female and male rhesus monkeys after a single injection of estrogen (Yamai *et al.*, 1971). However, when castrated rhesus monkeys were primed by estrogen implantations, an additional injection of estrogen induced an increase of LH secretion in males in a similar way as in females (Karsch *et al.*, 1973).

Hence, we concluded that the difference between the responses of male and female monkeys to the stimulatory action of estrogen appears to be a quantitative rather than a qualitative one, which may be abolished by prolonged exposure to low estrogen concentration. Moreover, the conclusion was drawn that the scheme for sexual differentiation of the central nervous system of rodents, related to the control of gonadotropin secretion, may not be applicable to primates, including men (Karsch *et al.*, 1973; Knobil, 1974).

Therefore, the evocability of a positive estrogen-feedback was reexamined in postpubertally castrated and estrogen- or androgen-primed male and female rats as well as in castrated and estrogen-primed men suffering from prostatic cancer.

Adult male and female rats were spayed and treated daily with 1 μg of EB or 200 μg of TP for 18 days (Dörner *et al.*, 1975b). On day 15 of sex hormone priming, an additional s.c. injection of 15 μg of EB per 100 gm body weight was administered at 8 AM. Blood samples were always taken at 4 PM, i.e., 40 and 16 hours before (initial values), and 8, 32, 56, and 80 hours after, the injection of 15 μg of EB. Serum LH levels were determined by radioimmunoassay (Niswender *et al.*, 1968).

The results are shown in Fig. 3. Castrated and estrogen-primed females showed a distinct surge of LH secretion, with a serum LH peak demonstrable 56 hours after the administration of 15 μg of EB. Castrated and androgen-primed females displayed a diminished and, in particular, a delayed surge of LH secretion, showing the highest serum LH level as late as at least 80 hours after EB administration. Cas-

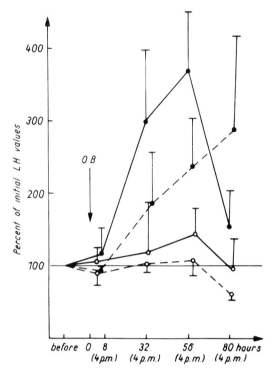

FIG. 3. Serum luteinizing hormone (LH) response to an s.c. injection of estradiol benzoate (OB) (15 μg/100 gm body weight) expressed as percentage of the mean initial LH values in postpubertally castrated and estrogen- or androgen-primed female and male rats (means and SEM). ●————●, Castrated and estrogen-primed female rats (N=8); ●---●, castrated and androgen-primed female rats (N=5); ○————○, castrated and estrogen-primed male rats (N=4); ○---○, castrated and androgen-primed male rats (N=5). From Dörner *et al.* (1975b).

trated and estrogen-primed males exhibited only a slight, but significant, increase of LH secretion ($p < 0.05$), with a serum LH peak demonstrable 56 hours after the administration of 15 μg of EB. The percentage increase of the serum LH level was significantly less in the estrogen-primed males than in the estrogen-primed females. Castrated and androgen-primed male rats, on the other hand, did not display any surge of LH secretion after EB administration.

In view of our findings obtained in rats, we drew the following conclusion: The evocability of a positive estrogen-feedback effect is dependent on the sex hormone levels during a critical differentiation phase and functional (priming) phase as well.

In case of a low androgen level during the differentiation period (e.g., in females or neonatally castrated males), a relatively strong positive estrogen-feedback action on LH secretion will be elicited after estrogen priming during the activation phase. On the other hand, after androgen priming a diminished and delayed positive estrogen feedback action on LH secretion will be evoked. In case of a high androgen level during the critical differentiation period (e.g., in males), a relatively slight positive estrogen-feedback action on LH secretion can be elicited only after estrogen priming during the activation phase.

These conclusions are consistent with findings obtained in humans (Dörner *et al.*, 1975d). Thus, castrated and estrogen-primed heterosexual men exhibited only a slight, but significant, increase of serum LH levels after an additional estrogen injection. On the other hand, intact heterosexual men did not display àny increase of LH values after an estrogen injection, in clear contrast to heterosexual women. Sex-specific differences in estrogen-induced gonadotropin release were also observed in hamsters (Buhl *et al.*, 1978), sheep (Clarke *et al.*, 1977), and pigs (Elsaesser and Parvizi, 1979).

3. *Sexual Dimorphism of the Brain*

Ifft (1964) had found in rats that the nucleolar size of specific hypothalamic neurons was changed after ovariectomy. Döcke and Koloczek (1966), from our group, then observed sex-specific differences in the nuclear size of anterior hypothalamic nerve cells between intact male and female rats. Finally, Pfaff (1966) described some differences in the nucleolar and nuclear sizes of nerve cells in specific brain regions between four male rats castrated at 7 days of age, and three intact male and two intact female littermates. Thus, some sex-specific differences of brain morphology had been observed, and they could be explained by different actual sex hormone levels during adulthood and, at least in part, during brain development as well.

Hence, we examined whether temporary changes of sex hormone levels produced during brain differentiation could lead, in fact, to permanent changes of brain structures associated with permanent changes of brain functions (Dörner and Staudt, 1968, 1969a).

Male rats of the Sprague-Dawley strain were castrated (or sham-operated) on the day of birth. Some of the neonatally castrated males were treated once with 1.25 mg of TP at 3 days of age. On the other hand, male and female rats were castrated after 14 days of age, i.e., after the critical period of brain differentiation. All of these animals were equally treated in adult life, i.e., 1.0 mg of TP was injected s.c. every day for 11 days followed by daily injections of 0.25 mg of TP for 18 days.

The following findings were obtained in the preoptic-anterior hypothalamic area and/or in the ventromedial hypothalamic nuclei, in contrast to the dorsomedial hypothalamic nuclei (Fig. 4). Postpubertally castrated plus androgen-treated female rats exhibited significantly larger nuclear sizes of the nerve cells in the preoptic-anterior and ventromedial hypothalamic region than male rats castrated after 14 days of age and equally treated in adulthood or intact males. Male rats orchidectomized on the day of birth also displayed significantly larger nuclear sizes of neurons than males castrated after 14 days of age or intact males. The nuclear size of females was approximately reached by the males castrated on the day of birth. These permanent structural changes caused by orchidectomy on the day of birth could be prevented by 1.25 mg of TP if administered at 3 days of age.

Furthermore, a significant correlation was demonstrated between the nuclear sizes of nerve cells in these brain regions and sexual behavior. The enlargement of nuclear volumes was correlated with an

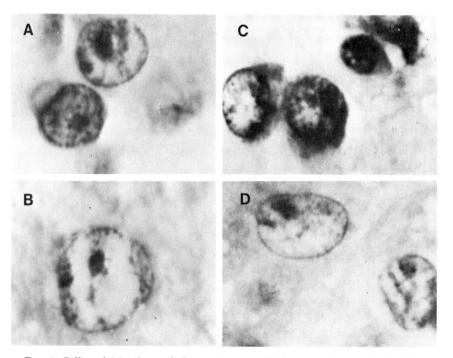

FIG. 4. Cell nuclei in the medial preoptic area: (A) intact male rat; (B) female rat castrated postpubertally and androgen-treated in adult life; (C) male rat orchidectomized after 14 days of life and androgen-treated in adulthood; (D) male rat orchidectomized on the day of birth and androgen-treated in adult life. From Dörner (1972, 1976).

increase of female, and decrease of male, sexual behavior (Dörner and Staudt, 1968).

Subsequently, the nuclear size of nerve cells in preoptic and hypothalamic regions as well as the ependyma matrix of these cells was investigated from day 16 of fetal life, in an attempt to find morphological indications for the beginning and ending of sexual differentiation of the brain (Dörner and Staudt, 1969b). While the medial preoptic area and the ventromedial nuclei were not yet clearly demarcated on day 16 of fetal life, they were well developed on day 18. Up to day 20, no significant morphological sex differences could be observed within these regions. During the last 2 days of gestation (days 20-22), however, a significant increase of the nuclear sizes in the preoptic area and the ventromedial nuclei took place in female fetuses only. Consequently, at the time of birth the nuclear volumes of nerve cells in these regions were significantly larger in females than in males.

The nerve cell nuclei of these regions further increased up to 2 weeks of age and then remained nearly unchanged up to adult life. In addition, at 2 weeks of age, there was a reduction of the ependyma matrix, which is responsible for the development of nerve cells in these brain regions, from about three cellular layers to a single ependyma layer. At this time, sex-specific brain differentiation appears to be ended, because the brain may be masculinized by sex hormones only as long as proliferating matrix ependyma bordering the third ventricle is present.

Ultrastructural differences in the preoptic area between intact male and female rats as well as between feminized males and masculinized females were then also observed (Raisman and Field, 1971, 1973). The number of synapses ending on dendritic spines of nonamygdaloid afferents in the preoptic area was found to be higher in intact females than in intact males. Moreover, castration of the males within 12 hours after birth (but not at 7 days of age) caused an increase to the female level. Conversely, females treated with 1.25 mg of TP at 4 days of age (but not at 16 days) showed a low number of spine synapses in the male range.

Permanent morphological alterations in the brain produced by perinatal exposure of rodents to sex hormones have included: (a) ultrastructural features of synaptic vesicles in the hypothalamic arcuate nucleus (Ratner and Adamo, 1971; King, 1972; Matsumoto and Arai, 1976); (b) dendritic branching patterns in the medial preoptic area (Greenough et al., 1977) as well as neuritic proliferation and branching in the preoptic area and infundibular-premammillary regions of in vitro preparations (Toran-Allerand, 1978); and (c) sex-specific differences in the gross extent of a component of the medial preoptic area, which is significantly larger in male and neonatally androgenized female rats than in normal female rats (Gorski *et al.*, 1977, 1978). Furthermore, Nottebohm and Arnold (1976) had described a similar sexual dimorphism in the brain of songbirds, i.e., in vocal control areas of the brain that participate in singing, a learned but clearly androgen-dependent behavior.

A clear sexual dimorphism that is dependent on sex hormone levels during brain differentiation was also observed in the medial and central part of the amygdala in rats (Staudt and Dörner, 1976). Morphological sex differences appear also to exist in the medial part of the amygdala in squirrel monkeys, since the nuclear sizes of these neurons are significantly different in normal males from those in ovariectomized females replaced with estrogen and progesterone (Bubenik and Brown, 1973).

4. *Neurotransmitters as Possible Mediators for Sexual Differentiation of the Brain*

As described above, neurotransmitters participate in the control of gonadotropin secretion and sexual behavior as well. Furthermore, permanent changes of gonadotropin secretion occur in rats after administration of the catecholamine-depletor reserpine in neonatal life (Kikuyama, 1961; Kawashima, 1964; Carraro *et al.*, 1965). In addition, we observed permanent changes of sexual behavior after such treatment (Dörner *et al.*, 1968a). Neonatally reserpinized male rats exhibited a significant decrease of male, combined with a significant increase of female, behavior in adulthood. After postpubertal castration and estrogen administration, they even displayed predominantly heterotypical, i.e., "homosexual" behavior, in contrast to equally treated but nonreserpinized control males.

We have obtained additional experimental data that suggest that neurotransmitters are not only temporary activators or inhibitors, but also organizers, of sexual behavior (Dörner, 1976; Dörner *et al.*, 1976b, 1977c).

Rats were treated with the monoamine oxidase inhibitor pargyline, the catecholamine-depletor reserpine, or the acetylcholinesterase-inhibitor pyridostigmine during the first 2 weeks of life. These animals showed significant permanent changes not only in their sexual behavior, but also in conditioned avoidance behavior, emotional reactivity, and exploratory activity, throughout life.

As shown in Fig. 5, male sexual activity was permanently decreased in males treated neonatally with pargyline, but permanently increased

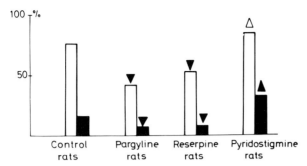

FIG. 5. Male sexual behavior in juvenile and adult male rats after treatment with pargyline, reserpine, or pyridostigmine during the first 2 weeks of life. Male sexuality was expressed as percentage of positive tests with mounting and ejaculation when exposed to castrated and estrogen-treated female rats; significantly decreased and significantly increased as compared to the controls (▼ and ▲, $p < 0.001$; △, $p < 0.05$). □, Tests with mounting; ■, tests with ejaculation. From Dörner (1977a).

in those treated with pyridostigmine. Male sexual activity was also increased in adult male rats treated neonatally with the serotonin synthesis inhibitor p-chlorophenylalanine. The mounting frequency in 8 adult males treated neonatally with p-chlorophenylalanine (0.5 mg on days 1 and 4 and 1.0 mg on days 7 and 10) was significantly higher than in 13 control males (means ± SD: 9.7 ± 1.8 and 6.3 ± 2.5 mountings per 5 minutes, respectively; t test: $p < 0.01$). Females treated neonatally with pargyline also showed a permanent decrease, and those given pyridostigmine showed a permanent significant increase, in male mounting behavior (Dörner *et al.*, 1977c).

The permanent behavioral changes produced by psychotropic drugs administered during the period of brain differentiation were associated with permanent structural and chemical changes in specific brain regions (Dörner *et al.*, 1977d; Staudt *et al.*, 1978). In the medial and central amygdalar regions, highly significantly increased nuclear volumes of the nerve cells were found in rats treated neonatally with reserpine and even more markedly in adult males treated neonatally with pargyline. Nuclear structures in the pargyline-treated males were more like those of control females than of control males. Furthermore, significantly decreased concentrations of norepinephrine (noradrenaline) and dopamine were found in the hypothalamus of adult rats treated neonatally with pargyline (Dörner *et al.*, 1977d).

Since sex hormones had been shown to exert similar effects during brain differentiation, we investigated whether the effects induced by psychotropic drugs may also be mediated by changes of sex hormone activities. Therefore, the organ weight of gonads and accessory sex glands of these animals were determined immediately after cessation of treatment (on day 15) or at 11 months of age. Hypoplasia of sex organs was found only in neonatally reserpinized, not in pargylinized, newborn males (Dörner and Hinz, 1978). In adulthood neither of these groups showed sex organ hypoplasia, although their sexual activity was significantly decreased. Furthermore, male sexual activity was found to be significantly increased in neonatally pyridostigminized males, which showed even a slight hypoplasia of seminal vesicles in neonatal life (Dörner et al., 1976b; Dörner and Hinz, 1978).

These findings suggest that changes of neurotransmitter concentrations and/or turnover rates apparently induced by psychotropic drugs can affect sex-specific brain differentiation in rats without mediation of sex hormones.

Several findings even speak in favor of the fact that neurotransmitters may act as mediators of sex hormones for sexual differentiation of the brain. Ladosky and Gaziri (1970) found a significant elevation of the brain serotonin content associated with a significant diminution of monoamine oxidase activity in 12-day-old female rats as compared to male rats. Androgen deficiency produced by castration in newborn males gave rise to an increased serotonin content in the brain (Gaziri and Ladosky, 1973). On the other hand, injections of androgens into females on day 1 resulted in reduced brain serotonin content on day 12 (Giulian et al., 1973). Furthermore, the main enzymes for serotonin synthesis, tryptophan hydroxylase and 5-hydroxytryptophan decarboxylase, were found to be higher in the brain of newborn and adult female rats than in that of male rats (Hardin, 1973; Vaccari et al., 1977).

Inhibition of the monoamine oxidase activity by pargyline, which might result in an increase of serotonin content in the brain, was observed to cause delayed onset and permanent decrease of male sexual behavior (Dörner et al., 1976b) associated with permanent female-like structural changes in the brain of male rats (Staudt et al., 1978). On the other hand, pargyline treatment of newborn females gave rise to precocious puberty (Dörner et al., 1977c). Moreover, treatment of newborn female rats with the serotonin precursor 5-hydroxytryptophan inhibited the induction of persistent estrus by androgen (Shirama et al., 1975). Thus, serotonin appears to inhibit male-like differentiation and maturation but to facilitate female-like differentiation and maturation of the brain.

Recently, Crowley et al. (1978) have described sex differences in the catecholamine content of discrete brain nuclei in adult rats that were permanently changed, at least in part, by alteration of the androgen level in neonatal life. The dopamine concentration in the hypothalamus was permanently reduced in male rats by neonatal castration (Crowley *et al.*, 1978) as well as by neonatal pargyline treatment (Dörner *et al.*, 1977d).

These findings suggest that neurotransmitters may act as mediators of sex hormones for sexual differentiation of the brain. Changes in neurotransmitter concentrations or turnover rates, or both, when they occur during brain development, may affect sexual behavior throughout life.

5. *Prenatal Stress and Sexual Differentiation of the Brain*

In animal experiments, we found the following correlations between the androgen level during brain differentiation and sexual behavior in adult life (Dörner, 1969): The higher the androgen (testosterone) level during sexual differentiation of the brain, the stronger—regardless of the genetic sex—was the male-like and the weaker the female-like sexual behavior in adulthood. In view of these findings, we suggest that a neuroendocrine predisposition to primary hypo-, bi-, and homosexuality can be based on different degrees of temporary androgen deficiency in males and androgen excess in females when they occur during brain differentiation (Fig. 6).

Since stress is known to decrease testicular testosterone secretion in adults, Ward (1972) performed experimental studies to find out if perinatal stress may also result in decreased testosterone levels of fetal or newborn rats, or both, and hence permanent changes of sexual be-

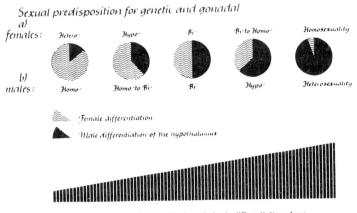

FIG. 6. Androgen-dependent sexual differentiation of the brain. From Dörner (1972, 1976).

havior. She observed that the male offspring of pregnant rats exposed to stress of restraint and high intensity light during days 14-21 of gestation displayed hyposexuality ("demasculinization") in adult life. After orchidectomy and estrogen plus progesterone administration these male rats exhibited significantly increased female-like lordotic behavior ("feminization") as compared to prenatally nonstressed and later equally treated males. Partial demasculinization in prenatally stressed male rats was confirmed by Masterpasqua et al. (1976), and partial feminization by Dahlöf et al. (1977). Dunlap et al. (1978) then described complete demasculinization, i.e., complete absence of male copulatory behavior, in male rats exposed to prenatal stress plus pre-pubertal social isolation, while copulatory behavior was only reduced, not abolished, by prenatal stress or prepubertal social isolation alone. This finding indicates that prenatal stress and prepubertal social isola-tion can interact to determine sexual potentials.

In 1977, Ward published data on parallel testing of homotypical (male-like) and heterotypical (female-like) behavior in prenatally stressed male rats after orchidectomy plus androgen treatment (1 mg of TP daily) in adult life. The homotypical (male-like) behavior of these males was tested with estrous lure females, and the heterotypical (female-like) behavior was tested with vigorous stud males. Ward found that most of the prenatally stressed males exhibited bisexual behavior after castration plus androgen treatment in adulthood, whereas the prenatally nonstressed but later equally treated males displayed heterosexual behavior.

Such combined behavioral tests were recommended by our group (Dörner and Hinz, 1968; Dörner et al., 1968a) for differentiation be-tween hetero-, bi-, and "homosexual" behavior. After androgen treat-ment in adult life (1 mg of TP daily) there were found (a) predomi-nantly heterotypical, i.e., "homosexual" behavior, in male rats cas-trated on the day of birth; (b) bisexual behavior in males castrated on the day of birth but replaced once with a low androgen dose (0.02 mg of TP) on day 3; and (c) heterosexual behavior in males castrated on the day of birth but treated once with a high androgen dose (1.25 mg of TP) on day 3 of life (Dörner, 1969).

Since bisexual behavior was also found in prenatally stressed males (Ward, 1977), we determined the plasma testosterone level in fetal and newborn male rats exposed to such prenatal stress (restraint and il-lumination of the mother animals). As shown in Fig. 7, the plasma testosterone values of the prenatally stressed males were significantly decreased in fetal and neonatal life and approached those of normal females (Stahl et al., 1978; Dörner, 1979b).

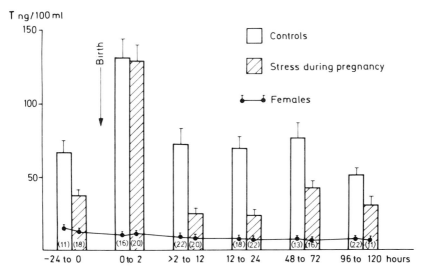

FIG. 7. Plasma testosterone (T) levels of rats in pre- and early postnatal life (means ± SEM). The mother animals were stressed by restraint and illumination three times daily for 45 minutes between days 14 and 21 of gestation. From Stahl *et al.* (1978).

The norepinephrine content in the hypothalamus of these prenatally stressed males was also found to be significantly decreased on the day of birth (Stahl *et al.*, 1978). Moreover, Moyer *et al.* (1978) reported that stress during pregnancy can permanently change norepinephrine concentrations in discrete brain regions of the male offspring.

Such permanent behavioral and chemical effects of prenatal stress may be induced, at least in part, by decreased testicular secretion of testosterone in male fetuses and newborns during brain differentiation. Hence, we drew the following conclusion: Stressful situations during pregnancy can result in elevation of maternal glucocorticoids that are transported via the placenta to the fetus, where they block the secretion of testicular testosterone. In agreement with this hypothesis, we have found, in fact, significantly increased plasma corticosterone levels in the stressed pregnant mother animals associated with significantly decreased organ weights of the adrenals and testes in their newborn offspring. Similar data were obtained by Dahlöf *et al.* (1978).

Most recently, we have observed predominantly heterotypical, i.e., "homosexual" behavior, in prenatally stressed male rats after castration plus estrogen treatment in adulthood, whereas prenatally nonstressed but later equally treated males displayed heterosexual behavior (Götz and Dörner, 1980). Hence, prenatal stress can predispose to the development of "homosexual" behavior in males.

In this context, it should be mentioned that in rats estrogens activate predominantly female behavior in (genetic female or male) animals with a female-differentiated brain, but predominantly male behavior in (genetic male or female) animals with a male-differentiated brain. By contrast, in primates not estrogens, but only androgens, activate male behavior in (genetic male or female) subjects with a male-differentiated brain, whereas androgens activate—even more strongly than estrogens—female-like behavior in (genetic female or male) primates with a female-differentiated brain. Thus it is possible that a predominantly female-differentiated brain in prenatally stressed male primates may be activated in adulthood by normal endogenous testosterone levels to predominantly female-like, i.e., "homosexual" behavior. This problem should be fully explored in primates, especially in human beings.

IV. Some Clinical Studies and Perspectives

1. Neuroendocrine Findings in Homosexuals and Transsexuals That Suggest Possible Discrepancies between the Genetic Sex and Sex-Specific Androgen Levels in Prenatal Life

Theories about the origins of homosexuality and transsexuality in the human now focus on the role of (a) sex hormone-dependent differentiation of the brain in prenatal life (Dörner, 1972, 1977a,b, 1979b) and/or (b) sex-specific development of the brain by postnatal psychosocial influences, i.e., by learning processes (Meyer-Bahlburg, 1977, 1979).

Our clinical studies on sex hormone-dependent differentiation of the brain were based on findings obtained in extensive animal experiments (Dörner, 1972, 1976):

1. Male rats castrated on the first day of life showed predominantly heterotypical behavior after androgen substitution in adulthood. In other words, genetic males exposed to a temporary androgen deficiency during sexual differentiation of the brain, but normal or approximately normal androgen levels in adulthood, were sexually stimulated preferentially by partners of the same sex.

2. The higher the androgen level during a critical differentiation phase, the stronger was the male-like and the weaker the female-like sexual behavior during the postpubertal activation phase, irrespective of the genetic sex. Even a complete inversion of sexual behavior was observed in male and female rats after androgen deficiency in males

and androgen excess in females during sexual differentiation of the brain. According to these findings a neuroendocrine predisposition to primary hypo-, bi-, and homosexuality may be based on different degrees of androgen deficiency in males and androgen excess in females during sex-specific brain differentiation.

3. In male rats castrated on the first day of life, a strong positive estrogen-feedback effect could be induced in a similar way as in normal females, but could not be induced in males castrated on day 14 of life or in neonatally androgenized females. In view of these findings, a positive estrogen-feedback effect appears to be evocable only in adulthood—without estrogen priming—if a low androgen level existed during brain differentiation.

Investigations carried out in the human produced the following data (Dörner *et al.,* 1972b, 1975c): A positive estrogen-feedback effect could be elicited in intact homosexual men in contrast to no such effect in intact heterosexual and bisexual men (Fig. 8). Thus, in homosexual men, an i.v. injection of estrogen (20 mg of Presomen, which is comparable to Premarin) produced primarily a decrease of the serum LH level followed secondarily by a significant increase above the initial serum LH level. On the other hand, in intact heterosexual men, the estrogen administration also produced a decrease of the serum LH level, but it was not followed, however, by an increase above the initial

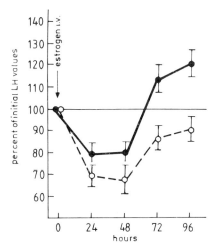

FIG. 8. Serum luteinizing hormone (LH) response to an i.v. estrogen injection (20 mg of Presomen) expressed as percentage of the mean initial LH values in homosexual (●—●) and hetero- or bisexual (○---○) men (means ± SEM). From Dörner (1976).

LH values. These findings suggested to us that homosexual men may possess—at least in part—a predominantly female-differentiated brain, which could be based on androgen deficiency in prenatal life.

In transsexual women with homosexual behavior, on the other hand, only a weak or at best moderate positive estrogen-feedback action on LH release could be evoked as compared to the evocability of a strong estrogen feedback action in heterosexual women (Dörner et al., 1976a). More recently, Seyler et al. (1978a,b) observed that the LH response to LH-RH after estrogen-priming also differed markedly in transsexual and/or homosexual women from that in heterosexual women. The LH response to LH-RH could not be clearly enhanced by estrogen-priming in transsexual and homosexual females, in contrast to heterosexual women. These data suggest that homosexual and transsexual women may possess, at least in part, a predominantly male-differentiated brain.

Meanwhile, the plasma basal levels of apparent free and total plasma testosterone as well as of FSH and LH were determined in homosexual and heterosexual males (Stahl et al., 1976b). As shown in Fig. 9, significantly lower free plasma testosterone levels were found in effeminate homosexual males than in heterosexual males. In contrast to free testosterone levels, no significant difference in total plasma testosterone levels was observed between homosexual and heterosexual males. Normal total plasma testosterone values in heterosexual males were also found by the majority of other investigators who used adequate control groups (Birk et al., 1973; Doerr et al., 1973; Barlow et al., 1974; Parks et al., 1974). However, the urinary excretion of conjugated testosterone, which may reflect the free plasma testosterone level, was found to be decreased in some homosexual males and increased in some homosexual females (Loraine et al., 1970, 1971).

Furthermore, the androsterone:etiocholanolone ratio showed a significant decrease in homosexual males, particularly in Kinsey 5 and 6 individuals, as compared to heterosexual males (Margolese, 1970; Evans, 1972; Margolese and Janiger, 1973). This finding may indicate a permanent shift in steroid metabolism to the female side, which could be induced by prenatal androgen deficiency.

In addition, higher plasma FSH and LH basal levels were found in homosexual males, but only in effeminate homosexual and transsexual males, than in heterosexual males (Rohde et al., 1978; Dörner, 1979a). Increased LH values were also observed in some homosexual males by other authors (Kolodny et al., 1972; Doerr et al., 1976).

From our experimental and clinical data, we advanced the following hypothesis. An androgen deficiency in genetic males during a critical

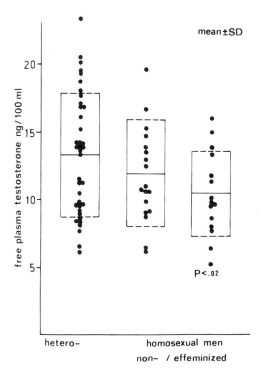

Fig. 9. Plasma free testosterone levels in heterosexual males and in noneffeminate and effeminate homosexual males. From Rohde *et al.* (1977).

period of brain differentiation gives rise to predominantly female differentiation of the brain. This androgen deficiency in early life could be compensated, at least in part, by increased hypophysial gonadotropin secretion in later life. Thus, the predominantly female-differentiated brain is postpubertally activated by an approximately normal androgen level for genetic males, leading to homosexual behavior. However, the approximately normal androgen level for a male-differentiated brain in heterosexual males does mean a markedly increased androgen level for a predominantly female-differentiated brain in homosexual males as compared to heterosexual females. The free plasma testosterone level was found to be 10.7 ± 3.3 ng/100 ml in 35 homosexual men, but only 0.52 ± 0.14 ng/100 ml in 6 heterosexual women near the time of ovulation and 0.36 ± 0.11 ng/100 ml at the beginning or ending of the menstrual cycle (Stahl *et al.,* 1976a,b). Therefore, it is also conceivable that the sexual drive toward male sex partners is found to be stronger in homosexual males than in heterosexual females.

In genetic females, on the other hand, the results of animal experiments in various species suggest that androgen excess during a critical period of brain differentiation can predispose to hypo-, bi-, or even homosexual behavior in postpubertal life.

Recently, we have observed increased plasma testosterone levels in lesbian women. However, a significant increase was found only in those (9 out of 21) lesbian females showing some virilism (Dörner, 1979a). Similar findings of increased testosterone values in about one-third to one-half of homosexual and/or transsexual women were obtained by other authors (Griffiths *et al.*, 1974; Gartrell *et al.*, 1977; Sipová and Starka, 1977).

In addition, Griffith *et al.* (1974) reported that the lesbians mostly looked older than their age, sometimes strikingly so. In this context it should be noted once more that perinatally androgenized female rats showed a significantly accelerated aging (Dörner, 1973; Dörner and Hinz, 1975).

Several experiments of nature are consistent with the hypothesis that in the human, as well as in other species, sex-specific sexual behavior is predetermined, at least in part, by the androgen level during brain differentiation.

1. Genetic females (46, XX) with congenital adrenal hyperplasia, who are exposed to a more or less increased androgen level in prenatal life, were observed to exhibit more frequently bi- or homosexual trends—even those with female assignment and/or postnatal normalization of androgen levels—than normal females (Hinman, 1951; Laron *et al.*, 1974; Money and Schwartz, 1977).

2. Individuals with Klinefelter's syndrome (47, XXY), who can be assumed to be exposed to a partial androgen deficiency in prenatal life (because of insufficient responsiveness of the fetal testes to hCG), were found to show an increased incidence of bi- and homosexuality in adult life (Freund, 1963; Johnson *et al.*, 1970; Meyer-Bahlburg, 1977).

3. Genetic males (46, XY) with testicular feminizing syndrome and primary insensitivity of their target organs (including brain) to androgen exhibit female-like sexual behavior, in contrast to their genetic and gonadal sex but in agreement with their somatic sex (Prader, 1978).

4. Most of all, genetic males (46, XY) with Imperato–McGinley syndrome are born with ambiguity of the external genitalia. Biochemical evaluation revealed a marked decrease in plasma 5α-dihydrotestosterone, which is secondary to a decrease in steroid 5α-reductase. The decrease in 5α-dihydrotestosterone in prenatal life resulted in more female-like differentiation of the external genitalia. Thus 18 of the

affected males (46, XY) were thought to be females at birth and raised as females. Their psychosexual orientation, however, was unequivocally male and their libido was clearly directed toward females. All but 2 out of the 18 affected postpubertal males even assumed the male gender role and male gender identity at the time of puberty. Only one subject has maintained a female gender identity and a female gender role postpubertally. Another subject has a male gender identity, but continues to dress as a female (Imperato-McGinley et al., 1974, 1979; Peterson et al., 1977).

These findings suggest that sexual differentiation of the brain, as well as sexual differentiation of the internal genitalia, is dependent on testosterone, whereas the sexual differentiation of the external genitalia is dependent on 5α-dihydrotestosterone. Furthermore, exposure of the developing brain to testosterone seems to be even more important for the sex-specific development of sexual orientation and even gender role than the sex of rearing, i.e., learning processes.

However, sexual differentiation of the brain in dependence on sex hormone levels and/or psychosocial conditions should no longer be considered as strictly alternative, but rather as complementary, effects, since neurotransmitters appear to represent common mediators of sex hormones and psychosocial influences as well for differentiation, maturation, and function of the brain (Dörner, 1978).

In the ontology of sexual differentiation, five steps may be distinguished in the human (Fig. 10). First, the gonosomal sex is determined by the sex chromosomes deriving from male and female germ cells. In a second step, the gonadal sex is differentiated under the control of the sex-determining genes and the H-Y antigen (Ohno, 1979). In a third step, the genital (somatic) sex and then, in a fourth step, the neuronal sex (mating and sex centers in the brain) are differentiated under the control of the androgen blood level in prenatal life. In a final fifth step, sexual differentiation in the human is completed by the development of gender role and gender identity, which are affected by the prenatally androgen-determined genital sex and neuronal sex as well as by postnatal psychosocial influences.

2. Search for Prenatal Discrepancies between Genetic Sex and Sex-Specific Androgen Levels

In view of the described data, sexual deviations in the human may be based, at least in part, on discrepancies between the genetic sex and a sex-specific androgen level during brain differentiation. Therefore, a genuine prophylaxis may become possible, if indeed it is desirable at

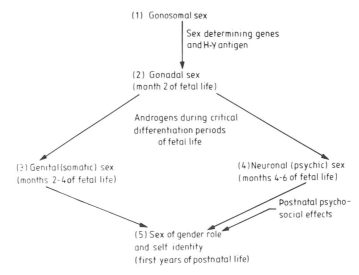

FIG. 10. Sexual differentiation in the human.

all, in the future by the prevention of such discrepancies during the period of sexual differentiation of the brain.

Three preconditions for this aim have already been achieved.

1. Our comparative studies of the morphogenesis of the hypothalamus in 84 human fetuses and hundreds of rats have led to the conclusion that the critical period of sex-specific brain differentiation occurs in the human between the fourth and seventh months of fetal life (Dörner and Staudt, 1972).

2. A simple and reliable method for the prenatal diagnosis of genetic sex was developed using fluorescence microscopy of amniotic fluid cells (Dörner et al., 1971b, 1973).

3. As shown in Fig. 11, levels of testosterone glucuronide (TG) and also of unconjugated testosterone were found to be significantly increased and FSH levels significantly decreased in the amniotic fluid of male fetuses as compared to that of female fetuses (Dörner, 1972, 1976; Dörner et al., 1972a, 1977b; Young-Lai, 1972; Giles et al., 1974; Clements et al., 1976; Judd et al., 1976; Robinson et al., 1977; Zondek et al., 1977; Künzig et al., 1977).

While sex-specific differences of testosterone levels in prenatal life were observed for the first time in amniotic fluids (Dörner, 1972; Dörner et al., 1972a), such sex-specific differences were then also found in fetal serum between weeks 9 and 25 of pregnancy (Reyes et al., 1974). More recently, we have found that the free plasma testosterone

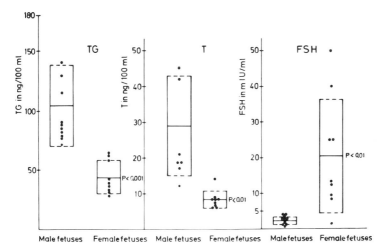

Fig. 11. Testosterone glucuronide (TG), testosterone (T), and follicle-stimulating hormone (FSH) levels in amniotic fluids of male and female human fetuses between weeks 15 and 26 of pregnancy (means ± SD). From Dörner *et al.* (1977d).

level in male fetuses at midpregnancy is even higher than in adult men (Stahl *et al.*, 1978; Dörner, 1979b).

Thus, the examination of amniotic fluids for genetic defects should be supplemented in the future by determination of hormone levels in order to find abnormalities that might lead to maldifferentiations, especially of the brain. Furthermore, to prevent iatrogenic sexual maldifferentiation, androgens and antiandrogens are contraindicated in pregnant women. In cases of adrenogenital syndrome, especially in female fetuses, glucocorticoid treatment should be started prenatally in order to inhibit adrenal overproduction of androgens. Moreover, sex hormone-producing adrenal or ovarian tumors should be removed in early pregnancy.

Preventive therapy of disturbances of sexual differentiation, if desirable at all, might also become possible in the future by administration of androgen to genetic male fetuses with clear evidence of androgen deficiency during critical differentiation periods. First of all, however, male fetuses with decreased testosterone levels as well as female fetuses with increased testosterone levels in amniotic fluids (or fetal blood) should be screened and followed up with respect to their sexual development in postnatal life. In my opinion, such a prospective study is the only possibility to give final conclusive evidence for the significance of prenatal discrepancies between genetic sex and sex-specific androgen level for a deviant sexual differentiation of the brain and hence for the development of sexual deviations in the human.

3. *Prenatal Maternal Stress as Possible Etiogenic Factor for Homosexuality in Human Males*

Male rats exposed to a transient androgen deficiency during sexual differentiation of the brain displayed a significantly increased sexual responsiveness to partners of the same sex in adult life (Dörner and Hinz, 1967; Dörner, 1976). Similar heterotypical (bi- or homosexual) behavioral patterns were then observed in adult male rats that had been exposed to prenatal maternal stress (Ward, 1977; Götz and Dörner, 1980). Furthermore, a significant decrease of plasma testosterone levels was found in male rat fetuses and newborns after prenatal maternal stress (Stahl *et al.*, 1978; Dörner, 1979b).

In view of these data, a study was carried out to attempt to answer the question whether stressful war or postwar situations may have irreversibly affected sexual differentiation of the brain in men who were born in Germany during or shortly after World War II. As shown in Fig. 12, out of 794 homosexual males who were registered by sexologists and venerologists in recent years, highly significantly more homosexuals were born during the stressful war and early postwar period between 1942 and 1947 (particularly in 1944 and 1945) than in the years before (1932-1939) or after (1948-1953) this period (Dörner *et al.*, 1980).

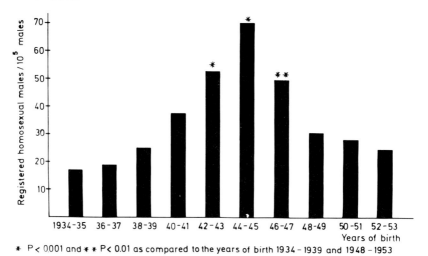

$*$ P < 0.001 and $**$ P < 0.01 as compared to the years of birth 1934 - 1939 and 1948 - 1953

FIG. 12. Relative frequency of homosexual males born in Germany before, during, or after World War II ($N = 794$). From Dörner (1979b).

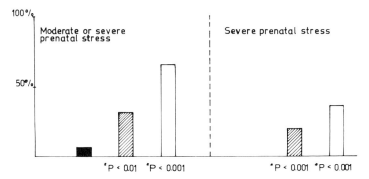

FIG. 13. Percentage of heterosexual (■, $N = 72$), bisexual (▨, $N = 25$), or homosexual (□, $N = 47$), men exposed to maternal stress during their prenatal life. *Indicates chi square test comparison with heterosexual men.

In addition, 72 bi- or homosexual men as well as 72 heterosexual men of similar age were asked about maternal stressful events that may have occurred during their prenatal life. As shown in Fig. 13, a highly significantly increased incidence of prenatal maternal stress was found in bisexual and, particularly, in homosexual men over that in heterosexual men. About one-third of the homosexual men reported that they had been exposed to severe maternal stress, such as bereavement, severe anxiety, rejection by the partner, or rape with severe psychological shock, and about an additional one-third to moderate maternal stress during their prenatal life. On the other hand, none of the heterosexual men was found to have been exposed to severe, and less than 10% of them to moderate, maternal stress during their prenatal life. These data also suggest that prenatal stress may represent an important risk factor for the etiogenesis of sexual deviations in later life.

V. Summary

In the mediobasal hypothalamus the gonadotropin-releasing hormone (GnRH) is secreted under the influence of neurotransmitters. It is transported by the hypothalamic–hypophysial portal vessels to the anterior pituitary, stimulating there the secretion of gonadotropins (FSH and LH). The gonadotropins control the generative and vegetative function of the gonads. The gonadal hormones, in turn, exert either only an inhibitory (negative) or, particularly estrogens, also a stimulatory (positive) feedback effect on gonadotropin secretion, depending on sex hormone levels during a critical pre- or perinatal period of brain differentiation and during the postpubertal priming period as well. In addition, sex hormones can sensitize mating centers in the brain to environmental sexual stimuli, mediated by neurotransmitters.

A "male mating center" located in the preoptic anterior hypothalamic area can be distinguished from a "female center" located in the hypothalamic ventromedial nuclei. In rats of either sex, predominantly male or female sexual behavior could be selectively stimulated or abolished either by intrahypothalamic implants of sex hormones or by electrolytic lesions in these regions. Furthermore, after bilateral or even unilateral lesions of the hypothalamic ventromedial nuclei, the decrease of female-like behavior was associated with an increase of male-like behavior. Similar findings were obtained by other authors in homosexual men.

In view of these data, different neuronal reflex circuits are responsible for male and female sexual behavior. In the medial preoptic anterior hypothalamic area a sex hormone-sensitive control center is located belonging to (or affecting) a neuronal reflex circuit responsible for male behavior, whereas in the ventromedial nuclei a sex hormone-sensitive control center is located belonging to (or affecting) a neuronal reflex circuit regulating female behavior. Some antagonistic interrelationships appear to exist between these male and female mating centers in the brain.

Male rats castrated on the day of birth exhibit predominantly heterotypical ("homosexual") behavior not only after estrogen treatment, but also after androgen treatment, in adulthood. In addition, an increased evocability of a positive estrogen feedback effect on LH secretion was observed in such genetic males. In homosexual men, an increased evocability of a positive estrogen-feedback action on LH secretion was also found as compared to heterosexual men, in which it was absent. These findings suggest that male homosexuality can be based, at least in part, on androgen deficiency during a critical period of brain differentiation. In addition, increased plasma FSH and LH levels associated with decreased plasma free testosterone levels were found in homosexual men, but only in effeminate homosexuals.

In genetic female animals, an androgen excess occurring during brain differentiation gives rise to a more or less male organization of the brain, i.e., a decreased evocability of a positive estrogen feedback action on LH secretion and/or a neuroendocrine predisposition for female hypo-, bi-, or homosexuality. Specific brain structures of these masculinized females are comparable to those of normal males. In some lesbian women, a decreased evocability of a positive estrogen-feedback action on LH secretion and/or increased plasma testosterone levels were observed.

In view of these data, sexual deviations in the human may be based, at least in part, on discrepancies between the genetic sex and a sex-specific androgen level during brain differentiation. This hypothesis is consistent with clinical findings obtained in several experiments of nature, e.g., in gonadal dysegenesis, testicular feminization, Klinefelter's syndrome, and, most of all, Imperato-McGinley's syndrome.

Therefore, a genuine prophylaxis may become possible in the future by prevention of such discrepancies during sexual differentiation of the brain. Three preconditions toward this aim have been achieved.

1. Comparative studies of hypothalamic biomorphosis in human fetuses and in rats have led to the conclusion that sexual differentiation of the brain may occur in the human between months 4 and 7 of fetal life.
2. A simple and reliable method for the prenatal diagnosis of genetic sex has been developed using fluorescence microscopy of amniotic fluid cells.
3. Significantly higher testosterone levels have been found in amniotic fluids of male fetuses than in those of female fetuses.

Sexual differentiation of the brain appears to be mediated, at least in part, by neurotransmitters, which may be regarded as local hormones of the brain. In rats, permanent changes in mating and nonmating behavior associated with permanent sex-specific structural and chemical changes in discrete brain regions were found after neonatal treatment with psychotropic drugs known to affect neurotransmitter metabolism in the brain.

The neurotransmitter metabolism of the developing brain may also be affected by stress. Thus, female rats that were exposed to stress during pregnancy gave birth to males exhibiting androgen deficiency in perinatal life and hypo-, bi-, or "homosexual" behavior in adult life. Finally, significantly more homosexual men were born in Germany during the stressful years of World War II than in the years before or after this period. Furthermore, we found that the incidence of prenatal maternal stress is significantly higher in bisexual and, particularly, in homosexual men than in heterosexual men. Thus, prenatal maternal stress may represent a possible etiogenic factor in the development of sexual deviations in males.

ACKNOWLEDGMENT

I would like to thank my wife for typing the manuscript.

REFERENCES

Alleva, F. R., Alleva, J. J., and Umberger, E. J. (1969). *Endocrinology* **85**, 312–318.

Anonymous (1970). *Nature (London)* **226**, 869–870.

Arai, Y., and Gorski, R. A. (1968). *Endocrinology* **82**, 1005–1014.

Aschheim, S., and Zondek, B. (1927). *Klin. Wochenschr.* **6**, 1322.

Aschner, B. (1912). *Pflueger's Arch. Gesamte Physiol. Menschen Tiere* **146**, 1–146.

Barlow, D. H., Abel, G. G., Blanchard, E. B., and Mavissakalian, M. (1974). *Arch. Sex Behav.* **3**, 571–575.

Barraclough, C. A. (1955). *Am. J. Anat.* **97**, 493–522.

Barraclough, C. A. (1961). *Endocrinology* **68**, 62–67.

Barraclough, C. A. (1966). *Recent Prog. Horm. Res.* **22**, 503–529.

Barraclough, C. A. (1967). *In* "Neuroendocrinology" (L. Martini and W. F. Ganong, eds.), Vol. 2, pp. 61–99. Academic Press, New York.

Barraclough, C. A., and Gorski, R. A. (1961). *Endocrinology* **68**, 68–79.

Barraclough, C. A., and Gorski, R. A. (1962). *J. Endocrinol.* **25**, 175–182.

Barraclough, C. A., and Leathem, J. H. (1954). *Proc. Soc. Exp. Biol. Med.* **85**, 673–674.

Barraclough, C. A., and Leathem, J. H. (1959). *Anat. Rec.* **134**, 239–255.

Beach, F. A., and Holz, A. M. (1946). *J. Exp. Zool.* **101**, 91–142.

Berthold, A. A. (1849). *Arch. Anat., Physiol. Wissensch. Med.* pp. 42–46.

Bignani, G. (1966). *Psychopharmacologia* **10**, 44–58.

Birk, L., Williams, G. D., Charsin, M., and Rose, L. I. (1973). *N. Engl. J. Med.* **289**, 1236–1238.

Booth, J. (1978). *J. Endocrinol.* **79**, 69–76.

Bradbury, J. T. (1941). *Endocrinology* **28**, 101–106.

Breuer, H., Schneider, H. T., Wandscheer, D. E., and Ladosky, W. (1978). *In* "Hormones and Brain Development" (G. Dörner and M. Kawakami, eds.), pp. 167–174. Elsevier/North-Holland Biomedical Press, Amsterdam.

Bronson, F. H., and Desjardins, C. D. (1969). *Endocrinology* **85**, 971–974.

Brookhart, J. M., and Dey, F. L. (1941). *Am. J. Physiol.* **133**, 551–554.

Brookhart, J. M., Dey, F. L., and Ranson, S. W. (1940). *Proc. Soc. Exp. Biol. Med.* **44**, 61–64.

Brookhart, J. M., Dey, F. L., and Ranson, S. W. (1941). *Endocrinology* **28**, 561–565.

Bubenik, G. A., and Brown, G. M. (1973). *Experientia* **29**, 619–621.

Buhl, A.E., Norman, R. L., and Resko, J. A. (1978). *Biol. Reprod.* **18**, 592–597.

Carraro, A., Corbin, A., Fraschini, F., and Martini, L. (1965). *J. Endocrinol.* **32**, 387–393.

Christensen, L. W., and Clemens, L. G. (1974). *Endocrinology* **95**, 984–990.

Christensen, L. W., and Clemens, L. G. (1975). *Endocrinology* **97**, 1545–1551.

Christensen, L. W., and Gorski, R. A. (1978). *Brain Res.* **146**, 325–340.

Christensen, L. W., Nance, D. M., and Gorski, R. A. (1977). *Brain Res. Bull.* **2**, 137–141.

Clark, G. (1942). *Am. J. Physiol.* **137**, 746–749.

Clarke, I. J., Scaramuzzi, R. J., and Short, R. V. (1977). *J. Endocrinol.* **73**, 385–389.

Clements, J. A., Reyes, F. I., Winter, J. S. D., and Faiman, C. (1976). *J. Clin. Endocrinol. Metab.* **42**, 9–19.

Crowley, W. R., Ward, I. L., and Margules, D. L. (1975). *J. Comp. Physiol. Psychol.* **88**, 62–88.

Crowley, W. R., Feder, H. H., and Morin, L. P. (1976). *Pharmacol., Biochem. Behavior* **4**, 67–71.

Crowley, W. R., O'Donohue, T. L., and Jacobowitz, D. M. (1978). *Acta Endocrinol. (Copenhagen)* **89**, 20–28.

Dahlöf, L. G., Hard, E., and Larsson, K. (1977). *Anim. Behav.* **25**, 958–963.

Dahlöf, L. G., Hard, E., and Larsson, K. (1978). *Physiol. Behav.* **20**, 193–195.

Dantchakoff, V. (1938). *Hebd. Seances Acad. Sci.* **206**, 945–947.

Davis, P. G., and Barfield, R. J. (1979a). *Neuroendocrinology* **28**, 217–227.

Davis, P. G., and Barfield, R. J. (1979b). *Neuroendocrinology* **28**, 228–233.

Denef, C. (1972). *Endocrinology* **91**, 374–384.

Dewsbury, D. A., and Davis, H. N., Jr. (1970). *Physiol. Behav.* **5**, 1331–1333.

Dieckmann, G., and Hassler, R. (1975). *Confin. Neurol.* **37**, 177–186.

Döcke, F., and Dörner, G. (1966). *Zentralbl. Gynaekol.* **88**, 273–282.

Döcke, F., and Dörner, G. (1975). *Endokrinologie* **65**, 375–377.

Döcke, F., and Koloczek, G. (1966). *Endokrinologie* **50**, 225–230.

Döcke, F., Smollich, A., Rohde, W., Okrasa, R., and Dörner, G. (1975). *Endokrinologie* **65**, 274–287.

Doerr, P., Kockott, G., Vogt, H. J., Pirke, K. M., and Dittmar, F. (1973). *Arch. Gen. Psychiatry* **29**, 829–833.

Doerr, P., Pirke, K. M., Kockott, G., and Dittmar, F. (1976). *Arch. Gen. Psychiatry* **33**, 611–614.

Dörner, G. (1962). *Zentralbl. Gynaekol.* **84**, 737–742.

Dörner, G. (1967). *Acta Biol. Med. Ger.* **19**, 569–584.

Dörner, G. (1968). *J. Endocrinol.* **42**, 163–164.

Dörner, G. (1969). *Dtsch. Med. Wochenschr.* **94**, 390–396.

Dörner, G. (1972). "Sexualhormonabhängige Gehirndifferenzierung und Sexualität." Fischer, Jena.

Dörner, G. (1973). *Z. Alternsforsch* **27**, 379–380.

Dörner, G. (1976). "Hormones and Brain Differentiation." Elsevier, Amsterdam.

Dörner, G. (1977a). *Endokrinologie* **69**, 306–320.

Dörner, G. (1977b). *In* "Handbook of Sexology" (J. Money and H. Musaph, eds.), pp. 227–244. Excerpta Med. Found. Amsterdam.

Dörner, G. (1978). *In* "Hormones and Brain Development" (G. Dörner and M. Kawakami, eds.), pp. 13–26. Elsevier/North-Holland Biomedical Press, Amsterdam.

Dörner, G. (1979a). *Ciba Found. Symp.* **62** (new ser.), 81–112.

Dörner, G. (1979b). *In* "Psycho-Neuroendocrinology in Reproduction" (L. Zichella and P. Pancheri, eds.), pp. 43–54. Elsevier/North-Holland Biomedical Press, Amsterdam.

Dörner, G., and Döcke, F. (1964a). *J. Endocrinol.* **30**, 265–266.

Dörner, G., and Döcke, F. (1964b). *Zentralbl. Gynaekol.* **86**, 1321–1327.

Dörner, G., and Fatschel, J. (1970). *Endokrinologie* **56**, 29–48.

Dörner, G., and Hinz, G. (1967). *Ger. Med. Mon.* **12**, 281–283.

Dörner, G., and Hinz, G. (1968). *J. Endocrinol.* **40**, 387–388.

Dörner, G., and Hinz, G. (1975). *Endokrinologie* **65**, 378–380.

Dörner, G., and Hinz, G. (1978). *Endokrinologie* **71**, 104–108.

Dörner, G., and Staudt, J. (1968). *Neuroendocrinology* **3**, 136–140.

Dörner, G., and Staudt, J. (1969a). *Neuroendocrinology* **4**, 278–281.

Dörner, G., and Staudt, J. (1969b). *Neuroendocrinology* **5**, 103–106.

Dörner, G., and Staudt, J. (1972). *Endokrinologie* **59**, 152–155.

Dörner, G., Döcke, F., and Hinz, G. (1968a). *Acta Biol. Med. Ger.* **21**, 577–580.

Dörner, G., Döcke, F., and Moustafa, S. (1968b). *J. Reprod. Fertil.* **17**, 173–175.

Dörner, G., Döcke, F., and Moustafa, S. (1968c). *J. Reprod. Fertil.* **17**, 583–586.

Dörner, G., Döcke, F., and Hinz, G. (1969). *Neuroendocrinology* **4**, 20–24.

Dörner, G., Döcke, F., and Hinz, G. (1971a). *Neuroendocrinology* **7**, 146–155.

Dörner, G., Rohde, W., and Baumgarten, G. (1971b). *Acta Biol. Med. Ger.* **26**, 1095–1098.

Dörner, G., Stahl, F., and Baumgarten, G. (1972a). *Endokrinologie* **60**, 285–288.

Dörner, G., Rohde, W., and Krell, L. (1972b). *Endokrinologie* **60**, 297–301.

Dörner, G., Rohde, W., Baumgarten, G., Herter, U., Halle, H., Gruber, D., Rössner, P., Bergmann, K. H., Götz, F., and Zillmann, R. (1973). *Zentralbl. Gynaekol.* **95**, 625–634.

Dörner, G., Döcke, F., and Götz, F. (1975a). *Endokrinologie* **65**, 133–137.

Dörner, G., Götz, F., and Rohde, W. (1975b). *Endokrinologie* **66**, 369–372.

Dörner, G., Rohde, W., Stahl, F., Krell, L., and Masius, W. G. (1975c). *Arch. Sex. Behav.* **4**, 1–8.

Dörner, G., Rohde, W., and Schnorr, D. (1975d). *Endokrinologie* **66**, 373–376.

Dörner, G., Rohde, W., Seidel, K., Haas, W., and Schott, K. (1976a). *Endokrinologie* **67**, 20–25.

Dörner, G., Hecht, K., and Hinz, G. (1976b). *Endokrinologie* **68**, 1–5.

Dörner, G., Hinz, G., and Schlenker, G. (1977a). *Endokrinologie* **69**, 347–350.

Dörner, G., Stahl, F., Rohde, W., Göretzlehner, G., Witkowski, R., and Saffert, H. (1977b). *Endokrinologie* **70**, 86–88.

Dörner, G., Hinz, G., Döcke, F., and Tönjes, R. (1977c). *Endokrinologie* **70**, 113–123.

Dörner, G., Staudt, J., Wenzel, J., Kvetnansky, R., and Murgas, K. (1977d). *Endokrinologie* **70**, 326–330.

Dörner, G., Döcke, F., Hinz, G., and Götz, F. (1979). *Int. Acad. Sex Res. 5th Annu. Meet., 1979* Abstracts, p. 4.

Dörner, G., Geier, T., Ahrens, L., Krell, L., Münx, G., Sieler, H., Kittner, E., and Müller, H. (1980). *Endokrinologie* **75**, 365–368.

Dorfman, R. I. (1967). *Anat. Rec.* **157**, 547–557.

Dunlap, J. L., Zadina, J. E., and Gougis, G. (1978). *Physiol. Behav.* **21**, 873–875.

Elsaesser, F., and Parvizi, N. (1979). *Biol. Reprod.* **20**, 1187–1193.

Ericsson, R. J., and Baker, V. F. (1966). *Proc. Soc. Exp. Biol. Med.* **122**, 88–92.

Evans, R. B. (1972). *J. Consult. Clin. Psychol.* **39**, 140–147.

Feder, H. H. (1967). *Anat. Rec.* **157**, 79–86.

Feder, H. H., and Whalen, R. E. (1965). *Science* **147**, 306–307.

Flerkó, B., Petrusz, B., and Tima, L. (1967). *Acta Biol. (Szeged)* **18**, 27–36.

Flerkó, B., Mess, B., and Illei-Donhoffer, A. (1969). *Neuroendocrinology* **4**, 164–169.

Foreman, M. M., and Moss, R. L. (1978). *Pharmacol., Biochem. Behavior* **9**, 235–241.

Foss, G. L. (1951). *Lancet* **1**, 667–669.

Freund, K. (1963). "Die Homosexualität beim Mann." Hirzel, Leipzig.

Fuxe, K., Everitt, B. J., and Hökfelt, T. (1977). *Pharmacol., Biochem. Behavior* **7**, 147–151.

Gartrell, N. K., Loriaux, D. L., and Chase, T. N. (1977). *Am. J. Psychiatry* **134**, 1117–1119.

Gawienowski, A. M., Merker, J. W., and Damon, R. A., Jr. (1973). *Life Sci.* **12**, 307–315.

Gaziri, L. C. J., and Ladosky, W. (1973). *Neuroendocrinology* **12**, 249–256.

Gerall, A. A. (1966). *J. Comp. Physiol. Psychol.* **62**, 365–369.

Gerall, A. A. (1967). *Anat Rec.* **157**, 97–104.

Gerall, A. A., and Ward, I. L. (1966). *J. Comp. Physiol. Psychol.* **62**, 370–375.

Gerall, A. A., McMurray, M. M., and Farrell, A. (1975). *J. Endocrinol.* **67**, 439–445.

Gerall, A. A., Dunlap, J. L., and Wagner, R. A. (1976). *Physiol. Behav.* **17**, 121–126.

Gessa, G. L., and Tagliamonte, A. (1975). *In* "Sexual Behavior: Pharmacology and Biochemistry" (M. Sandler and G. L. Gessa, eds.), pp. 117–128. Raven, New York.

Giles, H. R., Lox, C. D., Heine, M. W., and Christian, C. D. (1974). *Gynecol. Invest.* **5**, 317–323.

Giulian, D., Pohorecky, L. A., and McEwen, B. S. (1973). *Endocrinology* **93**, 1329–1335.

Goodman, L. (1934). *Anat. Rec.* **59**, 223–251.

Gordon, T. P., and Bernstein, I. S. (1973). *Am. Phys. Anthropol.* **38**, 221–226.

Gorski, R. A. (1963). *Am. J. Physiol.* **205**, 842–844.

Gorski, R. A. (1967). *Anat. Rec.* **157**, 63–69.

Gorski, R. A., and Wagner, J. W. (1965). *Endocrinology* **76**, 226–239.

Gorski, R. A., Harlan, R. E., and Christensen, L. W. (1977). *J. Toxicol. Environ. Health* **3**, 97–121.

Gorski, R. A., Gordon, J. H., Shryne, J. E., and Southam, A. M. (1978). *Brain Res.* **148**, 333–346.

Götz, F., and Dörner, G. (1976). *Endokrinologie* **68**, 275–282.

Götz, F., and Dörner, G. (1980). *Endokrinologie* **76**, 115–117.

Götz, F., Vedder, I., and Dörner, G. (1974). *In* "Endocrinology of Sex" (G. Dörner, ed.), pp. 75–77. Barth, Leipzig.

Goy, R. W., and Phoenix, C. H. (1963). *J. Reprod. Fertil.* **5**, 23–40.

Goy, R. W., Bridson, W. E., and Young, W. C. (1964). *J. Comp. Physiol. Psychol.* **57**, 166–174.

Goy, R. W., Phoenix, C. H., and Meidinger, R. (1967). *Anat. Rec.* **157**, 87–96.

Goy, R. W., Wolf, J. E., and Eisele, G. (1977). *In* "Handbook of Sexology" (J. Money and H. Musaph, eds.), pp. 139–176. Excerpta Med. Found., Amsterdam.

Grady, K. L., and Phoenix, C. H. (1963). *Am. Zool.* **3**, 482–483.

Grady, K. L., Phoenix, C. H., and Young, W. C. (1965). *J. Comp. Physiol. Psychol.* **59**, 176–182.

Greenough, W. T., Carter, C. S., Steerman, C., and DeVoogd, T. J. (1977). *Brain Res.* **126**, 63–72.

Griffiths, P. D., Merry, J., Browning, M. C. K., Eisinger, A. J., Huntsman, R. G., Lord, E. J. A., Polani, P. E., Tanner, J. M., and Whitehouse, R. H. (1974). *J. Endocrinol.* **63**, 549–556.

Gustafsson, J. A., and Stenberg, A. (1974). *Endocrinology* **95**, 891–896.

Hale, H. B. (1944). *Endocrinology* **35**, 499–506.

Hardin, C. M. (1973). *Brain Res.* **59**, 437–439.

Harris, G. W. (1963). *J. Physiol. (London)* **169**, 117–118.

Harris, G. W. (1964). *Endocrinology* **75**, 627–648.

Harris, G. W., and Jacobsohn, D. (1951). *J. Physiol. (London)* **113**, 35–36.

Harris, G. W., and Levine, S. (1962). *J. Physiol. (London)* **163**, 42–43.

Harris, G. W., and Levine, S. (1965). *J. Physiol. (London)* **181**, 379–400.

Harris, G. W., Michael, R. P., and Scott, P. P. (1958). *In Ciba Found. Symp., 1957 Neural Basis Behav.*, pp. 236–254.

Heimer, L., and Larsson, K. (1967). *Brain Res.* **3**, 248–263.

Herbert, J. (1974). *Prog. Brain Res.* **41**, 331–347.

Hillarp, N. A., Olivecrona, H., and Silverskiöld, W. (1954). *Experientia* **10**, 224–225.

Hinman, F. (1951). *J. Clin. Endocrinol. Metab.* **11**, 477–486.

Hohlweg, W. (1934). *Klin. Wochenschr.* **13**, 92–95.

Hohlweg, W., and Chamorro, A. (1937). *Klin. Wochenschr.* **16**, 196–197.

Hohlweg, W., and Junkmann, K. (1932). *Klin. Wochenschr.* **11**, 321–323.

Ifft, J. D. (1964). *Anat. Rec.* **148**, 599–603.

Imperato-McGinley, J., Guerrero, L., Gautier, T., and Peterson, R. E. (1974). *Science* **186**, 1213–1215.

Imperato-McGinley, J., Peterson, R. E., Gautier, T., and Sturla, E. (1979). *J. Steroid Biochem.* **11**, 637–645.

Jaffe, R. B. (1969). *Steroids* **14**, 483–498.

Johnson, H. R., Myhre, S. A., Ruvalcaba, R. H. A., Thuline, H. C., and Kelley, V. C. (1970). *Dev. Med. Child Neurol.* **12**, 454–460.

Judd, H. L., Robinson, F. J. D., Young, P. E., and Jones, O. W. (1976). *Obstet. Gynecol.* **48**, 690–692.

Kalra, S. P., and Sawyer, C. H. (1970). *Endocrinology* **87**, 1124–1128.

Kamberi, I. A. (1974). *In* "Endocrinology of Sex" (G. Dörner, ed.), pp. 166–184. Barth, Leipzig.

Karsch, F. J., Dierschke, D. J., and Knobil, E. (1973). *Science* **179**, 484–486.

Kawakami, M., and Terasawa, E. (1974). *In* "Biological Rhythms in Neuroendocrine Activity" (M. Kawakami, ed.), pp. 197–219. Igaku Shoin Ltd., Tokyo.

Kawashima, S. (1960). *J. Fac. Sci., Univ. Tokyo Sect. 4* **9**, 117–125.

Kawashima, S. (1964). *Zool. Jpn.* **37**, 79–85.

Kennedy, G. C. (1964). *J. Physiol. (London)* **172**, 383–392.

Kikuyama, S. (1961). *Zool. Jpn.* **34**, 111–116.

Kikuyama, S. (1963). *Zool. Jpn.* **36**, 145–148.

Kincl, F. A., and Maqueo, M. (1965). *Endocrinology* **77**, 859–862.

King, J. C. (1972). Ph.D. Dissertation, Tulane University, New Orleans, Louisiana.

Kinsey, A. C. (1941). *J. Clin. Endocrinol. Metab.* **1**, 424–428.

Knapstein, P., David, A., Wu, C. H., Anker, D. F., Flickinger, L., and Touchstone, J. C. (1968). *Steroids* **11**, 885–896.

Kniewald, Z., Massa, R., and Martini, L. (1971). *In* "Hormonal Steroids" (V. H. T. James and L. Martini, eds.), pp. 784–791. Excerpta Med. Found., Amsterdam.

Knobil, E. (1974). *Recent Prog. Horm. Res.* **30**, 1–46.

Kobayashi, F. (1967). *Folia Endocrinol. Jpn.* **43**, 20–26.

Kobayashi, F., and Gorski, R. A. (1970). *Endocrinology* **86**, 285–289.

Kolodny, R. C., Jacobs, L. S., Masters, W. H., Toro, G., and Daughaday, W. H. (1972). *Lancet* **2**, 18–20.

Koster, R. (1943). *Endocrinology* **33**, 337–348.

Kreuz, L. E., Rosé, R. M., and Jennings, J. R. (1972). *Arch. Gen. Psychiatry* **26**, 479–512.

Künzig, H. J., Meyer, U., Schmitz-Roeckerath, B., and Broer, K. H. (1977). *Arch. Gynaekol.* **223**, 75–84.

Kurcz, M., Nagy, I., Gerhardt, V., and Baranyoi, P. (1969a). *Acta Biol. Acad. Sci. Hung.* **20**, 163–170.

Kurcz, M., Maderspach, K., and Horn, G. (1969b). *Acta Biol. Acad. Sci. Hung.* **20**, 303–310.

Ladosky, W., and Gaziri, L. C. J. (1970). *Neuroendocrinology* **6**, 168–174.

Laron, Z., Pertzelan, A., Shurka, E., Galatzer, A., Gil, R., and Frisch, M. (1974). *In* "Endocrinologie sexuelle de la période périnatale" (M. G. Forest and J. Bertrand, eds.), pp. 407–420. INSERM, Paris.

Larsson, K. (1966). *Z. Tierpsychol.* **23**, 867–873.

Larsson, K. (1967). *Z. Tierpsychol.* **24**, 471–475.

Larsson, K., and Heimer, L. (1964). *Nature (London)* **202**, 413–414.

Law, T., and Meagher, W. (1958). *Science* **128**, 1626–1627.

Lax, E. R., Ghraf, R., Schriefers, H., Herrmann, M., and Petutschnigk, D. (1976). *Acta Endocrinol. (Copenhagen)* **82**, 774–784.

Levine, S., and Mullins, R. F. (1964). *Science* **144,** 185-187.

Levine, S., and Mullins, R. F. (1966). *Science* **152,** 1585-1592.

Lieberburg, I., and McEwen, B. S. (1975). *Brain Res.* **95,** 165-170.

Lieberburg, I., Maclusky, N. J., Roy, E. J., and McEwen, B. S. (1978). *Am. Zool.* **18,** 539-544.

Lindstrom, L., and Meyerson, B. J. (1966). *Acta Physiol. Scand.* **68,** Suppl. 277, 121.

Lisk, R. D. (1962). *Am. J. Physiol.* **203,** 493-496.

Lisk, R. D. (1967). *In* "Neuroendocrinology" (L. Martini and W. F. Ganong, eds.), Vol. 2, pp. 197-239. Academic Press, New York.

Lisk, R. D., and Suydam, A. J. (1967). *Anat. Rec.* **157,** 181-189.

Lodder, J., and Baum, M. J. (1977). *Behav. Biol.* **20,** 141-148.

Loraine, J. A., Ismail, A. A. A., Adamapoulos, D. A., and Dove, G. A. (1970). *Br. Med. J.* **4,** 406-408.

Loraine, J. A., Adamapoulos, D. A., Kirkham, K. E., Ismail, A. A. A., and Dove, G. A. (1971). *Nature (London)* **234,** 552-555.

Luttge, W. G., and Whalen, R. E. (1970). *Horm. Behav.* **1,** 265-281.

McDonald, P. G., and Doughty, C. (1974). *J. Endocrinol.* **61,** 95-103.

McDonald, P. G., Beyer, C., Newton, F., Brien, B., Baker, R., Tan, H. S., Sampson, C., Kitching, P., Greenhill, R., and Pitchard, D. (1970). *Nature (London)* **227,** 964-965.

McEwen, B. S., Lieberburg, I., Chaptal, C., and Krey, L. C. (1977). *Horm. Behav.* **9,** 249-263.

McEwen, B. S., Krey, L. C., and Luine, V. N. (1978). *In* "The Hypothalamus" (S. Reichlin, R. J. Baldessarini, and J. B. Martin, eds.), pp. 255-268. Raven, New York.

Malsbury, C. W. (1971). *Physiol. Behav.* **7,** 797-805.

Malsbury, C. W., Strull, D., and Davod, J. (1978). *Physiol. Behav.* **21,** 79-87.

Margolese, M. S. (1970). *Horm. Behav.* **1,** 151-155.

Margolese, M. S., and Janiger, O. (1973). *Br. Med. J.* **3,** 207-210.

Martinez, C., and Bittner, J. J. (1956). *Proc. Soc. Exp. Biol. Med.* **91,** 506-509.

Martini, L. (1978). *In* "Hormones and Brain Development" (G. Dörner and M. Kawakami, eds.), pp. 3-12. Elsevier/North-Holland Biomedical Press, Amsterdam.

Masterpasqua, F., Chapman, K. H., and Lore, R. K. (1976). *Dev. Psychobiol.* **9,** 403-411.

Matsumoto, A., and Arai, Y. (1976). *Neurosci, Lett.* **2,** 79-82.

Matsuyama, E., Weisz, J., and Lloyd, C. W. (1966). *Endocrinology* **79,** 261-267.

Mennin, S. P., and Gorski, R. A. (1975). *Endocrinology* **96,** 486-491.

Merari, A., and Ginton, A. (1975). *Brain Res.* **86,** 97-108.

Meyer-Bahlburg, H. F. L. (1977). *Arch. Sex. Behav.* **6,** 297-325.

Meyer-Bahlburg, H. F. L. (1979). *Arch. Sex. Behav.* **8,** 101-119.

Meyerson, B. J. (1964). *Psychopharmacologia* **6,** 210-218.

Meyerson, B. J. (1966). *Acta Physiol. Scand.* **67,** 411-422.

Meyerson, B. J. (1968). *Nature (London)* **217,** 683-684.

Meyerson, B. J., and Lewander, T. (1970). *Life Sci.* **9,** 661-671.

Mitskevich, M. S., and Borisowa, N. A. (1974). *In* "Endocrinology of Sex" (G. Dörner, ed.), pp. 106-113. Barth, Leipzig.

Mode, A., Skett, P., Eneroth, P., Sonnenschein, C., and Gustafsson, J. A. (1978). *In* "Hormones and Brain Development" (G. Dörner and M. Kawakami, eds.), pp. 139-146. Elsevier/North-Holland Biomedical Press, Amsterdam.

Money, J., and Schwartz, M. (1977). *In* "Congenital Adrenal Hyperplasia" (P. A. Lee, L. P. Plotnick, A. A. Kowarski, and C. J. Migeon, eds.), pp. 419-451. University Park Press, Baltimore, Maryland.

Moralli, G., Larsson, K., and Beyer, C. (1977). *Horm. Behav.* **9,** 203-217.

Moss, R. L., and McCann, S. M. (1973). *Science* **181,** 177-179.

Moss, R. L., Dudley, C., Foreman, M. M., and McCann, S. M. (1975). *In* "Hypothalamic Hormones: Chemistry, Physiology, Pharmacology and Clinical Uses" (M. Motta, P. G. Crosignanis and L. Martini, eds.). Academic Press, New York.

Moyer, J. A., Herrenkohl, L. R., and Jacobowitz, D. M. (1978). *Brain Res.* **144**, 173–178.

Müller, D., Orthner, H., Roeder, F., König, A., Bosse, K., and Kloos, G. (1974). *In* "Endocrinology of Sex" (G. Dörner, ed.), pp. 81–105. Barth, Leipzig.

Nadler, R. D. (1966). *Excerpta Med. Found. Int. Congr. Ser.* **111**, 363.

Naftolin, F., Ryan, K. J., and Petro, Z. (1971). *J. Endocrinol.* **51**, 795–796.

Naftolin, F., Ryan, K. J., and Davis, I. J. (1976). *In* "Subcellular Mechanisms in Reproductive Neuroendocrinology" (F. Naftolin and I. J. Davis, eds.), pp. 347–356. Elsevier, Amsterdam.

Nakashima, A., Koshiyama, K., Uozumi, T., Monden, Y., Hamanaka, Y., Kurachi, K., Aono, T., Mitsutani, S., and Matsumoto, K. (1975). *Acta Endocrinol. (Copenhagen)* **78**, 258–269.

Nance, D. M., Shryne, J., and Gorski, R. A. (1974). *Horm. Behav.* **5**, 73–81.

Nance, D. M., Christensen, L. W., Shryne, J. E., and Gorski, R. A. (1977). *Brain Res. Bull.* **2**, 307–312.

Neill, J. D. (1972). *Endocrinology* **90**, 1154–1159.

Neumann, F., and Elger, W. (1965). *Acta Endocrinol. (Copenhagen), Suppl.* **100**, 174.

Neumann, F., and Elger, W. (1966). *Endokrinologie* **50**, 209–224.

Neumann, F., and Kramer, M. (1966). *Excerpta Med. Found. Int. Cong. Ser.* **132**, 932–941.

Neumann, F., Elger, W., and Kramer, M. (1966). *Endocrinology* **78**, 628–632.

Neumann, F., Hahn, J. D., and Kramer, M. (1967). *Acta Endocrinol. (Copenhagen)* **54**, 227–240.

Niswender, G. D., Midgley, A. R., Jr., Monroe, S. E., and Reichert, L. E. (1968). *Proc. Soc. Exp. Biol. Med.* **128**, 807–811.

Noble, G. K., and Aronson, L. R. (1945). *Bull. Am. Mus. Nat. Hist.* **86**, 85–139.

Nottebohm, F., and Arnold, A. P. (1976). *Science* **194**, 211–213.

Nunez, E., Savu, L., Engelmann, F., Benassayag, C., Crépy, O., and Jayle, M. F. (1971). *C. R. Hebd. Seances Acad. Sci., Ser. D* **273**, 242–243.

Ohno, S. (1979). "Major Sex-Determining Genes." Springer-Verlag, Berlin and New York.

Palka, Y. S., and Sawyer, C. H. (1964). *Am. Zool.* **4**, 289.

Palka, Y. S., and Sawyer, C. H. (1966). *J. Physiol. (London)* **185**, 251–269.

Parks, G. A., Korth-Schütz, S., Penny, R., Hilding, R. F., Dumars, K. W., Frasier, S. D., and New, M. I. (1974). *J. Clin. Endocrinol. Metab.* **39**, 796–801.

Persky, H. (1978). *Proc. Int. Congr. Med. Sexol., 3rd, 1978* Abstracts p. 217.

Peterson, R. E., Imperato-McGinley, J., Gautier, T., and Sturla, E. (1977). *Am. J. Med.* **62**, 170–191.

Pfaff, D. W. (1966). *J. Endocrinol.* **36**, 415–416.

Pfaff, D. W., and Sakuma, Y. (1979). *J. Physiol. (London)* **288**, 189–202.

Pfeiffer, C. A. (1936). *Am. J. Anat.* **58**, 195–225.

Phoenix, C. H. (1974). *Physiol. Behav.* **12**, 1045–1055.

Phoenix, C. H., Goy, R. W., Gerall, A. A., and Young, W. C. (1959). *Endocrinology* **65**, 369–382.

Poppe, I., Stahl, F., and Dörner, G. (1974). *In* "Endocrinology of Sex" (G. Dörner, ed.), pp. 198–200. Barth, Leipzig.

Poppe, I., Stahl, F., Götz, F., and Dörner, G. (1975). *Endokrinologie* **65**, 227–228.

Powers, J. B., and Valenstein, E. S. (1972). *Science* **175**, 1003–1005.

Prader, A. (1978). *In* "Klinik der inneren Sekretion" (A. Labhart, ed.), pp. 654–688. Springer-Verlag, Berlin and New York.

Puig-Duran, E., Greenstein, B. D., and McKinnon, B. C. B. (1979). *J. Reprod. Fertil.* **56**, 707–714.

Raisman, G., and Field, P. M. (1971). *Science* **173**, 731–733.

Raisman, G., and Field, P. M. (1973). *Brain Res.* **54**, 1–29.

Ratner, A., and Adamo, N. J. (1971). *Neuroendocrinology* **8**, 26–35.

Raynaud, J. P. (1973). *Steroids* **21**, 249–258.

Revesz, C., Kernaghan, D., and Bindra, D. (1963). *J. Endocrinol.* **25**, 549–550.

Reyes, F. I., Boroditsky, R. S., Winter, J. S. D., and Faiman, C. (1974). *J. Clin. Endocrinol. Metab.* **38**, 612–617.

Robinson, J. D., Judd, H. L., Young, P. E., Jones, O. W., and Yen, S. S. C. (1977). *J. Clin. Endocrinol. Metab.* **45**, 755–761.

Rhode, W., Stahl, F., and Dörner, G. (1977). *Endokrinologie* **70**, 241–248.

Rhode, W., Stahl, F., Götz, F., and Dörner, G. (1978). *In* "Hormones and Brain Development" (G. Dörner and M. Kawakami, eds.), pp. 111–120. Elsevier/North-Holland Biomedical Press, Amsterdam.

Salaman, D. F. (1974). *Prog. Brain Res.* **41**, 349–361.

Salmon, M. J., and Geist, S. H. (1943). *J. Clin. Endocrinol. Metab.* **3**, 235–238.

Sawyer, C. H. (1963). *Anat. Rec.* **145**, 280.

Sawyer, C. H. (1979). *Can. J. Physiol. Pharmacol.* **57**, 667–680.

Schally, A. V., Kastin, A. J., and Arimura, A. (1971). *Fertil. Steril.* **22**, 703–721.

Schally, A. V., Coy, D. H., Arimura, A., Vilchez, J., Redding, T. W., and Kastin, A. J. (1978). *In* "Hypothalamic Hormones—Chemistry, Physiology and Clinical Applications (D. Gupta and W. Voelter, eds.), pp. 1–12. Verlag Chemie, Weinheim.

Schriefers, H., Lax, E. R., and Ghraf, R. (1979). *Acta Endocrinol. Congr., 12th, 1979* Advance Abstracts, pp. 463–465.

Schuetz, A. W., and Meyer, R. K. (1963). *Proc. Soc. Exp. Biol. Med.* **112**, 875–880.

Segal, S. J., and Johnson, D. C. (1959). *Arch. Anat. Microsc. Morphol. Exp.* **48**, 261–274.

Seyler, L. E., Jr., Canalis, E., Spare, S., and Reichlin, S. (1978a). *J. Clin. Endocrinol. Metab.* **47**, 176–183.

Seyler, L. E., Jr., Grace, K., Canalis, E., Spare, S., and Reichlin, S. (1978b). *Proc. Int. Congr. Med. Sexol.,3rd, 1978* Abstracts, p. 86.

Shay, H., Gershon-Cohen, J., Paschkis, K. E., and Fels, S. S. (1939). *Endocrinology* **25**, 933–943.

Sheridan, P. J., Sar, M., and Stumpf, W. E. (1975). *In* "Anatomical Neuroendocrinology" (W. E. Stumpf and L. D. Grant, eds.), pp. 134–141. Karger, Basel.

Shirama, K., Takeo, Y., Shimizu, K., and Maekawa, K. (1975). *Endocrinol. Jpn.* **22**, 575–579.

Simmons, J. E., and Lusk, M. (1969). *Acta Endocrinol. (Copenhagen)* **61**, 302–306.

Sipová, I., and Starka, L. (1977). *Arch. Sex. Behav.* **6**, 477–481.

Smith, P. E., and Engle, E. T. (1927). *Am. J. Anat.* **40**, 159–217.

Smith, W. N. A. (1967). *J. Embryol. Exp. Morphol.* **17**, 1–8.

Södersten, P. (1978a). *J. Endocrinol.* **76**, 233–240.

Södersten, P. (1978b). *J. Endocrinol.* **76**, 241–249.

Södersten, P., Larsson, K., Ahlenius, S., and Engel, J. (1976). *Pharmacol., Biochem. Behav.* **5**, 319–333.

Somana, R., Visessuwan, S., Samridtong, A., and Holland, R. C. (1978). *J. Endocrinol.* **79**, 399–400.

Soulairac, A., and Soulairac, M. L. (1970). *Probl. Actuels Endocrinol. Nutr.* **14**, 63–94.

Soulairac, M. L. (1963). *Ann. Endocrinol.* **24**, 26–53.

Soulairac, M. L., and Soulairac, A. (1975). *In* "Sexual Behavior: Pharmacology and Biochemistry" (M. Sandler and G. L. Gessa, eds.), pp. 99–116. Raven, New York.

Stahl, F., Dörner, G., Rohde, W., and Schott, G. (1976a). *Endokrinologie* **68**, 112–114.

Stahl, F., Dörner, G., Ahrens, L., and Graudenz, W. (1976b). *Endokrinologie* **68**, 115–117.

Stahl, F., Götz, F., Poppe, I., Amendt, P., and Dörner, G. (1978). *In* "Hormones and Brain Development" (G. Dörner and M. Kawakami, eds.), pp. 99–110. Elsevier/North-Holland Biomedical Press, Amsterdam.

Staudt, J., and Dörner, G. (1976). *Endokrinologie* **67**, 296–300.

Staudt, J., Stüber, P., and Dörner, G. (1978). *In* "Hormones and Brain Development" (G. Dörner and M. Kawakami, eds.), pp. 35–41. Elsevier/North-Holland Biomedical Press, Amsterdam.

Stumpf, W. E., and Sar, M. (1978). *In* "Hormones and Brain Development" (G. Dörner and M. Kawakami, eds.), pp. 27–33. Elsevier/North-Holland Biomedical Press, Amsterdam.

Swanson, H. H. (1966). *J. Endocrinol.* **36**, 327–328.

Swanson, H. H. (1970). *J. Reprod. Fertil.* **21**, 183–186.

Swanson, H. H., and van der Werff ten Bosch, J. J. (1963a). *Acta Physiol. Pharmacol. Neerl.* **12**, 82–83.

Swanson, H. H., and van der Werff ten Bosch, J. J. (1963b). *J. Endocrinol.* **26**, 197–207.

Swanson, H. H., and van der Werff ten Bosch, J. J. (1964). *Acta Endocrinol. (Copenhagen)* **47**, 37–50.

Swanson, H. H., Brayshaw, J. S., and Payne, A. P. (1974). *In* "Endocrinology of Sex" (G. Dörner, ed.), pp. 62–75. Barth, Leipzig.

Swartz, S. K., and Soloff, M. S. (1974). *J. Clin. Endocrinol. Metab.* **39**, 589–594.

Takasugi, N. (1963). *Endocrinology* **72**, 607–619.

Takewaki, K. (1962). *Experientia* **18**, 1–6.

Toran-Allerand, C. D. (1978). *Am. Zool.* **18**, 553–565.

Turner, C. D. (1940). *J. Exp. Zool.* **83**, 1–31.

Vaccari, A., Brotman, S., Cimino, J., and Timiras, P. S. (1977). *Brain Res.* **132**, 176–185.

Vandenburgh, J. G. (1969). *Physiol. Behav.* **4**, 261–264.

Vaughan, E., and Fisher, A. E. (1962). *Science* **137**, 758–760.

Vértes, M., Varga, P., Göcze, P., Vértes, Z., and Kovacz, S. (1977). *Acta Physiol. Acad. Sci. Hung.* **50**, 307–315.

Vreeburg, J. T., van der Vaat, P. D., and van der Schoot, P. (1977). *J. Endocrinol.* **74**, 375–382.

Wagner, J. W., Erwin, W., and Critchlow, B. V. (1966). *Endocrinology* **79**, 1135–1142.

Ward, I. L. (1972). *Science,* **175**, 82–84.

Ward, I. L. (1977). *J. Comp. Physiol. Psychol.* **91**, 465–471.

Waxenberg, S. E., Drellich, M. G., and Sutherland, A. M. (1959). *J. Clin. Endocrinol. Metab.* **19**, 193–202.

Weisz, J., and Gibbs, C. (1974). *Endocrinology* **94**, 616–620.

Whalen, R. E., and Edwards, D. A. (1966). *J. Comp. Physiol. Psychol.* **62**, 307–310.

Whalen, R. E., and Edwards, D. A. (1967). *Anat. Rec.* **157**, 173–180.

Whalen, R. E., and Nadler, R. D. (1963). *Science* **141**, 273–274.

Whalen, R. E., and Olsen, K. L. (1978). *Brain Res.* **152**, 121–132.

Whalen, R. E., Peck, C. K., and Lo Piccolo, J. (1966). *Endocrinology* **78**, 965–970.

Wilson, J. G. (1943). *Anat. Rec.* **86**, 341–363.

Wilson, J. G., Young, W. C., and Hamilton, J. B. (1940). *Yale J. Biol. Med.* **13**, 189–202.

Wilson, J. G., Young, W. C., and Hamilton, J. B. (1941a). *Endocrinology* **29,** 779–783.

Wilson, J. G., Hamilton, J. B., and Young, W. C. (1941b). *Endocrinology* **29,** 784–789.

Wollman, A. L., and Hamilton, J. B. (1967). *Endocrinology* **81,** 350–356.

Wrenn, T. R., Wood, J. R., and Bitman, J. (1969). *J. Endocrinol.* **45,** 415–420.

Yamai, T., Dierschke, D. J., Hotchkiss, J., Bhattacharya, A. H., Surve, A. H., and Knobil, E. (1971). *Endocrinology* **89,** 1034–1041.

Yamomachi, K., and Arai, Y. (1975). *Endocrinol. Jpn.* **22,** 243–246.

Yazaki, I. (1960). *Annot. Zool. Jpn.* **33,** 217–225.

Yazaki, I. (1970). *Annot. Zool. Jpn.* **43,** 19–22.

Young, W. C., Goy, R. W., and Phoenix, C. H. (1964). *Science* **143,** 212–218.

Young-Lai, E. V. (1972). *J. Endocrinol.* **54,** 515–516.

Zemlan, F. P., Ward, I. L., Crowley, W. R., and Margules, D. L. (1973). *Science* **179,** 1010–1011.

Zondek, T., Mansfield, M. D., and Zondek, L. H. (1977). *J. Obstet. Gynaecol. Br. Commonw.* **84,** 714–716.

Index

A

Adenoma, toxic, 122–123
Adenosine triphosphatase, Na$^+$, K$^+$ aldosterone and, 79–84
Adenylate cyclase
  activation by TSaab, 163–164
  activity in bone and bone cells, 241–242
  mechanism of coupling and activation in kidney, 234
Aldosterone
  action in target epithelia
    antagonists, 104–109
    cation secretion, 70–77
    cellular targets, 98–104
    historical, 57–59
    interaction with antidiuretic hormone, 68–70
    mineralocorticoid receptor, 59–65
    protein induction, 77–88
    RNA and protein synthesis, 65–68
    two models of action, 88–98
Antagonists, of aldosterone, 104–109
Antidiuretic hormone, interaction with aldosterone, 68–70
Autoimmune disease, pathogenesis of
  forbidden clone theory, 187–191
  genetic predisposition to, 192–196
  less likely concepts of, 191–192
  toward a general principle of therapy, 196
Autoimmune thyroiditis, horror autotoxicus and, 123

B

Blood
  retinol transport in, 40–42
  steroid hormone transport in, 35
Bone, mechanism of action of PTH and calcitonin in, 239–240
  adenylate cyclase activity, 241–242
  calcitonin receptors, 241
  cell types involved, 240–241
  cyclic AMP responses in skeletal tissue, 242–243

cyclic nucleotide phosphodiesterase and, 243
  protein kinases, 242
Brain
  sex hormone-dependent differentiation, animal experiments on, 341–360
  sexual differentiation
    clinical studies and perspectives, 360–369
    gonadotropin secretion, 33–338
    sexual behavior, 338–341

C

Calcitonin
  mechanism of action, identification of receptors, 236–239
  receptors in bone, 241
  role of cyclic nucleotides in secretion
    C-cell anatomy and physiology, 228
    direct evidence for role of cAMP, 230
    experimental systems for study, 229
    indirect evidence for role of cAMP, 229–230
Cation(s), secretion, aldosterone and, 70–77
Cellular targets for aldosterone, 98–104
Citrate synthase, aldosterone and, 77–79
Clonal variation, in TSaab specificity, 180–181
Complement, LATS action and, 163
Cyclic adenosine monophosphate, LH-RH and, 309–310
Cyclic nucleotide(s)
  in extracellular fluids
    effects of PTH, 244–245
    pseudohypoparathyroidism, 245–247
  role in calcitonin secretion
    C-cell anatomy and physiology, 228
    direct evidence for role of cAMP, 230
    experimental systems for study, 229
    indirect evidence for role of cAMP, 229–230